WHIPLASH INJURIES

Current Concepts in Prevention, Diagnosis, and Treatment of the Cervical Whiplash Syndrome

WHIPLASH INJURIES

Current Concepts in Prevention, Diagnosis, and Treatment of the Cervical Whiplash Syndrome

Editors

Robert Gunzburg, M.D., Ph.D.
Senior Consultant
Department of Orthopaedics
Centenary Clinic
Antwerp, Belgium

Marek Szpalski, M.D.
Senior Consultant
Department of Orthopaedics
Centre Hospitalier Molière Longchamp
Brussels, Belgium

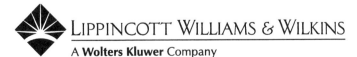

LIPPINCOTT WILLIAMS & WILKINS
A **Wolters Kluwer** Company
Philadelphia • Baltimore • New York • London
Buenos Aires • Hong Kong • Sydney • Tokyo

Acquisitions Editor: Kathey Alexander
Developmental Editor: Emilie Linkins
Manufacturing Manager: Dennis Teston
Production Manager: Maxine Langweil
Production Editor: Rita Madrigal
Indexer: Victoria Boyle
Compositor: Lippincott–Raven Electronic Production
Printer: Maple Press

Printed in the United States of America

9 8 7 6 5 4 3 2

Library of Congress Cataloging-in-Publication Data
Whiplash injuries : current concepts in prevention, diagnosis, and treatment of the cervical whiplash syndrome / [edited by] Robert Gunzburg, Marek Szpalski.
    p.   cm.
   Includes bibliographical references and index.
   ISBN 0-397-51856-0
   1. Whiplash injuries. I. Gunzburg, Robert. II. Szpalski, Marek.
   [DNLM: 1. Whiplash Injuries—therapy. Whiplash Injuries—diagnosis. 3. Whiplash Injuries—physiopathology. WE 725 W5728 1997]
RD531.W48 1997
617.5′3—dc21
DNLM/DLC
For Library of Congress   97-30023
                                              CIP

Contents

Basics

Definition of the Whiplash Injury

Contributing Authors

Michael A. Adams, Ph.D.
Senior Research Fellow
Department of Anatomy
University of Bristol
Southwell Street
Bristol BS2 8EJ,
United Kingdom

A. Aleksiev, M.D., Ph.D.
Department of Orthopaedics
Iowa Spine Research Center,
University of Iowa
200 Hawkins Drive
Iowa City, IA 52242

Klaus F. Augustiny, M.A.
Clinical Psychologist
Department of Psychiatry
University of Berne
Inselspital
CH-3010 Berne, Switzerland

Lawrence Brett Babat, M.D.
Department of Orthopaedic Surgery
Brown University
Providence, RI 02912

Georges Bauherz, M.D.
Department of Neurology
Centre Hospitalier Molière Longchamp
Rue Marconi 142
1180 Brussels, Belgium

Christiane Beauchemin, M.D.
Société de l'assurance automobile
du Québec
333 Jean Lesage
G1K 8A2 Quebec, Canada

Michel Benoist, M.D.
Department of Orthopaedic Surgery
Section of Rheumatology
Hôpital Beaujon
University of Paris VII
113 Avenue Victor Hugo
75116 Paris, France

Stefan Bergré, M.D.
Department of Internal Medicine
Psychosomatic Unit
University of Berne
Inselspital
CH-3010 Berne, Switzerland

Nikolai Bogduk, M.D., Ph.D., D.Sc.,
Dip. Anat., F.A.F.R.M.
Professor of Anatomy and
Musculoskeletal Medicine
University olf Newcastle
Newcastle Bone and Joint Institute
Royal Newcastle Hospital
Newcastle, NSW 2300, Australia

William Castro
Academy for Manual Medicine
University of Münster
Germany

Jacek Cholewicki, Ph.D.
Assistant Professor
Biomechanics Laboratory
Yale University School of Medicine
333 Cedar Street, LSOG 217
New Haven, CT 06510

Monique J.B. Cordonnier, M.D.
Department of Ophthalmology
Erasme Hospital
Free University of Brussels
Route de Lennik 808
1070 Brussels, Belgium

Henry Vernon Crock, M.D., F.R.C.S.,
F.R.A.C.S.
Consultant Spinal Surgeon
Spinal Disorders Unit
Cromwell Hospital
Cromwell Road
London SW5 OTU,
United Kingdom

Arthur C. Croft, D.C., M.S.
Assistant Adjunct Professor
Department of Orthopaedics
Los Angeles College of Chiropractics
16200 Amber Valley Drive
Whittier, CA 90609-1166

Marie A. Dayton
Claims Manager
Insurance Corporation of British Columbia
Bodily Injury and Rehabilitation Services
301 ESP 151 West Esplanade
North Vancouver, B.C. V7M 3H9, Canada

Anne de Heering, M.S.
Licenieé en Neurolinguistique
Centre Hospitalier Molière Longchamp
Rue Marconi
1180 Brussels, Belgium

Jacques de Moor, M.D.
Department of Radiology
Universitair Ziekenhuis Antwerpen
University of Antwerp
Wilrijkstraat 10
B2650 Edegem, Belgium

Arthur M. A. De Schepper, M.D., Ph.D.
Professor of Radiology
Universitair Ziekenhuis Antwerpen
University of Antwerp
Wilrijkstraat 10
B2650 Edegem, Belgium

Claire Desbiens
Chargée de Projet sur L'Entorse Cervicale
Société de l'assurance automobile du Québec
333 Jean Lesage
G1K 8J6 Québec, Canada

E. Jeffrey Donner, M.D.
The Spine Institute
Rocky Mountain Associates in Orthopaedics
1900 N. Boise Ave. 110
Loveland, CO 80538

Jiři Dvořák, M.D.
Professor of Neurology
Spine Unit
Schulthess Clinic
Lengghalde 2
CH 8008 Zürich, Switzerland

Michael D. Freeman, D.C., M.P.H., Ph. D.
Epidemiologist, Accident Reconstructionist
Deaprtment of Public Health
Oregon State University
4747 River Road North
Salem, OR 97303

**Charles S.B. Galasko, M.Sc., M.B.,
 Ch.M., F.R.C.S. (Eng.), F.R.C.S. (Ed)**
Professor of Orthopaedic Surgery
University of Manchester
Clinical Sciences Building
Hope Hospital
Eccles Old Road
*Salford, Manchester, M6. 8HD,
 United Kingdom*

Marc Giroux, M.D.
*Directeur des Politiqueset Programmes
 pour les Accidentes*
*Société de l'assurance automobile
 du Québec*
333 Jean Lesage
G1K 8A2 Québec, Canada

Jonathan N. Grauer, M.D.
Resident
Department of Biomechanics
Yale University Medical School
333 Cedar Street, LSOG 217
New Haven, CT 06510

**Charles G. Greenough, M.D., MChir,
 F.R.C.S.**
Consultant Orthopaedic Surgeon
Middlesbrough General Hospital
Ayresome Green Lane
*Middlesbrough, Cleveland TS5 5AZ,
 United Kingdom*

Dieter Grob, P.D. D.med
Assistant Professor
Spine Unit
Schulthess Clinic
Lengghalde 2
CH 8008 Zürich, Switzerland

Robert Gunzburg, M.D., Ph. D.
Senior Consultant
Department of Orthopaedics
Eeuwfeestkliniek (Centenary Clinic)
Harroniestraat 68
2018 Antwerpen, Belgium

Leif Hasselquist, M.A., A.T.C.
Department of Biomedical Engineering
University of Iowa
Spine Research Center
Department of Orthopaedics
200 Hawkins Drive
Iowa City, IA 52242

Jean-Pierre Hayez, M.D.
Teaching Hospital
Free University of Brussels
Rue Marconi 142
1180 Brussels, Belgium

Lotta Jakobsson, M.Sc.E.
Senior Research Engineer
Volvo Safety Center
Volvo Car Corporation
S-405 08 Göteborg, Sweden

Halldór Jónsson, Jr., M.D., Ph.D.
Department of Orthopaedic Surgery
National University Hospital
P.O. Box 10
121 Reykjavik
Iceland

Peter M. Klara, M.D., Ph.D.
Associate Professor
Department of Neurosurgery
Eastern Virginia Medical School
Spinal Research and Education Foundation
Norfolk, VA 23501

Pierre Lucas, M.D.
Professor of Legal Medicine
Free University of Brussels
22 Avenue de Jardins
B-1030 Brussels, Belgium

Willem F. Luitjes, M.D.
Department of Neurosurgery
Slotervaart Hospital
Louwesweg 6
1066 EC Amsterdam, The Netherlands

Marianne L. Magnusson, Dr.Med.Sc.
Research Associate, Adjunct Professor
Departments of Orthopaedic Surgery and
  Biomedical Engineering
University of Iowa
200 Hawkins Drive
Iowa City, IA 52242-1088

Jean-Yves Maigne, M.D.
Head of the Department of Physical Medicine
Hôtel-Dieu University Hospital
1 Place Notre-Dame
75004 Paris, France

Didier H. Martin, M.D., Ph.D.
Chef de Clinique Adjoint
Department of Neurosurgery
University Hospital
University of Liège
Sart Tilman B35
4000 Liège , Belgium

H. Michael Mayer, M.D.
Associate Professor
Department of Orthopaedic Surgery/
  Oskar-Helene-Heim
Free University of Berlin
Clayallee 229
D-14195 Berlin, Germany

Stefan Meyer
Diplom-Ingenieur
Ingenieurbüro Schimmelpfennig und Becke
Münsterstrasse 101
48155 Münster, Germany

Francoise Michel, P.T.
Department of Orthopaedic Surgery
Centre Hospitalier Molière Longchamp
Rue Marconi 142
1180 Brussels, Belgium

Kimio Nibu, M.D.
Department of Orthopaedics
Yamaguchi University School of Medicine
1144 Kogushi, Ube City
Yamaguchi Pref. 755, Japan

Margareta Nordin, Dr. Sci.
Research Associate Professor
Occupational and Industrial Orthopaedic Center
Hospital for Joint Diseases Orthopaedic
  Institute;
and Department of Environmental Medicine
New York University School of Medicine
63 Downing Street
New York, NY 10014

Manohar M. Panjabi, Ph.D. Dr. Tech.
Full Professor
Biomechanics Laboratory
Yale University Medical School
333 Cedar Street, LSOG 217
New Haven, CT 06510

Paul M. Parizel, M.D., Ph.D.
Prof. Dr.
Department of Radiology
University of Antwerp
University Hospital
Wilrijkstraat 10
B 2650 Edegem, Belgium

Philippe Petroons, M.D.
Department of Radiology
Centre Hospitalier Molière Longchamp
Rue Marconi 142
B 1180 Brussels, Belgium

Kenneth A. Pettine, M.D.
The Spine Institute
Rocky Mountain Associates in Orthopaedics
1900 N. Boise Ave. 110
Loveland, CO 80538

Christoph Peuker
Department of Radiology
Clemens-Hospital
Münster, Germany

Malcolm H. Pope, Dr.Med.Sc., Ph.D.
Distinguished Professor
Department of Orthopaedics
Iowa Spine Research Center
University of Iowa Hospital and Clinic
200 Hawkins Drive
Iowa City, IA 52242

Bogdan P. Radanov, M.D.
Associate Professor of Psychiatry
Department of Psychiatry
University of Berne
Inselpital
3010 Berne, Switzerland

Wolfgang Rauschning, M.D., Ph.D.
Research Professor, Clinical Anatomy
Department of Orthopaedic Surgery
Academic University Hospital
S-751 85 Uppsala, Sweden

Markus Schilgen
Academy for Manual Medicine at the
*   Westfalian Wilhelms University*
Von-Esmarchstrasse 56
Münster, Germany

Mary Louise Skovron, Ph.D.
Genentech, Inc.
Mailstopp 88
460 Point San Bruno Blvd.
South San Francisco, CA 94080

Mireille Soeur, M.D.
Department of Neurology
Centre Hospitalier Molière Longchamp
Rue Marconi 142
B 1180 Brussels, Belgium

Kevin Spratt, Ph.D.
Department of Orthopaedics
Iowa Spine Research Center, University of Iowa
200 Hawkins Drive
Iowa City, IA 52242

Matthias Sturzenegger, M.D.
Associate Professor of Neurology
Department of Neurology
University of Berne
Inselspital
CH-3010 Berne, Switzerland

Michael F. Sullivan, M.B., B.Chem.,
**   F.R.C.S.**
Consultant Surgeon
Department of Orthopaedics
London University
Royal National Orthopaedic Hospital
95 Harley Street
WIN 1DF London, United Kingdom

Mats Y. Svensson, Ph.D.
Assistant Professor
Department of Injury Prevention
Chalmers University of Technology
S-412 96 Göteborg, Sweden

Marek Szpalski, M.D.
Senior Consultant
Department of Orthopaedics
Centre Hospitalier Molière Longchamp
Rue Marconi 142
1180 Brussels, Belgium

Luc van den Hauwe, M.D.
Department of Radiology
Universitair Ziekenhuis Antwerpen
University of Antwerp
Wilrijkstraat 10
B2650 Edegem, Belgium

Pieter F. van Akkerveeken, M.D.,
**   Ph.D.**
Orthopaedic Surgeon
Rug Advies Centrum
Utrechtseweg 92
3702 AD Zeist, The Netherlands

Johan W. M. Van Goethem, M.D.
Department of Radiology
University Hospital of Antwerp
Wilrijkstraat 10
B2650 Edegem, Belgium

Christian Van Nechel, M.D.
Neuro-Ophthalmology Unit
Free University of Brussels Hospital
808 Route de Lennik
B 1070 Brussels, Belgium

Michael Weber
Engineer
Ingenieurbüro Schimmelpfennig und Becke
Münsterstrasse 101
48155 Münster, Germany

Jacques S. Widelec, M.D.
Department of Radiology
Centre Hospitalier Molière Longchamp
Rue Marconi 142
B 1180 Brussels, Belgium

Kristina Wiklund
Saab Automobiles AB
Traak Al-7
S- 46180 Trollhättan,
Sweden

Hidezo Yoshizawa, M.D., Ph.D.
Professor of Medicine
Department of Orthopaedic Surgery
Fujita Health University
*   School of Medicine*
1-98 Dengakugakubo
Tyoake City, Aichi 470-11,
Japan

Andre Zanen, Ph.D.
Erasme Hospital
Free University of Brussels
Neuro-Ophthalmology Unit
Route de Lennik 808
B 1070 Brussels, Belgium

Preface

The reporting of accidents involving a whiplash mechanism and the incidence of whiplash associated disorders (WAD) are increasing at an alarming rate. It can account for up to 85% of compensated claims for injuries in motor vehicle collisions. The cost in the United Kingdom is estimated at £2.5 billion, which represents 0.4% of the gross national product.

However, we know very little about the mechanism of the whiplash injury, the anatomical lesions sustained are undefined, and the pathogenesis of the subsequent disorders are quite obscure. Furthermore, the psychosocial issues linked to the pathology represent controversial issues, and recently the reality of WAD has even been questioned. The presumed injury is a soft-tissue sprain which limits diagnostic efficacy.

The handling of whiplash injuries concerns many different disciplines: biomechanicians for the study of mechanics of the injury, a wide range of medical specialists in diagnosis and treatment, and automotive engineers in primary prevention.

Many medical specialties are involved in the treatment of WAD: orthopaedic surgeons, neurosurgeons, neurologists, rheumatologists, physiatrists, chiropractors, physical therapists, psychiatrists, pain specialists, medicolegal and insurance practitioners, as well as general practitioners. The latter are often confronted in their family practices with the long-term consequences of WAD.

In this book, we have tried to concisely summarize the current knowledge about this pathology in order to provide valuable information to any health professional confronted with patients presenting with WAD. It should give readers a global view and a better understanding of all of the aspects surrounding WAD, and will help them provide efficient treatment modalities. It should also help readers to inform their patients objectively about all the consequences of their condition. To achieve this goal, the foremost specialists in this matter cover a wide range of subjects: anatomy and biomechanics, epidemiology, diagnosis, medical and surgical treatment, neurological and psychological consequences, long-term follow-up, disability assessment, and automobile seat design.

Some new biomechanical experiments and theories are described regarding collision velocity and the protective role of neck muscles. The importance of sometimes hidden osteoligamentous injuries is stressed. The acute care measures, efficacy of medical treatments, manipulation and cognitive therapies, as well as different surgical techniques are discussed. Some lesser-known, but quite common, consequences like oculomotor and neurolinguistic troubles are analyzed and treatments proposed.

An important part of the book deals with the costs of WAD and legislative issues, a new method for impairment ratings of spinal injuries is described which takes into account objective lesions, pain, function, and quality of life. The aspects of primary prevention in automobile design is dealt with by engineers from major automobile manufacturers with a traditionally high involvement in security.

This book tries to assemble state-of-the-art knowledge about a common and difficult condition that many practioners are likely to encounter.

Robert Gunzburg, M.D., Ph.D.
Marek Szpalski, M.D.

Introduction

Whiplash exemplifies the irony of musculoskeletal medicine. For a condition that affects so many people in the Western World, the knowledge base is quite incomplete. We have relied on opinions and consensus instead of science. This irony was brought into stark relief by the report of the Québec Task Force on Whiplash-Associated Disorders (1), which had every intention of providing a meta-analysis on the diagnosis and treatment of whiplash, but could find no literature worthy of such an analysis. By default, it had to resort to consensus, not science.

This book is a step toward correcting our ignorance and misconceptions about whiplash, and it is pleasing to see that this problem has now attracted concerted and responsible research by eminent individuals.

Whiplash is a biomechanical event that occurs in a motor vehicle accident. It involves an excursion of the head and neck without any direct blow to the head. Some victims are injured; others are not. Some develop symptoms; others do not. Most symptoms are resolved, but many persist and become chronic. Neck pain and headache are the cardinal symptoms, but many patients also suffer from visual disturbances, disturbed balance, and altered cerebral function. Conventional diagnostic techniques by and large fail to identify any responsible lesion or to pinpoint the source of pain. Some authorities claim that there is no injury, and ascribe chronicity and peculiar symptoms to behavioral disorders, if not to malingering. Without a structural diagnosis, most treatments are empirically based and either do not work or are of unproven value.

For each of these components of the whiplash problem there are unresolved issues, mythologies, and controversies. In this book, we find some answers, several resolutions, encouraging directions, and some admission of remaining deficiencies.

The chapter by Adams, on biomechanics of the cervical spine, is conspicuous by what it does not say than by what it does say. We are learning increasingly more about the lumbar spine, but lack equivalent data on the structure and properties of the cervical discs, ligaments, joints, and muscles. Nevertheless, Panjabi has revitalized cadaver studies to demonstrate the kinematics of the cervical spine. Pope has revisited the reaction time of the neck muscles during whiplash.

Injuries do occur, even though they may not be demonstrable by contemporary imaging techniques. The postmortem studies of Rauschning reveal the many injuries that can occur, but that are undetectable by plain x-rays. Svensson has demonstrated that the dorsal root ganglia can be injured, echoing earlier studies in this regard (2,3). Meyer, Weber and colleagues have started to explore the biomechanical threshold for mechanical injuries. Benoist reviews the variable data on the natural history of whiplash and, like Holm, underscores that for the majority of patients the prognosis is benign; only a minority of patients are disabled by chronic pain, but it is these patients who constitute the challenge in management and research. Freeman and Croft dispel the erroneous conclusions of the Schrader study (4). Galasko confirms that some 80% of patients remain disabled four years later.

Greenough dispels the notion that chronic patients are malingering and ascribes chronicity to an iatrogenic disorder stemming from the lack of recognition that these patients do suffer. Similarly, Sullivan ascribes the problem to the adversarial legal system in which patients find themselves. Radanov echoes his previous work, showing that personality factors do not predict chronicity. What underlies chronicity is the lack of recognition, diagnosis, and treatment of the persisting pain and other symptoms.

No matter how intangible or how bizarre they may seem, the symptoms of whiplash are real. Grob emphasizes the need for meticulous diagnosis. He, Dvořák, and Donner highlight the need for special investigations, such as zygapophysial joint blocks and disc stimulation in order to pinpoint the source of pain. Van Nechel and de Heering show that peculiar oculomotor and neurolinguistic problems can be diagnosed, but only if special techniques are used. These symptoms are all-too-easily dismissed as malingering if physicians rely simply on clinical examination and their own lack of knowledge of what can be done to diagnose them.

It is with respect to treatment that major deficiencies remain. Nordin advocates early mobilization, but acknowledges that there is little data to prove the efficacy of any conservative therapy. Maigne advocates spinal manipulation, but likewise acknowledges the absence of any study on this proposition. Van Akkerveeken and Vendrig advocate cognitive behavioral therapy, but still lack conclusive data. Szpalski and Gunzburg acknowledge the lack of data on the efficacy of medications, but present the results of a controlled trial of nonsteroidal anti-inflammatory agents.

Crock, Klara, and Luitjes describe a variety of surgical options, but the key lies in matching diagnosis with therapy. The challenge for surgery lies not with the treatment of spinal cord injuries (Mayer and Martin), but with the treatment of neck pain. Crock champions the use of provocation discography, and Donner reports considerable success with cervical fusion based on discography. Bogduk demonstrates that accurate diagnosis with zygapophysial joint blocks predicates the complete relief of pain with percutaneous radiofrequency neurotomy.

Coming full circle, away from diagnosis and treatment, Jakobsson introduces the role for prevention, and Wiklund demonstrates the success of appropriately designed headrests.

In essence, we now have good data on the mechanics and epidemiology of whiplash. Diagnostic tools are emerging which demonstrate that the symptoms are real and should not be dismissed. We recognize that denying this reality is as much a contributor to the problem as the injuries themselves. Where medical practice is still lagging is in applying appropriate treatment. But this problem should not be insoluble; it requires only continued effort with inspired and disciplined research.

Nikolai Bogduk
Newcastle Bone and Joint Institute,
and Faculty of Medicine and Health Sciences
University of Newcastle
Newcastle, New South Wales, Australia

REFERENCES

1. Spitzer WO, Skovron ML, Salmi LR, et al. Scientific monograph of the Quebec task force on whiplash-associated disorders: redefining "whiplash" and its management. *Spine* 1995;20:1S–73S.
2. Taylor JR, Twomey LT. Acute injuries to cervical joints: an autopsy study of neck sprain. *Spine* 1993;9:1115–1122.
3. Taylor JR, Taylor MM. Cervical spine injuries: an autopsy study of 109 blunt injuries. *J Musculoskeletal Pain* 1996;4:61–79.
4. Schrader H, Obelieniene D, Bovim G, Surkiene D, Mickeviciene D, Miseviciene I, Sand T. Natural evolution of late whiplash syndrome outside the medicolegal context. *Lancet* 1996;347:1207–1211.

WHIPLASH INJURIES

Current Concepts in
Prevention, Diagnosis, and Treatment of
the Cervical Whiplash Syndrome

SECTION 1

Basics

*Whiplash Injuries: Current Concepts in
Prevention, Diagnosis, and Treatment
of the Cervical Whiplash Syndrome,*
edited by Robert Gunzburg and Marek Szpalski.
Lippincott–Raven Publishers, Philadelphia © 1998.

1

The Vascular Supply of the Cervical Spine and the Cervical Spinal Cord*

Henry Vernon Crock and Hidezo Yoshizawa

*H. V. Crock: Spinal Disorders Unit, Cromwell Hospital, London SW5 OTU, United Kingdom.
H. Yoshizawa: Department of Orthopaedic Surgery,
Fujita Health University School of Medicine, Toyoake City, Aichi 470-11, Japan.*

In discussions about the clinical aspects of cervical spine injuries and diseases, attention is still largely focused on the mechanical implications of spinal deformity after injury and on the mechanical aspects of spinal cord or cervical nerve root compression resulting from degenerative diseases. Apart from a general acceptance of the importance of the vertebral arteries in syndromes attributed to insufficiency of blood flow in these vessels, the significance of the vascular supply to the cervical spine and cervical spinal cord is, sadly, often ignored. It has practical relevance not only to surgical technique in the cervical spine but also to the interrelation of clinical syndromes, such as cervical radiculomyelopathy and brachial neuralgia. This chapter is designed to present a brief account of the blood supply to the cervical vertebral column and cervical spinal cord that is accurate in its essentials yet easy to remember (1,2).

THE VASCULAR SUPPLY TO THE CERVICAL SPINE

The cervical vertebral column is supplied predominantly by branches of the vertebral arteries. In the region of the craniocervical junction, arteries supplying C1 and C2 are often derived from branches of the external carotid arteries, such as the ascending pharyngeal arteries. At the level of the cervicothoracic junction, the vessels of origin are derived in part from branches of the thyrocervical trunk and from ascending intercostal branches of the thoracic aorta. Although there are regional variations in the origins of the arteries supplying the vertebrae, the actual vessels that supply the bone are applied immediately to the periosteum, and there is a striking uniformity in the patterns of distribution of the arteries on the surfaces and within the substance of each vertebra (Fig. 1).

---

*Figures in this chapter © H. V. Crock.

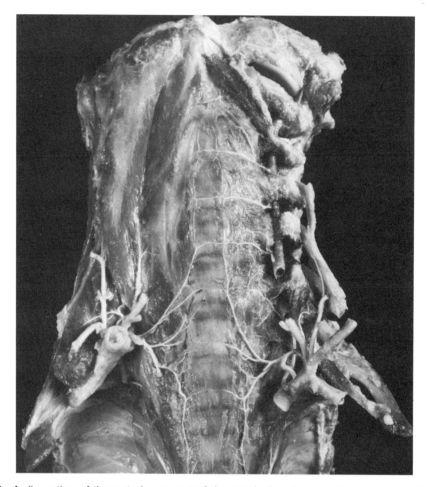

FIG. 1. A dissection of the anterior aspect of the cervical and upper thoracic spine of a 3¹/₂-year-old girl, showing the origins and courses of arteries supplying the anterolateral aspects of the vertebral bodies. The longus colli muscle group is intact on the right side of the specimen but has been removed on the left side to expose the anterior vertebral branches of the vertebral arteries, which are analogous to the posterior intercostal and lumbar arteries. Branches of the thyrocervical trunk contribute to the blood supply of the lower cervical and upper thoracic vertebral bodies.

THE BLOOD SUPPLY TO THE CERVICAL VERTEBRAL BODIES

When looking at cervical angiograms, there appears to be an overwhelming complexity to the orientation of vessels in the neck. In fact, there is an underlying simplicity in the patterns of vessels supplying individual vertebrae and the cervical spinal cord.

When each vertebral body is viewed from the front and sides, a prominent branch of the vertebral artery can be seen to course around the waist between the superior and inferior vertebral endplates. Three sets of branches arise from this vessel, the first penetrating the vertebral body to form an arterial grid in the centrum (Figs. 2,3). The second and third sets of branches pass upward and downward on the periosteum toward the respec-

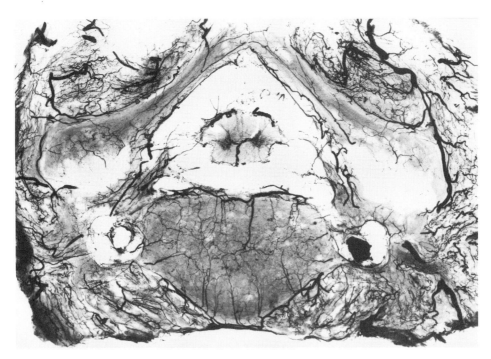

FIG. 2. A radiograph of a thin transverse section through the centrum area of a typical cervical vertebral body, from a 20-year-old woman. Radiate arteries contribute to the centrum grid. The surface vessels on the anterolateral and posterior surfaces of the vertebral bodies, from which the centrum arterial grid derives its branches, take their origin from anterior and posterior branches of the vertebral arteries on each side.

tive metaphyseal zones of the vertebral body, where branches penetrate the bone and contribute to the capillary networks of the vertebral endplates.

At the level of the intervertebral foramina, three sets of branches enter the spinal canal. The first of these is distributed to the floor of the spinal canal. It bifurcates immediately on entering the canal into ascending and descending branches that contribute to the formation of an arcuate grid in the floor of the canal, from which three sets of branches arise. These are analogous to those seen on the anterolateral aspects of the vertebral bodies (Fig. 4). The second set of arteries entering the spinal canal is destined to supply the cervical spinal cord and dural sac. It will be described in detail later.

The third set of branches form an arcuate pattern in the roof of the spinal canal, mirroring the pattern in its floor. These vessels lie on the periosteum and ligamenta flava, on the anterior aspects of the cervical laminae. From this arcuate system, vessels penetrate the lamina, contributing to its blood supply and to that of the spinous processes, pedicles, and zygapophyseal joints (see Fig. 2).

The dorsal aspects of the laminae are crossed by single terminal branches of the vertebral arteries, which extend to the tips of the spinous processes, applied to the periosteum. These give rise to intraosseus branches that supply the spinous processes, laminae, and zygapophyseal joints on the one hand, and to branches that pass into the paravertebral muscles on the other. The origins of these vessels are usually from the vertebral arteries but may spring from tributaries of the ascending cervical or pharyngeal arteries.

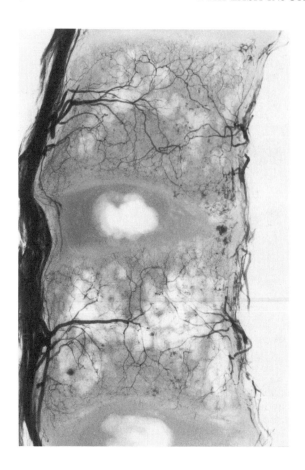

FIG. 3. A radiograph of a thin mid-sagittal section from a lumbar vertebral body of a young adult. The vessels contributing to the formation of the arterial grid in the centrum are analogous to those seen in the cervical vertebra in Figure 2.

THE BLOOD SUPPLY OF THE DURAL SAC AND CERVICAL SPINAL CORD

The second set of vessels that enter the intervertebral foramina, as outlined, are the neural branches of the vertebral arteries, which give rise segmentally to anterior and posterior radicular arteries. These vessels course along the nerve roots, penetrating the dural root sleeves to pass on to the anterior or posterior surfaces of the cervical cord in a subpial position, where they join, respectively, the anterior longitudinal arterial channel of the spinal cord and the posterolateral longitudinal arterial channels (Fig. 5). Fine branches of the deep cervical and ascending cervical arteries course along the dural root sleeves toward the dural sac, on the surface of which they are arranged in patterns resembling those of the periosteal arteries on the shafts of long bones.

The first illustrated account of the arterial supply of the human spinal cord was prepared by Thomas Willis, with illustrations by Sir Christopher Wren. It was published in Latin, in London, in 1663 (3). Willis illustrated an anterior view of a human fetal cervical spinal cord demonstrating the segmental distribution of anterior radicular arteries joining the anterior longitudinal arterial channel (Fig. 6). That channel is formed classically by right- and left-sided branches arising from the vertebral arteries near their termination in the basilar trunk. His description of this segmental distribution of radicular arteries has been challenged by many authors but confirmed in special anatomic preparations in the human adult (2) (see Fig. 5).

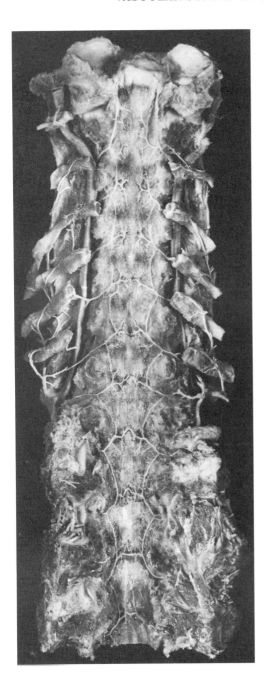

FIG. 4. A dissection of the posterior aspect of the cervical and upper thoracic spine of a 34-year-old man. The posterior aspects of the vertebral bodies have been exposed and portions of the posterior longitudinal ligament have been removed from a number of the vertebral bodies in the lower part of the specimen. This exposes the arterial connections between the arcuate vessels on both sides of the midline, from which centrum branches penetrate the posterior vertebral cortex to join the arterial grid in the center of the vertebral bodies. In the upper part of the specimen, on both sides, the anterior spinal canal branches take their origins from the vertebral arteries. In the neck, these vessels form a familiar arcuate arterial pattern on the anterior surface of the spinal canal, which is repeated along its length as far distally as the sacrum.

THE DORSAL ASPECT OF THE CERVICAL SPINAL CORD

The arrangement of arteries on the dorsal aspect of the spinal cord is distinct from that on its anterior aspect. Posterolateral longitudinal arterial channels take their origins from branches of the posterior inferior cerebellar arteries and vertebral arteries on both sides, and they course along the lateral longitudinal sulci of the spinal cord in close relationship with the entry points of the dorsal nerve rootlets.

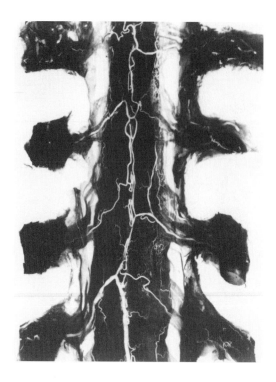

FIG. 5. The anterior surface of the cervical spinal cord from a 20-year-old woman. The anterior median longitudinal arterial trunk of the spinal cord is duplicated in a number of areas, whereas in the lower cervical segment it is a single large vessel. Unretouched, this arterial injection of the spinal cord provides evidence supporting the claim that radicular artery contributions to the anterior median longitudinal arterial trunk of the spinal cord are segmental. The size of individual radicular arteries varies considerably.

The surface of the cervical spinal cord carries three main vessels: the anterior median longitudinal arterial channel and the posterolateral longitudinal arterial channels. Between these three main channels there are circumferential and vertically orientated tributaries, which form the vasa corona of the spinal cord.

INTRAMEDULLARY DISTRIBUTION OF ARTERIES

Sulcal branches from the anterior median longitudinal arterial channel enter the spinal cord at regular intervals in the midline, penetrating the gray matter and arborizing alternately into its right and left sides around the central canal of the spinal cord (Fig. 7). Radiate branches penetrate its dorsolateral aspects directly from the posterolateral longitudinal arterial channels and from the vasa corona around the circumference, supplying predominantly the white matter of the cord and overlapping to some extent with the central blood supply of the gray matter.

The arterial network within the spinal cord is dense and gives rise to a complex capillary system from which prominent veins arise and pass out radially to join veins on the surface of the spinal cord (Fig. 8).

The orientation of veins on the surface of the cervical spinal cord differs from that of the arteries. There are principal median longitudinal venous channels, on both the anterior and the posterior surfaces of the cord, lying, as do the other vessels, in a sub-pial position. Between these two main channels there is a complex arrangement of vasa corona, with transverse and longitudinally orientated branches giving rise to anterior and posterior radicular veins that run along the nerve roots and emerge in the epidural space to join the bulky venous radicles of the internal vertebral venous plexus.

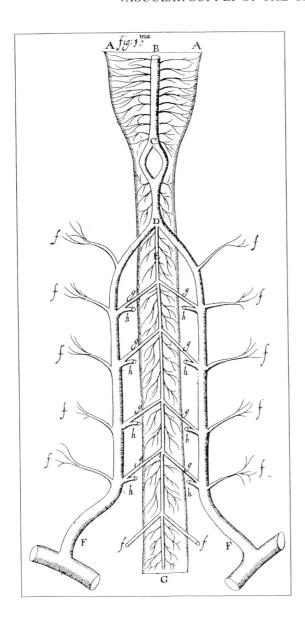

FIG. 6. A reproduction of the drawing from Thomas Willis' book, *Cerebri Anatome* (London, 1664), illustrating the segmental nature of the arterial supply of the cervical spinal cord viewed from the front.

THE VENOUS DRAINAGE OF THE VERTEBRAL COLUMN

In each vertebral body, a capillary bed is formed in the region of the vertebral endplates. This gives rise to an intraosseous complex of veins. First, a horizontal subarticular collecting vein system develops. The main stems of this network drain posteriorly into the spinal canal to join the anterior internal vertebral venous plexus, and peripherally around the vertebral margins to join ascending and descending veins, which course toward the center of the vertebral body on its surface to join the external vertebral veins. The intraosseous veins of the second group course upwards or downwards from the vertebral endplate capillary beds toward the centrum grid known as Batson's plexus. Tribu-

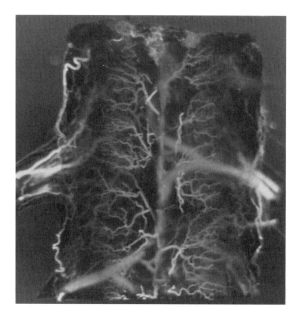

FIG. 7. A coronal section of a segment of the cervical spinal cord from a 13-year-old child. The section is cut just posterior to the bulbous anterior horns of gray matter. In the midline, the anterior median longitudinal arterial trunk of the spinal cord is out of focus. The specimen has been prepared to illustrate the manner of branching of the central sulcal arteries of the spinal cord. Adjacent individual sulcal central arteries deviate to one side of the cord or the other, and they branch laterally in patterns resembling closely cropped leafless trees. Occasionally, a single central sulcal artery bifurcates to form a treelike pattern on both the right and left sides of the midline.

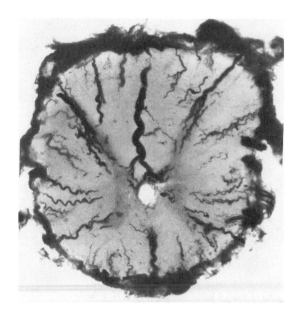

FIG. 8. A thin transverse section from the thoracic spinal cord of a 13-year-old boy. The overall pattern of venous drainage is radiate. Centrally placed veins drain anteriorly and posteriorly into median longitudinal veins on the respective surfaces of the cord. The other radiate branches join the tributaries of the vasa corona on the surface of the cord, lying beneath the pia mater.

taries of this plexus drain posteriorly into the anterior internal vertebral venous plexus and circumferentially into the external vertebral veins on the surface of the waist of the vertebral body. The external vertebral veins join the venous plexus that surrounds the vertebral arteries or tributaries of the jugular venous system in the neck.

REFERENCES

1. Crock HV. *An atlas of vascular anatomy of the skeleton and spinal cord*. London: Martin Dunitz, 1996.
2. Crock HV, Yoshizawa H. *The blood supply of the vertebral column and spinal cord in man*. New York: Springer-Verlag, 1977.
3. Willis T. *Cerebri anatome*. London: Fo. Martyn & Fa. Alleftry, 1664.

Whiplash Injuries: Current Concepts in Prevention, Diagnosis, and Treatment of the Cervical Whiplash Syndrome, edited by Robert Gunzburg and Marek Szpalski. Lippincott–Raven Publishers, Philadelphia © 1998.

2

Biomechanics of the Cervical Spine

Michael A. Adams

M. A. Adams: Department of Anatomy, University of Bristol, Bristol BS2 8EJ, United Kingdom.

The purpose of this chapter is to give a general introduction to the mechanical properties of the cervical spine. Intervertebral disc function and failure are discussed, and some suggestions are made regarding the nature of whiplash injuries. However, a detailed mechanical analysis of whiplash is left for other chapters.

MOVEMENTS OF THE CERVICAL SPINE

Almost 40% of the height of the cervical spine from C2 to C7 is made up of intervertebral discs (21), so it is not surprising that this is the most mobile region of the spine. Each motion segment has approximately 20° of flexion/extension movement, 14° of side-to-side lateral bending, and 10° to 15° of side-to-side axial rotation (Table 1).

Cadaveric experiments on cervical motion segments demonstrate the high intrinsic mobility of the cervical spine. Bending moments (stresses) required to produce small angular movements of the cervical spine are only 15% to 35% of those required to produce the same movement in the lumbar spine, even after the bending moments have been adjusted to account for the greater size of the lumbar specimens (27).

Large movements are guided by the uncovertebral "joints" and by the articular facets, which, in the cervical spine, are relatively broad and orientated at approximately 45° to the vertical and sagittal planes. These oblique articular surfaces cause a high degree of movement coupling in different planes as indicated in Figure 1. For example, 10° of axial rotation of a cervical motion segment is accompanied by 5° of lateral bending, and 10° of lateral bending produces 3° of axial rotation (36). "Pure" rotation or bending of the head about the shoulders therefore requires complex compensatory movements in the upper cervical spine.

The C1-C2 articulation, which has no intervertebral disc, can be axially rotated by more than 80°. According to Kapandji (21), flexion and extension of this joint involve rolling and sliding of the lateral masses in a manner similar to the movements of the femoral condyles on the tibial plateau. The curved shape of the lateral masses ensures that axial rotation is accompanied by a vertical separation of the two vertebrae, resulting in a slight helical movement rather than pure rotation. (It is not clear, however, to what extent Kapandji's observations are based on experimental measurements.)

TABLE 1. *Range of movement (in degrees) of cervical motion segments in vivo, as determined in experiments on healthy individuals*

	C1-C2	C2-C3	C3-C4	C4-C5	C5-C6	C6-C7
Flexion and extension[a]	15	12	17	21	23	21
Lateral bend[b]		14	14	14	14	14
Axial rotation[c]	83	6	13	13	14	11

[a] Data from Dvořák J, Froehlich D, Penning L, Baumgartner H, Panjabi MM. Functional radiographic diagnosis of the cervical spine: flexion/extension. *Spine* 1988;13(7):748–755.
[b] Data from Penning L. Normal movements of the cervical spine. *Am J Roentgenol* 1978;130:317–326.
[c] Data from Dvořák J, Panjabi MM, Gerber M, Wichman W. CT-functional diagnostics of the rotary instability of the upper cervical spine. *Spine* 1987;12:197–205.

STABILITY OF THE CERVICAL SPINE

The wide range of movement of the cervical spine can create problems of stability. The neutral zone is that range of movement in which the discs and ligaments provide practically no resistance to movement (26,30), and in the cervical spine the neutral zone is approximately 7° (from one side to the other) for each motion segment (36). This applies to axial rotation as well as to flexion/extension and lateral bending, and it is greater than in any other region of the spine. Rotational and bending stability of the cervical spine within the neutral zone is therefore left very much to the paraspinal musculature, so muscle injuries might be expected to lead to rotational instability. Beyond the neutral zone, ligaments play a larger role. Sectioning of the posterior ligaments doubles the range of forward flexion (37) and of axial rotation (35).

Translational movements, such as forward or lateral slipping of one vertebra relative to the one below, are more than doubled when the neural arch is removed (27), so the facet joints and intervertebral ligaments must play a large role in resisting horizontal forces between cervical vertebrae. None of the longitudinal neck muscles are well suited to prohibit such small transverse movements: the anterior-posterior shear displacements remain less than 2 mm in a three-vertebra specimen, even when the shear force rises to 150 newtons (33). Translational stability probably depends on the integrity of the intervertebral ligaments and facet joints.

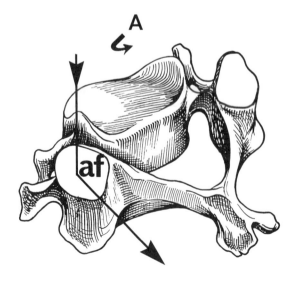

FIG. 1. In the cervical spine, the broad oblique articular facets of the apophyseal joints and uncovertebral joints serve to couple movements of axial rotation and lateral bending. The *arrows* indicate how lateral flexion of a superincumbent vertebra (not shown) would cause its descending left inferior articular process to be deflected posteriorly by the articular facet (*af*), creating an axial rotation movement (*A*) in the direction of the arrow. (Adapted from Kapandji IA. *The physiology of the joints, vol. 3. The trunk and the vertebral column.* Edinburgh: Churchill Livingstone, 1974.)

A high proportion of the compressive force on the cervical spine appears to be resisted by the apophyseal joints. The axial deformation caused by compressive loading is doubled when these joints are removed (27), and the compressive strength of sections of cervical spine is halved if they are flexed so that the apophyseal joints are unable to resist a proportion of the applied compressive force (24).

INJURY TO THE CERVICAL SPINE

The precise mechanisms of injury to the osteoligamentous cervical spine have received less attention than injuries to the lumbar spine. Many early experiments involved impact loading of whole cadavers to simulate automobile injuries, but the results are difficult to interpret because of the absence of muscle forces, which in life can act to reduce bending moment on the spine while at the same time greatly increasing compression (Fig. 2). As will be discussed, the ratio of bending to compression has a large effect in determining the site and nature of spinal injuries. Tests on whole cadavers, or on large multibone specimens, have the added difficulty of allowing unphysiologic movements of intermediate "floating" bones that are held in position neither by muscle activity, as in life, nor by the experimental apparatus, as in motion segment experiments. Large specimens also increase the difficulty in identifying the site of first injury, or the precise forces responsible for it. Other, more controlled experiments have applied only small loads (30) or have used fixation systems that lead to premature damage to the specimens being tested (27).

Shea et al. (33) avoided many of these problems and applied high, controlled loads to three-vertebra sections of human cervical spine. They found that flexion injuries damaged the discs most frequently, but they also caused a variety of injuries to ligaments and bones. Failure occurred at an average bending moment of 7 newton-meters (Nm) (for the upper cervical specimens) and 12.5 Nm (for the lower cervical specimens). Flexion

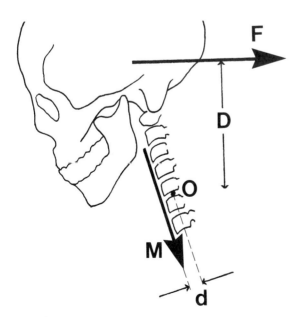

FIG. 2. When the head is thrown into flexion or extension, very high forces (*M*) are required in the neck muscles to prevent injury. This is because the paravertebral muscles lie close to the centers of rotation near the cervical discs (*O*), whereas the inertial force acting on the head (*F*) acts on a much greater lever arm. Approximately, $M \times d = F \times D$. In many incidents, the muscle force (*M*) will be much greater than the weight of the head.

angles at failure corresponded to 12° to 13° for each motion segment. Living people experience discomfort if only 10 Nm of bending moment (or even less) is applied to their cervical spine while their neck muscles are fully relaxed (25). The similarity between these *in vitro* and *in vivo* results emphasizes the importance of muscle action in protecting the osteoligamentous cervical spine in bending.

An axial torque (twisting) pre-load appears to increase the cervical spine's strength in bending, but it also ensures more widespread damage in the disc and ligaments when failure does eventually occur (33). The viscoelastic nature of spinal tissues may increase the spine's strength in bending during high-velocity injuries, but experiments on cadaveric *lumbar* motion segments suggest that this effect will not be large: bending stiffness increases by only 10% to 15% when the duration of loading falls from 5 seconds to 0.5 second (1).

Forced hyperextension has not been investigated as thoroughly as flexion, but the data of Moroney et al. (27) suggest that it involves high loading of the neural arch. The high contribution of the apophyseal joints to compressive strength (see later) provides additional evidence that these joints are often the site of failure in forced hyperextension.

Compressive failure of the cervical spine occurs at approximately 3.6 kN (24), but compressive strength falls to 1.8 to 2.2 kN if the specimens are positioned in a flexed position (24,33), as occurs in certain impacts. This may be because flexion unloads the apophyseal joints and stretches the posterior intervertebral ligaments [at least in the lumbar spine (5)], and both of these effects will increase loading of the vertebral body. Head-on collisions simulated on large cadaver head-and-neck specimens showed that high compressive forces can cause the cervical spine to buckle in a rather unpredictable manner, often with extension in the mid cervical spine and flexion in the lower (28). It is not clear if this buckling behavior would persist if the neck were stabilized by muscle action.

Compressive injuries to the disc–vertebral body unit have been studied closely in *lumbar* motion segments, but results may be applicable to the cervical spine also, because discs in both regions have a similar ratio of height to anteroposterior diameter. Pure compression always damages the vertebral body before the disc, regardless of whether the force is applied once or many times during cyclic loading (10–12,23,32). The site of damage is normally the vertebral body endplate, or the vertically oriented trabeculae that lie just behind it (11,32). In either case, the nucleus is able to bulge more into the vertebral body, increasing the space available for the nucleus and reducing the hydrostatic pressure within it (6). Because less compressive force is resisted by the nucleus pulposus, more must be resisted by the annulus fibrosus and apophyseal joints, so high concentrations of compressive stress can appear in the annulus, particularly posterior to the nucleus (6). Effectively, the disc behaves like a flat (i.e., deflated) tire (9). There is some evidence that high compressive stresses cause the lamellae of the annulus to collapse into the depressurized nucleus during subsequent repetitive loading (7). Internal disruption of this sort, involving reverse bulging of the lamellae of the inner annulus, is a common feature of disc degeneration (13,19,34).

The strength in anteroposterior shear of cadaveric cervical spine specimens has been found to be approximately 200 N, but the site and nature of failure were not recorded (33).

INTERVERTEBRAL DISC PROLAPSE

Posterior herniation of intervertebral discs is a common injury in both cervical and lumbar spines (22,34), but the mechanisms of prolapse have been studied only in the latter. Controlled loading experiments on human cadaveric lumbar motion segments (3) show that posterior disc prolapse occurs when high compressive forces are combined with high forward bending stresses, as they often are in whiplash injuries. An additional component of lateral bending makes prolapse more likely and moves the site of failure from the midline posterior annulus to the opposite posterolateral corner of the disc, which is stretched the most by the component of lateral bending (3). Repetitive loading in bending and compression can create radial fissures in the posterolateral corners of discs, allowing small quantities of nuclear material to escape (4,17). Once out of the disc, fragments of nucleus pulposus (and to a lessor extent, annulus fibrosus) absorb tissue fluid and swell to 2 to 3 times their size in a few hours (14). Furthermore, this displaced material exhibits an inflammatory response (18) that may influence surrounding tissue (29). These effects mean that symptoms associated with disc prolapse may not occur with full severity at the time of initial injury but will become more severe over a period of hours or days, hiding the essentially mechanical nature of the underlying problem.

A combination of high backwards bending moment and high compressive force appears to increase posterior bulging of lumbar discs and, in rare cases, causes anterior disc prolapse (2). Similar events may occur when the cervical spine is thrown into forced extension.

BIOMECHANICS AND WHIPLASH

Although this subject is dealt with in more detail in other chapters, we can say that there does appear to be a fundamental lack of experimental evidence showing just which cervical structures are damaged and how. Therefore, a few suggestions will be made here, based on experimental evidence from the lumbar spine.

In most whiplash injuries, the cervical spine is subjected to forced flexion or extension movements, or both in quick succession (Fig. 3). High bending stresses (bending "moments") will be accompanied by compressive forces arising from the neck muscles as they contract in an attempt to limit the bending (see Fig. 2). If the injured person is warned of the impending collision (perhaps by the sound of breaking, or by the brake lights of the car in front), then the neck muscles will have time to contract vigorously, and the ratio of compression to bending will probably be high. As discussed above, damage

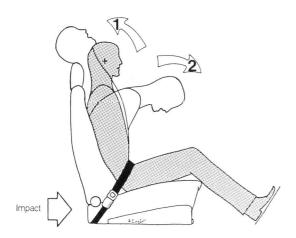

FIG. 3. During a typical whiplash injury, the head is effectively thrown backward and then forward relative to the shoulders. Adapted from Foreman SM, Croft AC. *Whiplash injuries. The cervical acceleration/deceleration syndrome.* Baltimore: Williams and Wilkins, 1988;64.

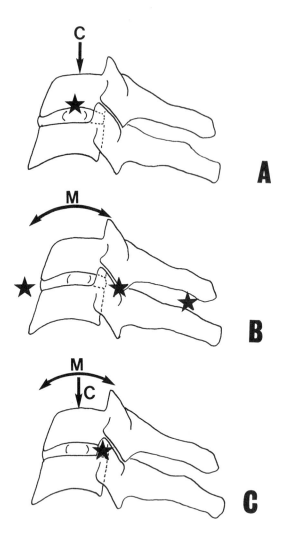

FIG. 4. The effects of bending and compression on the cervical spine can be estimated from experiments on cadaveric lumbar motion segments. **A:** A high compressive force (*C*) creates high pressure in the center of intervertebral discs, and this can damage the vertebral body and endplates. **B:** A high bending moment (*M*), either in flexion or extension, creates high forces in those muscles and ligaments that lie farthest from the centers of rotation near the discs and may injure them. **C:** Compression and bending acting together can cause disc prolapse, as the pressurized central region of the disc is displaced through the stretched and weakened annulus.

may then occur in the vertebral body and endplate (Fig. 4A). Alternatively, if the collision is entirely unexpected, then the muscles may not be able to contract in time to protect the neck, and bending moment will greatly dominate the compressive force. The muscles and ligaments are then more likely to sustain injury, with anterior structures being at risk during the hyperextension phase and posterior structures during the hyperflexion phase (see Fig. 4B). If the collision is *partially* anticipated, or if it is fully anticipated but the neck muscles are unable to hold the head steady, then the accident may result in high compressive *and* bending stresses acting at the same time. During the flexion phase of whiplash, this may cause posterior disc prolapse in the manner discussed (see Fig. 4C). In a recent study of 50 consecutive patients with whiplash (20), eight were found to have recent posterior disc herniations at surgery.

A second important factor in whiplash injuries may be the extent to which the victim is turning around to look over his or her shoulder at the time of impact. Axial rotation stretches the capsular ligaments on the side of the neck that the head is turning to and compresses the apophyseal joint surfaces on the contralateral side. Conversely, the lateral bending movements that are always coupled with axial rotation (as discussed) load the facet surfaces on the ipsilateral side and stretch the capsule on the contralateral side. It is easy to see, therefore, that any turning of the head at impact may increase the risk of injury to the apophyseal joint surfaces (in the hyperextension phase) and capsular ligaments (in the hyperflexion phase). In another study on 50 patients with whiplash, apophyseal joint pain was identified in 54% of patients on the basis of successful pain blocking on two separate occasions (8).

CONCLUSIONS

The high mobility of the cervical spine leads to problems of rotational and bending instability if the muscles are injured or weak, and translational instability if the ligaments are weak. The site of injury during whiplash will depend on the extent to which the victim was contracting his neck muscles at the time of impact, and on whether he or she was turning to look over one shoulder.

ACKNOWLEDGMENTS

This work of the author is supported by the Arthritis and Rheumatism Council of Great Britain.

REFERENCES

1. Adams MA, Dolan P. Time dependent changes in the lumbar spine's resistance to bending. *Clin Biomech* 1996; 11:194–200.
2. Adams MA, Dolan P, Hutton WC. The lumbar spine in backward bending. *Spine* 1988;13(9):1019–1026.
3. Adams MA, Hutton WC. Prolapsed intervertebral disc. A hyperflexion injury. *Spine* 1982;7:184–191.
4. Adams MA, Hutton WC. Gradual disc prolapse. *Spine* 1985;10:524–531.
5. Adams MA, McNally DS, Chinn H, Dolan P. Posture and the compressive strength of the lumbar spine. International Society of Biomechanics Award paper. *Clin Biomech* 1994;9:5–14.
6. Adams MA, McNally DS, Wagstaff J, Goodship AE. Abnormal stress concentrations in lumbar intervertebral discs following damage to the vertebral body: a cause of disc failure. European Spine Society (Acromed) Award paper. *Eur Spine J* 1993;1:214–221.
7. Adams MA, Morrison HP, Dolan P. Internal disruption of an intervertebral disc can be caused by previous minor damage to an adjacent vertebral body. Presented to the International Society for the Study of the Lumbar Spine, Helsinki, Finland, June 1995.
8. Barnsley L, Lord SM, Wallis BJ, Bogduk N. The prevalence of chronic cervical zygapophysial joint pain after whiplash. *Spine* 1995;20(1):20–26.
9. Brinckmann P, Grootenboer H. Change of disc height, radial disc bulge and intradiscal pressure from discectomy: an in vitro investigation on human lumbar discs. *Spine* 1991;16:641–646.
10. Brinckmann P. Injury of the annulus fibrosus and disc protrusions. An in vitro investigation on human lumbar discs. *Spine* 1986;11(2):149–153.
11. Brinckmann P, Biggemann M, Hilweg D. Fatigue fracture of human lumbar vertebrae. *Clin Biomech* 1988;3 (Suppl 1):S1–S23.
12. Brinckmann P, Biggemann M, Hilweg D. Prediction of the compressive strength of human lumbar vertebrae. *Spine* 1989;14:606–610.
13. Crock HV. Internal disc disruption: a challenge to disc prolapse 50 years on. *Spine* 1986;11:650–653.
14. Dolan P, Adams MA, Hutton WC. The short-term effects of chymopapain on intervertebral discs. *J Bone Joint Surg* 1987;69B:422–428.
15. Dvořák J, Froehlich D, Penning L, Baumgartner H, Panjabi MM. Functional radiographic diagnosis of the cervical spine: flexion/extension. *Spine* 1988;13(7):748–755.
16. Dvořák J, Panjabi MM, Gerber M, Wichmann W. CT-functional diagnostics of the rotatory instability of the upper cervical spine. *Spine* 1987;12:197–205.
17. Gordon SJ, Yang KH, Mayer PJ, Mace AH, Kish VL, Radin EL. Mechanism of disc rupture—a preliminary report. *Spine* 1991;16(4):450–456.

18. Gronblad M, Virri J, Tolonen J, et al. A controlled immunohistochemical study of inflammatory cells in disc herniation tissue. *Spine* 1994;19:2744–2751.
19. Gunzburg R, Parkinson R, Moore R, et al. A cadaveric study comparing discography, MRI, histology, and mechanical behaviour of the human lumbar disc. *Spine* 1992;17:417–423.
20. Jonsson H, Cesarini K, Sahlstedt B, Rauschning W. Findings and outcome in whiplash-type neck distortions. *Spine* 1994;19(24):2733–2743.
21. Kapandji IA. *The physiology of the joints, vol. 3. The trunk and the vertebral column.* Edinburgh: Churchill Livingstone, 1974.
22. Kokubun S, Sakurai M, Tanaka Y. Cartilaginous endplate in cervical disc herniation. *Spine* 1996;21(2):190–195.
23. Liu YK, Njus G, Buckwalter J, Wakano K. Fatigue response of lumbar intervertebral joints under axial cyclic loading. *Spine* 1983;8:857–865.
24. Maiman DJ, Sances A, Myklebust JB, et al. Compression injuries of the cervical spine: a biomechanical analysis. *Neurosurgery* 1983;13:254–260.
25. McGill SM, Jones K, Bennett G, Bishop PJ. Passive stiffness of the human neck in flexion, extension, and lateral bending. *Clin Biomech* 1994;9(3):193–198.
26. Moller J, Nolte L-P, Visarius H, Willburger R, Crisco JJ, Panjabi MM. Viscoelasticity of the alar and transverse ligaments. *Eur Spine J* 1992;1:178–184.
27. Moroney SP, Schultz AB, Miller JAA, Andersson GBJ. Load-displacement properties of lower cervical spine motion segments. *J Biomech* 1988;21:769–779.
28. Nightingale RW, McElhaney JH, Richardson WJ, Best TM, Myers BS. Experimental impact injury to the cervical spine: relating motion of the head and the mechanism of injury. *J Bone Joint Surg* 1996;78A(3):412–418.
29. Olmarker K, Blomquist J, Stromberg J, Nannmark U, Thomsen P, Rydevik B. Inflammatogenic properties of nucleus pulposus. *Spine* 1995;20(6):665–669.
30. Panjabi MM, Summers DJ, Pelker RR, Videman T, Friedlaender GE, Southwick WO. Three-dimensional load-displacement curves due to forces on the cervical spine. *J Orthop Res* 1986;4:152–161.
31. Penning L. Normal movements of the cervical spine. *Am J Roentgenol* 1978;130:317–326.
32. Perey O. Fracture of the vertebral endplate. A biomechanical investigation. *Acta Orthop Scand* 1957(suppl 25).
33. Shea M, Edwards WT, White AA, Hayes WC. Variations of stiffness and strength along the human cervical spine. *J Biomech* 1991;24:95–107.
34. Tanaka M, Nakahara S, Inoue H. A pathologic study of discs in the elderly. *Spine* 1993;18(11):1456–1462.
35. Ulrich C, Woersdoerfer O, Kalff R, Claes L, Wilke H-A. Biomechanics of fixation systems to the cervical spine. *Spine* 1991;16:S4–9.
36. Wen N, Lavaste F, Santin JJ, Lassau JP. Three-dimensional biomechanical properties of the human cervical spine in vitro. I. Analysis of normal motion. *Eur Spine J* 1993;2:2–11.
37. Wen N, Lavaste F, Santin JJ, Lassau JP. Three-dimensional biomechanical properties of the human cervical spine in vitro. II. Analysis of instability after ligamentous injuries. *Eur Spine J* 1993;2:12–15.
38. Foreman SM, Croft AC. Whiplash injuries. The cervical acceleration/deceleration syndrome. Baltimore: Williams and Wilkins, 1988;64.

Whiplash Injuries: Current Concepts in Prevention, Diagnosis, and Treatment of the Cervical Whiplash Syndrome, edited by Robert Gunzburg and Marek Szpalski. Lippincott–Raven Publishers, Philadelphia © 1998.

3

Normal Imaging of the Cervical Spine: Roentgen Anatomy, Variants, and Pitfalls

Johan W. M. Van Goethem, Jacques Widelec, Jacques de Moor, Luc van den Hauwe, Paul M. Parizel, Philippe Petroons, and Arthur M. A. De Schepper

J. W. M. Van Goethem, J. de Moor, L. van den Hauwe, P. M. Parizel, and A. M. A. De Schepper: Department of Radiology, University of Antwerp, Edegem, Belgium. J. Widelec and P. Petroons: Department of Radiology, Centre Hospitalier Molière Longchamp, Brussels, Belgium.

The cervical spine can be divided into two mechanically and anatomically different units. The first unit is the upper cervical spine, consisting of the occiput, sometimes referred to as C0, the atlas (C1), and the axis (C2). Sometimes this unit is called the cervicocranium. The second unit is the middle and lower cervical spine, extending from C3 through C7.

THE UPPER CERVICAL SPINE

Anatomy

Bony Elements

The atlas is a unique ringlike structure without vertebral body. It has an anterior arch from which arises the anterior tubercle on the midline, a lateral mass on each side, and a posterior arch. It has neither pedicles nor laminae as do other cervical bodies, and it has no true spinous process.

The axis is the largest cervical vertebra. It differs from all other vertebrae by the existence of its dens or odontoid process, which embryologically corresponds to the body of the atlas. Also, the pedicle of C1 is represented by that portion of the axis body that extends from its prominent anterior convexity to the mass of bone supporting its superior articulating surface.

Joints

The occipitoatlantal joints are formed by the convex articulating surface of the occipital condyles and the concave superior facets of the lateral masses of the atlas.

The atlas and axis articulate through four joints. The posterior surface of the anterior arch of C1 and the anterior surface of the dens form the anterior median atlantoaxial joint. The posterior part is formed between the posterior surface of the dens and the transverse atlantal ligament. The lateral atlantoaxial joints are formed by the contiguous articulating surfaces of the lateral masses of C1 and C2 (Fig. 1).

Ligaments

Anteriorly, the anterior longitudinal ligament (ALL) extends upward from C2 as the atlantoaxial membrane to C1 (superficial and deep anterior atlantoaxial ligament), and from there on as the atlanto-occipital membrane to the anterior surface of the clivus.

The alar ligaments extend from the superolateral aspect of the dens to the occipital condyles.

The transverse (atlantal) ligament is situated posteriorly to the dens and separated from it by a true synovial membrane. It connects the medial surfaces of the lateral masses of the atlas.

The apical dental ligament extends from the tip of the dens to the basion (the tip of the clivus). Usually, a small amount of fat is interposed between the tip of the dens and the tip of the clivus. Absence of this fat tissue should be considered abnormal.

The posterior longitudinal ligament (PLL) extends upwards as the membrana tectoria to the anterior lateral aspect of the foramen magnum.

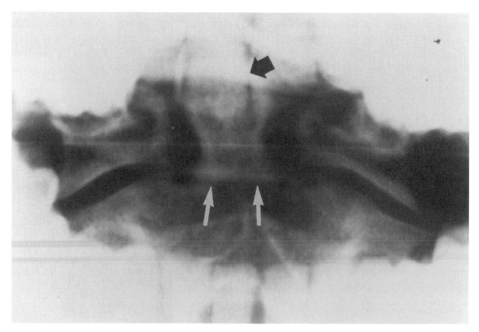

FIG. 1. Frontal view of the atlantoaxial articulation. Superposition of the maxillary incisors may create the image of a vertical lucency over the dens axis *(black arrow)*, not to be mistaken for a fracture. Projection of the posterior arch of C1 over the base of the odontoid may simulate a horizontal dens fracture *(white arrows)*. Symmetry of the lateral atlantoaxial articulations and equal distance of the lateral articular masses of C1 to the dens axis is a sign of neutral position of the head.

Roentgen Anatomy: Normal Findings and Pitfalls

Bone

All anatomic bony elements are readily visible on plain radiographs, computed tomography (CT), and magnetic resonance imaging (MRI). It is however important to recognize the normal projections of these structures on plain radiographs and to understand their normal anatomic relationships.

The atlanto-occipital articulation is usually visible only on the frontal radiograph. In the lateral projection, there is superimposition of the left and the right articulation and usually the mastoids. Hence, fractures of the occipital condyles and the lateral masses of C1 are not readily visible on lateral radiographs.

In the frontal open-mouth projection, the lateral masses of C1 have a greater vertical height laterally than medially (see Fig. 1). At the inner third of this articular mass there is an area of increased density where the transverse ligament attaches. This should not be mistaken for a fracture of the lateral mass of C1.

The lateral masses of C1 normally show an equal distance to the odontoid process at a given height (see Fig. 1). This distance, however, may vary throughout the vertical lining of this space. On the frontal view, the lines joining the articular space C0-C1 on one side with the articular space C1-C2 on the other side cross each other, always on the midline precisely at the center of the dens (19).

Even very slight rotation can produce asymmetry in the distance between the dens and C1 on the left and right side. This can be derived from the off-center projection of the spinous process of C2.

On neutral lateral radiographs, the distance between the anterior arch of the atlas and the dens should not exceed 3 mm in adults. In flexion, this distance can be larger, especially in children (9,16).

Frequently, the lower margin of the posterior arch of C1 projects over the base of the dens in the frontal radiograph, creating an illusion of a slightly high dens fracture (2).

Also, the overlapping shadow of the maxillary incisors may produce pseudofractures of the dens (see Fig. 1). This should be differentiated from real closure defects of the anterior arch of C1 (1) and from congenital schisis of the dens in which a vertical cleft persists in adult life (Fig. 2).

Normally, the medial margins of the facets of C2 are aligned with the inferior facets of C1 on a frontal radiograph in neutral position. With rotation of the head, the displacement of the facets of C1 relative to C2 will be in the same direction on both sides. This is opposed to the bilateral lateral displacement of the lateral masses of C1 in the Jefferson burst fracture of C1. In children, however, this finding may caused by a disparity in growth between atlas and axis. It is most commonly seen about the age of 4 years (15).

During rotation of the head, the atlas pivots about the dens (5). The lateral mass of the atlas at the contralateral side rotates forward and medially in relationship to the axis. It becomes more rectangular in appearance and projects closer to the dens on frontal radiographs. The other lateral mass moves posteriorly. Its distance to the dens first remains unaltered and then decreases. With further rotation, the joint spaces appear narrower on radiographs and the total height of the atlantoaxial complex decreases.

On a lateral radiograph, the dens usually extends vertically from the body of C2. Sometimes, it may incline backwards as much as 30° to 40° (17) (Fig. 3). The posterior lining of the dens may be irregular and not aligned with the other posterior vertebral cortical linings.

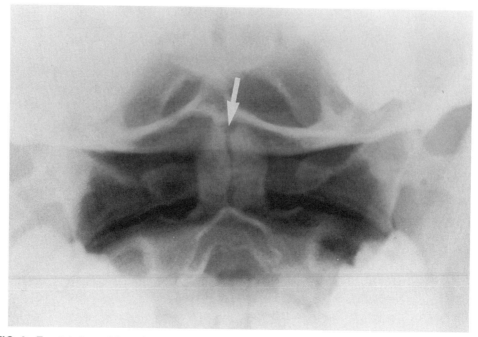

FIG. 2. Frontal view of the atlantoaxial articulation. A striking vertical cleft is noted in the odontoid *(white arrow)*. It represents a developmental nonunion known as schisis. It should not be mistaken for a traumatic lesion.

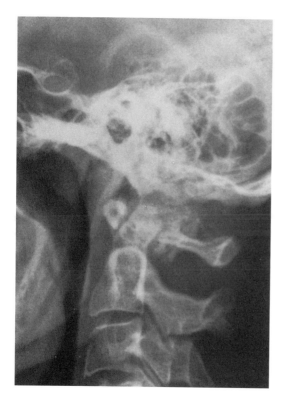

FIG. 3. Lateral view of the upper cervical spine. The dens axis may tilt as far backward as 30° to 40° in normal adults. The spinolaminar line, however, should remain intact, as is the case here.

Soft Tissues

Air in the pharynx normally outlines the uvula, the tongue, and the posterior nasopharyngeal wall on lateral radiographs. The soft-tissue shadow in front of the upper cervical spine principally represents the anterior atlanto-occipital and atlantoaxial ligament, the constrictor muscles, and the mucosal lining of the pharynx. Usually, it closely adheres to C1 and C2. The contour of the normal cervicocranial prevertebral soft-tissue shadow is that of posterior concavity, except at the level of the anterior tubercle of C1.

Roentgen Variants That May Simulate Traumatic Lesions

Sometimes, accessory bony elements can be seen between the base of the skull and C1. They may present as third occipital condyles or occipital vertebrae (11). Sometimes, they are still attached and arise as bony spurs from the base of the skull.

The posterior arch of C1 shows a normal cleft in children up to 6 years old. It may close asymmetrically and sometimes persists in adult life. The laminae or posterior arch of C1 can be absent (uni- or bilaterally) (3,10), which is not necessarily an innocent lesion (14) (Fig. 4). The absence of the posterior arch is often associated with hypertrophy of the anterior arch.

Arcuate foramina are formed by calcification of the oblique atlanto-occipital ligaments. Through these foramina pass the vertebral arteries (Fig. 5).

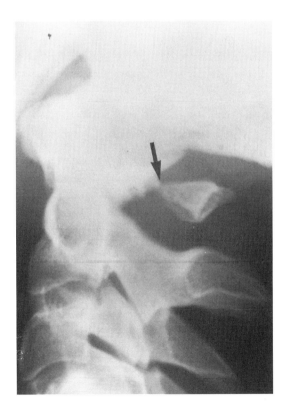

FIG. 4. Lateral view of the upper cervical spine. Congenital/developmental hypoplasia or aplasia of (a part of) the posterior arch of C1 is not uncommon. It may be bilateral and incomplete as is presented here *(black arrow)*, but it can also be unilateral and/or complete. It is not always an innocent finding, but it should be differentiated from acute traumatic lesions.

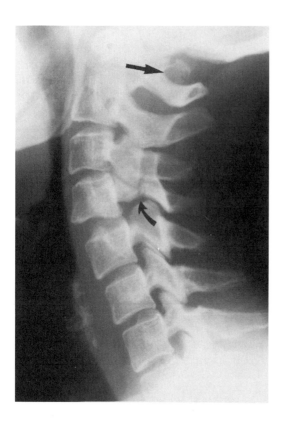

FIG. 5. Lateral view of the upper cervical spine. Foramina arcuata are formed by the posterior arch of C1 and the calcified oblique atlanto-occipital ligaments *(straight arrow).* Through these foramina pass the vertebral arteries. Also note partial fusion of the posterior elements of C3 and C4 with bilateral spondylolysis of C4 *(curved arrow).* Concomitant anomalies are a key in the diagnosis of a developmental malformation rather than a traumatic lesion.

The dens has a normal ossification center (or more than one) at the tip. It appears at age 2 and fuses at 12 years of age. The synchondrosis at the base of the odontoid may be mistaken for a fracture in children. The junction closes by age 7, but it may persist in adult life. Failure of union of the odontoid leads to a separate os odontoideum (Fig. 6). It can be difficult to differentiate from an old dens fracture (13).

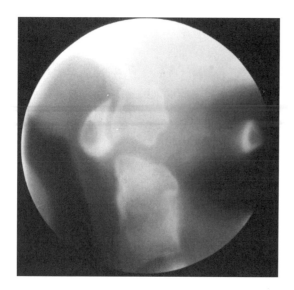

FIG. 6. Lateral tomography of the upper cervical spine. The os odontoideum embryologically represents the body of C1. It is not uncommon that it does not fuse with the body of C2, forming a separate os odontoideum instead of a normal (fused) dens axis. It is sometimes very difficult to differentiate between this and an old dens fracture.

THE LOWER CERVICAL SPINE

Anatomy

Bony Elements

The lower cervical spine includes C3 through C7. The vertebral bodies are uniform in configuration but increase gradually in size. Each vertebra consists of a body, paired pedicles and articular masses, laminae, and a single spinous process. The transverse process projects laterally from each side of the vertebral body and articular mass. It contains the transverse foramen through which the vertebral artery passes.

Joints

The vertebral bodies are bounded by their endplates. In between the endplates, the disc forms the intervertebral joint. The superior endplate laterally forms the uncinate process, which forms the uncovertebral joint (the joint of Luschka) with the immediately superior vertebral inferior endplate.

The articular or pillar masses are rhomboid-shaped structures lined by their articulating surfaces. They form the facetal or apophyseal joints. The plane of these joints is angled approximately 35° anteriorly from the vertical. The superior facets of the joints (the inferior facets of the vertebrae) are above and behind the lower inferior facets. The posterior margins of the articulating facets are parallel, symmetrical, and close to the same vertical plane on all levels in neutral position.

Neural Foramina

The cervical neural foramina are formed by the vertebral bodies anteriorly, the pedicles above and below, and the articular pillars and the ligamentum flavum posteriorly. These foramina are well seen on oblique views. Normally, the foramina C2-C3 through C6-C7 are visible.

Ligaments

The dense, strong ALL and the PLL extend from the axis to the sacrum. They are closely adherent to the vertebral bodies and intervertebral disks. The ligamentum nuchae attaches to the spinous process of the cervical segments. The interspinous ligament is a thin membranous structure; the supraspinous ligament is a strong fibrous component of the ligamentum nuchae that connects the apices of the spinous processes to the external occipital protuberance.

Roentgen Anatomy: Normal Findings and Pitfalls

Bone

On the lateral radiograph, the vertebral bodies are almost square. The transverse process forms a U-shaped mass superimposed on the vertebral body.

The articular masses from left and right should coincide on the lateral radiograph, which is an indicator of neutral cervical position (i.e., no rotation). The facetal joints are not normally visualized on frontal radiographs because of their inclination in the vertical plane. As a result, the lateral margins of the articulating masses form a smooth, continuous, and sharply demarcated density.

On lateral radiographs, the thin vertical strip of internal cortical bone at the base of the spinous processes forms the spinolaminar line, which marks the posterior extent of the spinal canal.

From the level of C3 downward, the spaces between the spinous processes are approximately the same height. The spinous processes themselves, however, may differ considerably in size. This is not true for the laminae, which are more homogeneous, and therefore the interlaminar spaces are more uniform in height. An increase in interlaminar space (fanning) may occur in posterior ligament tears (18).

Flexion and extension occur in a gradual fashion, with the highest amount of rotation and translation in the upper segments (4,18). Horizontal translation of two vertebral bodies can be as much as 4 mm between flexion and extension (20) (Fig. 7). The stature of the cervical spine should not be interpreted on CT or MRI examinations, because these are performed with the patient supine.

In oblique radiographs, the relationship of the laminae to each other is likened to shingles on a roof, with the lamina above covering the one below.

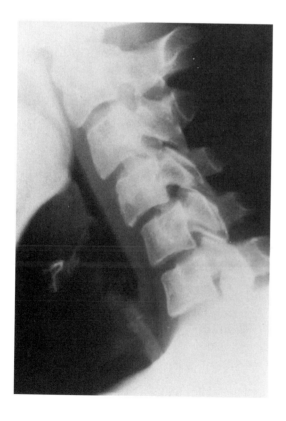

FIG. 7. Lateral view of the cervical spine in anterior flexion. Especially in young adults, there is an important anterior translation of the vertebral bodies in anterior flexion. This should be gradual, with the greatest movement at the highest levels, and it should not exceed 4 mm. Otherwise, one should think about abnormal ligamentous laxity or rupture.

Soft Tissues

The prevertebral soft-tissue shadow of the lower cervical spine is larger than that of the upper cervical spine by virtue of a high amount of fatty tissue in the prevertebral fascial space, and the presence of the esophagus. The esophagus usually gives an abrupt change (approximately a twofold increase) in the thickness of the prevertebral soft tissues, and its upper limit can be found between C3 and C6, depending on the amount of flexion/extension of the spine and the phase of swallowing (12). The width of the prevertebral soft-tissue shadow should not exceed 4 mm anterior to the midpoint of the anterior cortex of C3 in normal adults (6).

Roentgen Variants That May Simulate Traumatic Lesions

Anomalous articulations and (partial) fusions (incomplete segmentation) often occur at the C2-C3 level (see Fig. 5).

In flexion, pseudosubluxation in regularly seen in children, especially at the C2-C3 level (8). However, it may also occur in adults (7) or at lower cervical levels. The posterior cervical line is often not disturbed.

Upturned spinous processes should not be mistaken for a sign of ligamentous injury or fracture (Fig. 8). Their configuration does not change with flexion/extension.

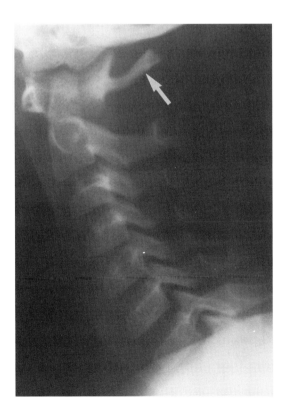

FIG. 8. Lateral view of the upper cervical spine in a normal child. Upturned spinous processes, or an upturned posterior arch of C1 as in this case, is a normal variant *(white arrow)*. Its configuration should not alter during flexion/extension. In children, the vertebral bodies are wedge shaped at all levels, and they should not be confused with compression fractures.

In children, the vertebral bodies are wedge shaped, which should not be confused with compression fracture (see Fig. 8). This wedge shape can persist in adult life.

The normal secondary ossification centers of the vertebrae close around the age of 16. Sometimes, persistent ring apophyses or limbus vertebrae can be noted. These ununited ossification centers can also be found at the articular processes or at the tip of the spinous process.

Finally, bifid spinous processes should not be mistaken for fracture.

REFERENCES

1. Chalmers AG. Spondyloschisis of the anterior arch of the atlas. *Br J Radiol* 1985;58:761–763.
2. Daffner RH. Pseudofracture of the dens: Mach bands. *Am J Roentgenol* 1977;128:607–612.
3. Dalinka MK, Rosenbaum AE, Van Houten F. Congenital absence of the posterior arch of the atlas. *Radiology* 1972;103:581–583.
4. Dvořák J, Panjabi MM, Grob D, Novotny JE, Antinnes JA. Clinical evaluation of functional flexion/extension radiographs of the cervical spine. *Spine* 1993;18:120.
5. Fielding JW. Cineroentgenography of the normal cervical spine. *J Bone Joint Surg* 1957;39:1280.
6. Harris JH Jr. Abnormal cervicocranial retropharyngeal soft-tissue contour in the detection of subtle acute cervicocranial injuries. *Emerg Radiol* 1994;1:15.
7. Harrison RB, Keats TE, Winn HR, et al. Pseudosubluxation of the axis in young adults. *J Can Assoc Radiol* 1980;31:176–177.
8. Jacobson G, Beeckler HH. Pseudosubluxation of the axis in children. *Am J Roentgenol* 1959;82:472.
9. Locke GR, Gardner JI, Van Epps EF. Atlas-dens interval in children. *Am J Roentgenol* 1966;97:135–140.
10. Logan WW, Stuard ID. Absent posterior arch of the atlas *Am J Roengenol* 1973;118:431–434.
11. Lombardi G. The occipital vertebra. *Am J Roentgenol* 1961;86:260.
12. Penning L. Roentgenographic evaluation: obtaining and interpreting plain films in cervical spine injury. In: Bailey RW, ed. *The cervical spine*. The Cervical Spine Research Society. Philadelphia: JB Lippincott, 1983.
13. Roback DL. Topics in radiology. *JAMA* 1981;245:963.
14. Schultze P, Buurman R. Absence of the posterior arch of the atlas. *Am J Roentgenol* 1980;134:178–180.
15. Suss RA, Zimmerman RD, Leeds NE. Pseudospread of the atlas: false sign of Jefferson fracture in children. *Am J Roentgenol* 1983;140:179–182.
16. Swischuk LE. The cervical spine in childhood. *Curr Prob Diagn Radiol* 1987;13:98.
17. Swischuk LE, et al. The posterior tilted dens: normal variation simulating fracture. *Pediatr Radiol* 1979;8:27.
18. Van Goethem JWM, Biltjes IGGM, van den Hauwe L, Parizel PM, De Schepper AMA. Whiplash injuries: is there a role for imaging? *Eur J Radiol* 1995;22:8.
19. Wackenheim. *Imagerie du rachis cervical.* Berlin: Springer-Verlag, 1989.
20. White AA III, Panjabi MM. *Clinical biomechanics of the spine*, 2nd ed. Philadelphia: JB Lippincott, 1990.

SECTION 2

Definition of the Whiplash Injury

*Whiplash Injuries: Current Concepts in
Prevention, Diagnosis, and Treatment
of the Cervical Whiplash Syndrome,*
edited by Robert Gunzburg and Marek Szpalski.
Lippincott–Raven Publishers, Philadelphia © 1998.

4

Injuries of the Cervical Spine
in Automobile Accidents: Pathoanatomic
and Clinical Aspects*

Wolfgang Rauschning and Halldór Jónsson, Jr.

*W. Rauschning: Department of Orthopaedic Surgery, Academic University Hospital,
Uppsala, Sweden.
H. Jónsson, Jr.: Department of Orthopaedic Surgery, Landspítalinn University Hospital,
Reykjavik, Iceland.*

This chapter is based on two journal articles: Our paper on hidden cervical spine injuries in traffic accident victims (27) is a pathoanatomic study in subjects who were killed by contact head injuries, whereas our paper on findings and outcome in whiplash-type neck distortions (28) is a clinical study on 50 consecutive automobile occupants who, wearing seat belts, were subjected to non-contact-type indirect deceleration forces in car accidents.

PATHOANATOMIC STUDY

The rationale for our first investigation was the increasing number of reports on traumatic cervical spine soft-tissue injuries that are notoriously missed on plain radiograms (2,5,14,16,38,39). Several forensic studies have borne out a high incidence of cervical spine injuries in fatal traffic accidents associated with head injuries (2,12,16,26). "Hidden" lesions of the cervical spine have also been produced in human cadavers and in animals that had been subjected to biomechanical experiments involving high deceleration forces and a variety of impact modes (25,33,40,47). There also appears to be an increasing incidence of neck injuries after the use of seat belts became compulsory (29,45,48).

For our forensic study, we selected traffic accident victims with skull fractures (by definition, nonwhiplash!), hypothesizing that forces of the head impact would be transmitted (and dissipated) to the cervical spine, causing a spectrum of injuries that then could be studied radiographically and pathoanatomically to ascertain the accuracy of plain radiographs in detecting such injuries. We studied 22 forensic specimens of traffic accident victims with skull fractures from 19 men and three women with a mean age of 26 years (range, 14 to 55 years). Five of these had survived the accident in neurointensive care for up to 3 days, and 17 had been killed on site. The police reports were scrutinized for the cause and type of the accident and also for probable direction of the impact. At autopsy, all external injuries were recorded and the sites of the impact lesion to the head and face and of the skull fractures were recorded in great detail following a strict protocol. The

---

*Illustrations and figures in this chapter © W. Rauschning and H. Jónsson.

cervical spines and the brachial plexus were inspected for injuries. The spines, including the paraspinal soft tissues, were then frozen *in situ* and removed.

Radiographic Technique

Fine-focus radiographs were taken in anteroposterior (AP), lateral, and 45-degree oblique planes, using fluoroscopy for precision alignment. The tube was tilted 30° from superiorly or inferiorly to separately visualize the articular pillars on both sides. Lateral radiographs were taken both in the straight lateral view with the articular pillars projecting over each other and in the 10-degree tilted images that separated the joint outlines. Several exposures were usually necessary to obtain an accurate view of all cervical segments. An average of ten films were taken of each specimen. Figure 1 shows examples of the radiographic views. The radiographs were evaluated segment by segment for fractures, dislocations, and any signs of soft-tissue injuries.

Cryosectioning Technique

After freeze-embedding of the specimens in high viscosity carboxymethylcellulose gel, the specimens were serially sectioned in the sagittal plane on a heavy-duty sledge

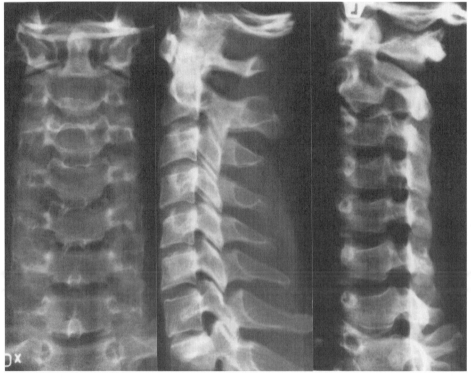

A–C

FIG. 1. Radiographs of an experimental *in vitro* specimen . **A:** An AP view. **B:** A straight lateral view. **C:** A 45-degree oblique view showing the foramina, pedicles, and uncinate processes. No injuries are seen on these radiographs. The pathoanatomic analysis showed multiple disc and facet joint injuries, a nerve root avulsion, and a subdural hematoma.

cryomicrotome. This surface cryoplaning technique has been described in detail elsewhere (42). At intervals of 1 mm or less, the specimen surface was cleaned, thawed, and photographed on high-resolution color reversal film. Because of the hardness of the bone in these young individuals, only 5- to 10-μm thin sections could be removed at each stroke; it took an average of 20 minutes to trim off 1 mm of tissue.

Radioanatomic Correlation

The slides were studied at high magnification and all injuries were listed and then correlated with the initial ("first-look") radiographic evaluation. Radiographs with discrepancies between radiographic and pathoanatomic findings were classified as either false positive or false negative and were resubmitted to the radiologist for a "second-look" reassessment, indicating only the ambiguous level, not the exact location of the injury. Finally, all radiographs were scrutinized in view of the pathoanatomic lesion by directly comparing the radiographs with the slides.

Occiput-Atlas-Axis Injuries

Probably because of the skull base fractures, no injuries were reported at the craniocervical junction during forensic autopsy. Initial assessment of the radiographs indicated one atlanto-axial asymmetry and three odontoid process fractures (one type B and two

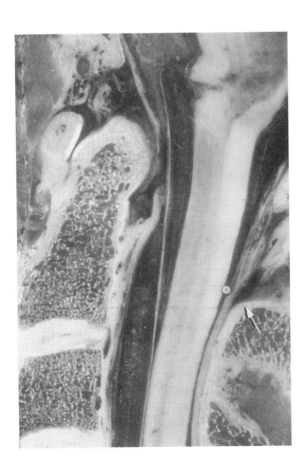

FIG. 2. Gross disruption of all occipito-atlanto-axial ligaments. Specimen radiographs showed only a slight atlanto-axial asymmetry. Note the subluxation and anterior rotation of the atlas, the complete ruptures of the anterior atlanto-occipital membrane, the apical and cruciate ligament, the tectorial membrane, and the avulsion of the ligamentum flavum from the C2 lamina *(arrow)*. In addition, two uncovertebral and two disc ruptures, three transverse process fractures, three facet joint and three ligamentum flavum ruptures were found in this specimen.

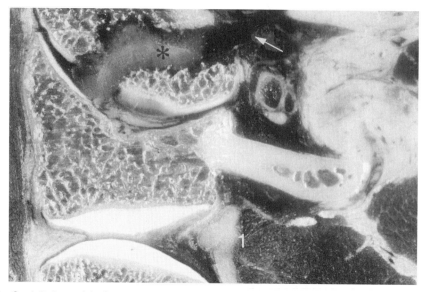

FIG. 3. Occipital condyle fracture that was detected only at second look on the radiographs. The lower fragment is displaced posteriorly and medially. Embedding medium fills the wide fracture gap and the bone defect caused by the avulsion of the alar ligament insertion *(asterisk).* Note the torn joint capsule *(white arrow),* the muscle rupture under the posterior arch of the atlas, and the vertebral artery with the underlying C1 nerve. All are surrounded by wide venous sinuses. The posterior meniscoid and the joint capsule of the atlanto-axial joint are torn, pulling the C2 nerve *(1)* into the joint space. In addition, this specimen displayed one anterior annulus and two root ruptures.

type C). The asymmetry was caused by a complete rupture of all major ligaments in the occiput-atlas-axis complex (Fig. 2). All odontoid process fractures were associated with ruptures of the cruciate ligament and the tectorial membrane. One occipital condyle fracture was detected (Fig. 3). This fracture was missed at first look, but it was detected at second look on one of the 45-degree oblique radiographs. A total of 44 ruptures of the joint capsules and ligaments were found in the upper cervical spine. There were 15 ruptures of the atlanto-occipital joints, five complete ruptures of the alar ligaments, and 24 ruptures of the apical and cruciate ligaments and of the tectorial membrane.

Cervical Spine Injuries, C2 to T1

At autopsy, four hematomas of the prevertebral muscles were found, two extending along the brachial plexus. Cryosectioning revealed four large hematomas deep in the posterior neck musculature, eight ligamentum flavum ruptures (Fig. 4), and 69 facet joint injuries. In most of these, a combination of hemarthrosis, rupture or displacement of meniscoid synovial folds, and partial or complete ruptures of the joint capsules were present. There were three comminuted transverse process fractures (Fig. 5) with bruising of the ganglia and brachial plexus hemorrhage.

We found most injuries at the discovertebral junction. Such discoligamentous lesions have also been reported by other authors (21,24,25,33). We found 77 lesions on the uncovertebral joints, usually bilaterally and at multiple levels (Fig. 6). In specimens from adults, the discs were invariably torn in their substance (Fig. 7). Fourteen discs displayed

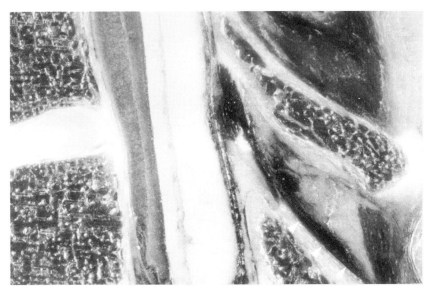

FIG. 4. Avulsion of the ligamentum flavum from the lower border of the C7 lamina. The interspinous soft tissues are stripped from the superior aspect of the spinous process of T1 *(arrowheads)*. The posterior annulus of the C7-T1 disc is intact. Both facet joints were torn at this level. In addition, both atlanto-axial joints, the cruciate ligament, and the tectorial membrane were ruptured, and a massive hematomyelia was found anteriorly in the spinal cord between C3 and C6. Note also the cartilage cap on the tip of the C7 spinous process.

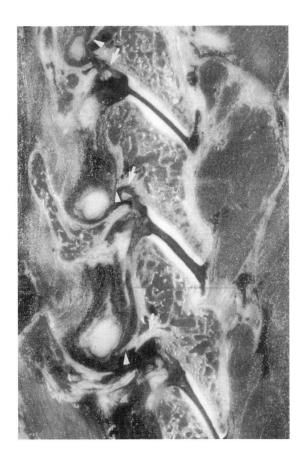

FIG. 5. Multiple facet joint ruptures and transverse process fractures from C4 to C6. Autopsy showed a hematoma at these levels that extended along the brachial plexus into the axilla. The fractures were detected at second look on the specimen radiographs. The fractures run posteriorly through the intertransverse bar *(arrows)*, tearing the joint capsules and the meniscoids. Note the hemarthroses and the perineural hematomas. Sharp bony spikes puncture the nerves *(arrowheads)*.

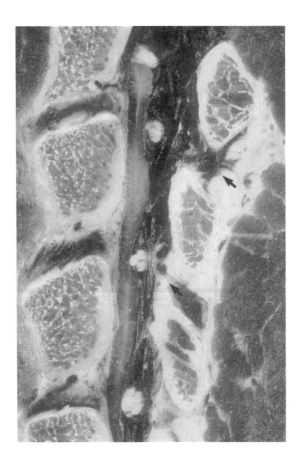

FIG. 6. Multiple uncovertebral injuries between C2 and C5. At autopsy, a rupture of the brain stem was seen. The ligamentum flavum is ruptured at C2-C3 and C3-C4 *(arrows).* The anterior epidural space is filled with the embedding medium. Venous sinuses surround the root sleeves. The C3 root is avulsed and displaced anteriorly and inferiorly. In addition, there were multiple-level facet joint injuries and posterior annulus avulsions, a large disc herniation, and several ligamentum flavum ruptures.

avulsion of the annulus only from the apophyseal rim, three anteriorly and 11 posteriorly, and in eight discs the ruptures extended into the center of the discs. In two specimens from adolescents, we observed a different pattern of disc injury: there were eight partial or complete separations of the cartilaginous endplates from the bony vertebral endplates without any macroscopic signs of injuries in the disc substance (Fig. 8). These disc avulsions resembled epiphysiolyses of the appendicular skeleton and occurred either at one endplate or at both endplates of the same vertebra. It is known that the cartilaginous endplates fuse with the bony endplates at the age of 24. Similar distraction injuries have been reproduced in animals in deceleration-type impact experiments (32,41). At present, we do not know the clinical significance of these endplate separations. In one specimen with posterior annulus ruptures at five levels, the nucleus pulposus had herniated into the spinal canal through an avulsion of the annulus fibrosus from the lower rim of C5 (Fig. 9). This herniation completely obliterated the anterior epidural and subarachnoid spaces, severely compressing the spinal cord against the unyielding lamina.

In the spinal canal, we found one epidural and two subarachnoid hematomas, one spinal cord hematoma, and four avulsions of nerve rootlets from the spinal cord. Three transverse process fractures were initially missed but later verified. One upper articular process fracture could not be detected on any of the radiographs. One nerve root avulsion and the three transverse process fractures were seen in the two specimens with brachial plexus hematomas. The segmental distribution of the soft-tissue injuries is shown in Figure 10.

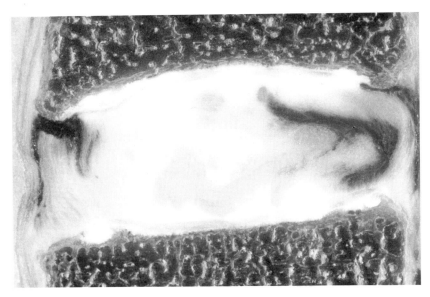

FIG. 7. Multiple ruptures in the C5-C6 disc. No injuries were seen at autopsy. Anteriorly *(left)*, the annulus is torn from the apophyseal rim. The anterior longitudinal ligament is intact but severed from the outer annulus. Posteriorly *(right)*, a smaller annulus avulsion is associated with a large rupture of the inner annulus and nucleus pulposus. A hematoma extends under the intact posterior longitudinal ligament. In addition, a C6 facet joint fracture and multiple-level uncovertebral injuries were found, although all radiographs were negative.

Summarizing these findings, there was a 100% incidence of cervical spine injuries in traffic accident victims with fatal craniocerebral trauma. Although hematoma in the prevertebral tissues is the most significant indicator of an underlying spinal lesion (12), the absence of hematoma does not preclude serious injury; only four of our cases had such muscle hematomas. Current autopsy techniques are likely to miss the vast majority of cervical spine injuries (12,16,43). In the upper cervical spine, even major injuries are difficult to detect because this region is hidden under the skull base and behind the facial skeleton. Unlike emergency and bedside radiographs, our specimen radiographs were taken under optimal experimental conditions (without motion artifacts and obscuring mandible and shoulders). It is reasonable to assume that these injuries would be overlooked in clinical situations and that plain radiographs cannot detect the vast majority of injuries, unless they are associated with vertebral malalignment or with avulsions of bony insertion sites (1,25,33,50).

Early recognition of cervical spine injuries is essential for identifying lesions that warrant surgical intervention both to alleviate acute neurovascular compromise and to prevent late disabling sequelae (11,30). Targeted radiographic examinations in the acute stage are necessary to detect hidden or occult soft-tissue injuries that may be impossible to diagnose in the later course of the disease (14,15,50). Abnormal spinal curvatures, segmental malalignment, and disturbance in the normal motion pattern in the injured segments on flexion/extension radiographs are indicative of soft-tissue injuries (19). Magnetic resonance imaging carries a high promise in diagnosing acute spinal soft-tissue lesions (6,7,20).

In comatose neurotraumatized patients, even gross fracture dislocations are not infrequently overlooked, and unfortunately there numerous reports of fatalities caused by

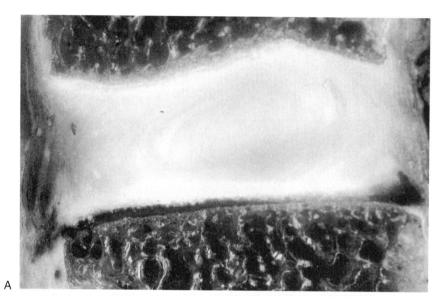

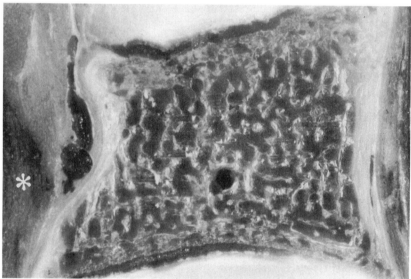

FIG. 8. A: Complete avulsion of the lower cartilaginous endplate of the C6-C7 disc from C7. Autopsy showed an anterior hematoma at this level and the radiographs were normal. There is no macroscopic injury of the disc substance. The annulus is torn from C7 anteriorly *(left)* but not posteriorly. The longitudinal ligaments are not seen in this paramedian section. In addition, we found multiple partial cartilaginous endplate avulsions, uncovertebral and facet joint injuries, and complete ruptures of all the atlanto-occipital joints and ligaments in this specimen. **B:** Subtotal avulsions of the cartilaginous endplates bordering C5. At autopsy, hematomas were found in the prevertebral muscles at these levels. The annulus fibrosus is intact. Note the hematoma in the longus colli muscle *(asterisk).* Several partial and one total cartilaginous endplate avulsion, several uncovertebral and facet joint injuries, and complete ruptures of the atlanto-occipital joints and ligaments were found in this specimen despite normal radiographs.

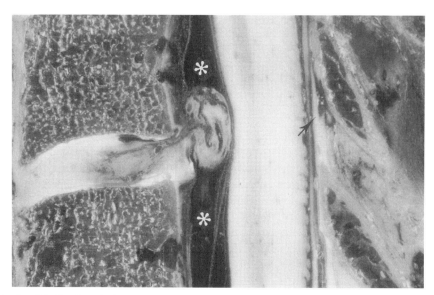

FIG. 9. C5-C6 disc herniation. Autopsy showed a brain-stem rupture but no injuries of the cervical spine. The nucleus pulposus is extruded through the annulus rupture, pushing the spinal cord against the lamina and compressing the spinal cord and anterior spinal artery. Above and below the herniation, the epidural spaces are widened, forming large triangular venous sinusoids *(asterisk)*. Note the avulsion of the ligamentum flavum from the lamina of C5 *(arrow)*. In addition, we found multiple uncovertebral and facet joint injuries and posterior annulus and ligamentum flavum ruptures, although all specimen radiographs were normal.

inappropriate handling of neurointensive care patients (10,30). We therefore recommend that cervical spine injuries be suspected in patients with craniocerebral trauma until proven otherwise (5,12,16,38) and that computed tomography of the skull and brain should be extended throughout the entire cervical spine to detect those small bone avul-

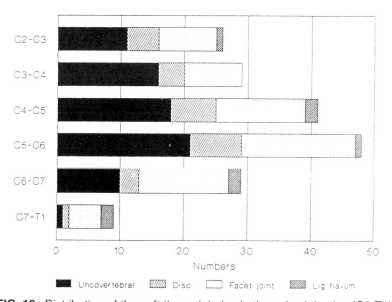

FIG. 10. Distribution of the soft-tissue injuries in the subaxial spine (C2-T1).

sions and subtle asymmetries that may be the only signs of discoligamentous injuries (9,49,50). Whereas most patients with skull-base fractures survive the accident (30), ligamentous ruptures at the craniocervical junction are almost invariably fatal. All odontoid process fractures in our series were associated with ruptures of the cruciate ligaments and of the tectorial membrane, reflecting the severity of these injuries.

CLINICAL STUDY

Patients with neck distortions frequently develop severe and disabling symptoms such as neck pain and radicular pain, sometimes long time after the accident (18,22). These symptoms can persist over years and may become bizarre and disabling (4,22,34–36), and entail cumbersome and costly insurance litigations (23). A significant increase in cervical spine injuries has been reported after the introduction of seat belts (32,36,46). Radiologic and pathoanatomic studies in recent years have shown that craniocerebral trauma commonly is associated with cervical spine injuries (14,27). Most physicians are unaware of the potential severity of these injuries and only few patients are routinely reassessed for possible missed lesions after the emergency examination. Plain radiographs are almost invariably normal and may contribute to the physician's notion of whiplash as a benign, self-limiting condition.

Patients

Fifty consecutive patients who had been involved in whiplash-type automobile accidents during a 13-month period were studied prospectively. Most had been injured in city traffic accidents. The majority of patients (17 men, 33 women; mean age, 33 years) were students; 37 were drivers, 8 front seat passengers, and 5 rear seat passengers. All patients claimed to have worn seat belts at the time of the accident.

Emergency Examination

The patients were examined by orthopedic surgeons on duty. Clinical examination included assessment of neck mobility and tenderness, and of the sensor, motor, and reflex functions. Plain radiographs were taken in the lateral, AP, and 45-degree oblique views. Sick-leave, analgesics, and a soft collar were prescribed when necessary. All 50 patients were then reexamined after 6 weeks. The intensity of neck pain and/or radiating pain was mapped on a 10-grade visual analog scale (VAS), and the dermatomal pain pattern was drawn on sketch forms. Radiating symptoms were defined as pain radiating into the upper extremity within anatomically defined dermatomes and sensory disturbances, paresis, and reflex changes; sensor and motor functions and tendon reflexes were also tested. Neck mobility was measured with inclinometers and goniometers and the neck muscles were palpated for tenderness. In addition to a second set of plain radiographs, flexion/extension films were obtained and evaluated according to the Yale criteria.

Examination after Six Weeks

After six weeks, 26 patients had made a complete recovery and had resumed their previous work, sports, and leisure activities without any restrictions. All radiographs were normal.

However, 24 patients now had developed persistent or aggravated neck pain (Table 1). Of these, 19 also had radiating pain, including the six patients who had presented with

TABLE 1. Clinical, radiographic, and MRI findings in the 24 patients with persisting neck and/or radicular pain, 6 weeks after the car accident

Patient number	Age (yr)	Sex	Collision	Radicular symptoms[a]				Pain intensity[b]			Instability (flexion/extension radiograms)	Protrusion of the disc on MRI	Treatment (mo after the injury)
				Acute	6 weeks	1 year	5 years	6 weeks	1 year	5 years			
1	21	F	Front					9n	3n	3n	C5-C6	0	Surgical (3)
2	22	F	Rear		C8 bilat	*C8 left*	*C8 left*	9	7r	4r		0	Nonsurgical
3	23	F	Rear					9n	3n	5n	C3-C4	0	Surgical (6)
4	26	F	Front					8n	5n	2n	C5-C6	2	Nonsurgical
5	27	F	Rear	C8 bilat	C8 bilat	*C8 right*	*C8 right*	7	2	6		0	Nonsurgical
6	29	F	Front					8n	4n	1n	C5-C6	1	Nonsurgical
7	30	F	Rear		C6+C7 left	*C6+C7 left*		8n	3n	6n	C5-C6	0	Nonsurgical
8	31	M	Rear					8	1n	0		3	Surgical (8)
9	31	M	Side	C6 right	C6 right			9	1	0		4	Surgical (1.5)
10	31	M	Side	C6 left	C6 left			9	0	0		3	Surgical (1.5)
11	34	F	Front		C6 right	C6 right	C6 right	8	3r	4r		0	Nonsurgical
12	36	M	Front		C7 bilat	*C7 left*	*C7 left*	8	3n	2n		0	Nonsurgical
13	37	M	Rear		C8 left	*C8 left*	C8 left	6	4n	4n		0	Nonsurgical
14	39	M	Side		C6 bilat	*C6 bilat*	C6 bilat	8	3n	3n		0	Nonsurgical
15	41	F	Rear	C6 left	C6 left			8	0	0		3	Surgical (1.5)
16	42	F	Front		C6 right	*C6 right*	C6 right	6	4r	1r		1	Nonsurgical
17	43	M	Rear	C6 bilat	C6 bilat	*C6 bilat*		7	4n	1n		3	(Declined surgery)
18	43	F	Side		C6 right	*C6 right*	*C6 right*	8	3n	3n		0	Nonsurgical
19	43	F	Front		C6 bilat			8	0	0		3	Surgical (7)
20	44	M	Rear		C6 left	C6 left	C6 left	7	3n	1n		0	Nonsurgical
21	45	M	Rear	C8 right	C8 right			8	0	0		3	Surgical (3)
22	47	M	Side		C7 right	C7 right	C7 right	6	5r	6r		3	(Declined surgery)
23	55	F	Front		C6 left	*C7 left*		7	0	0		3	Surgical (12)
24	55	M	Front		C5 bilat	*C5 left*		7	2n	0		4	Surgical (11)

[a] Italics denote sensory disturbances (numbness, paresthesia, dysesthesia).

[b] Neck and radicular pain were graded together from 0 to 9 on the visual analog scale. The suffixes n and r designate isolated neck or radicular pain, respectively.

M, male; F, female; bilat, bila:eral.

radiating pain initially. Several patients had some difficulty in distinguishing their neck pain from radiating pain. Fourteen of the 24 patients had either milder symptoms or diffuse clinical findings that were not in complete agreement with the diagnostic imaging results. The flexion/extension radiographs were normal in all 19 patients with radiating pain. Five patients complained of incessant deep neck pain and tenderness of VAS intensity 8 to 9 and had unequivocal segmental instability.

Magnetic Resonance Imaging

The patients with persisting neck pain and/or radiating pain were examined with magnetic resonance imaging (MRI) (Figs. 11,12). For better delineation of the disc protrusions, gadolinium contrast was administered (see Fig. 12C). The disc protrusions were graded from grade 0 to 4 on the T1-weighted sagittal images. Our proposed grading system is based on tracings of cryosectional images from specimens with actual traumatic disc herniations (see Fig. 11). The disc signal intensities were classified as normal or reduced on the T2-weighted sagittal images; signal intensity was reduced in 49 of the 144 discs (34%). At 27 levels, these signal abnormalities were associated with disc protrusions: grades 1 and 2 in 16, and grades 3 and 4 in 11 (see Fig. 12). Seven of the grade 3 and 4 protrusions were lateral, four were midline or paramedian. Half of our patients with grades 3 and 4 disc protrusions had onset of radiating pain within days, the others developed symptoms within a few weeks. Ten of the 19 patients with persistent and severe radiating pain had grade 3 and 4 symptomatic disc protrusions (see Table 1). In the nine

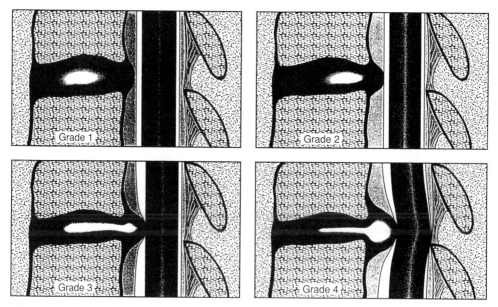

FIG. 11. Grading system of disc protrusions on the MRI-scans based on analysis of 15 *in vivo* incurred disc herniations in other specimens. Grade 0: straight contour of the posterior annulus fibrosus. Grade 1: small annulus fibrosus protrusion. Grade 2: medium-size annulus fibrosus protrusion obliterating two-thirds of the anterior epidural and subarachnoid spaces. Grade 3: large disc protrusion dislocating the spinal cord posteriorly. Grade 4: large disc protrusions compressing the spinal cord.

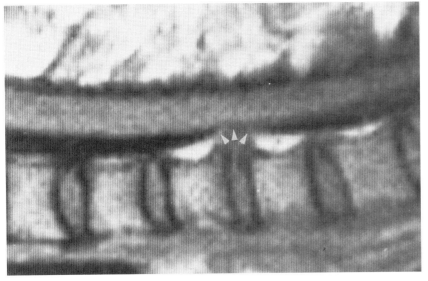

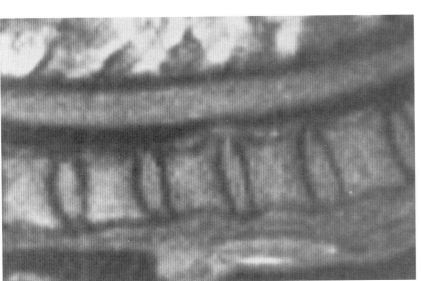

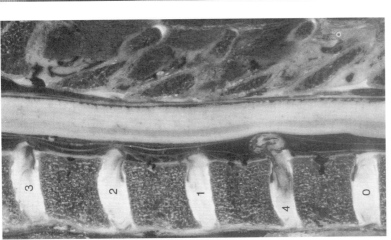

A–C

FIG. 12. A: Anatomic specimen from a young car-accident victim showing a normal *disc (0)*, and herniated discs of grades 1, 2, 3, and 4 at the levels marked with the corresponding numbers. **B,C:** Patient 9, a 31-year-old man with radiating pain after a car collision. **B:** The T2-weighted, nonenhanced MRI scan showing multilevel reduced disc signals but relatively poor detail delineation of the intraspinal soft tissues. **C:** The gadolinium-enhanced, T1-weighted MRI scan shows a distinct delineation of a large disc protrusion that completely obliterates the anterior combined epidural and subarachnoid spaces and pushes the spinal cord against the lamina, also compressing the spinal cord *(arrowheads)*.

patients with radiating pain, there was no unequivocal correlation between neurologic and MRI findings.

Although disc protrusions are quite common in asymptomatic subjects (7), we found a good correlation between the severity of radicular symptoms and the large size of the disc protrusions (see Table 1). Late changes in disc signal intensity may reflect not only loss of water (hydrogen), but also internal disc disruption and degeneration after the primary traumatic lesions. Our anatomic studies in normal and pathologic spine specimens have shown that the posterior annulus fibrosus of the cervical discs is straight and that even grade 1 bulges are associated with fragmentation and tearing of the annular lamellae (see Figs. 9,12A). Most authorities recommend that MRI be done within a few weeks of the injury to diagnose soft-tissue injuries (6,17,20). By contrast, MRI studies did not show any of the posterior injuries.

Surgical Findings

Indications for surgery were strictly clinical: severe and prolonged incessant neck pain and/or radiating pain, corroborated by the diagnostic imaging findings. Discectomy and fusion with tricorticate autogenous bone grafts and anterior plating were employed (Fig. 13). Eight patients had anterior fusions between 6 weeks and 12 months

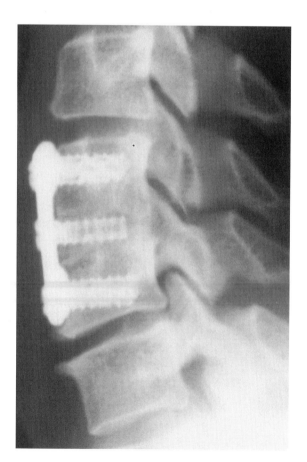

FIG. 13. The patient in Figure 12, 6 months postoperatively. The fusion is healed in good position and with restored intervertebral height. The plate has purchase in both the vertebrae and the bone graft.

after the accident. At all levels, blood-imbibed disc ruptures were found. All midline disc protrusions were in continuity with the discs and were easily extracted. By contrast, all lateral disc herniations, although seemingly in continuity with the disc on the MRI scans, were sequestrated fragments that were dislodged behind the uncinate processes. Distraction of the disc space and diligent inspection of the uncinate process region under good illumination were necessary to detect the small crevices in the posterior annulus by probing. Only after widening of these annular rents was it possible to extract the sequesters. Two elderly patients had disc protrusions associated with uncovertebral spondylosis that compressed the root and the ganglion. Radiating pain subsided immediately after the operation in all patients. Two patients with severe persistent neck pain and marked posterior gaping on the flexion radiographs had posterior fusions. Surgery confirmed ruptures of the facet joints, the ligamenta flava, and the deep neck musculature.

Follow-Up

One and 5 years after the accident, the 50 patients answered a questionnaire comprising 41 questions about site and intensity of neck pain and radiating pain, weakness, sensory disturbances, headache, daily living and leisure activities, workplace situation, periods and degree of sick-leave, and the effects of treatment and rehabilitation. Pain was graded on a 10-grade VAS, and the distribution and intensity of the radiating pain were drawn on sketch forms. Neck mobility was measured with inclinometers and goniometers and a complete neurologic examination was conducted by an independent neurologist. A fourth and fifth set of radiographs, including functional radiographs, were evaluated for abnormal mobility adjacent to the fused levels and spondylosis changes.

Clinical Outcome

Of the 26 patients who were asymptomatic 6 weeks after the accident, all had resumed full work and leisure activities. Nineteen of these were completely asymptomatic at follow-up. Among the remaining seven, one woman had developed bizarre vertigo, dizziness, and headache after a 6-month asymptomatic interval and was still on sick-leave after 5 years. Six patients had developed minor neck stiffness, tiredness, and tenderness that necessitated lighter work and occasional physiotherapy. Among the 24 symptomatic patients, 14 with pain persisting over 6 weeks had ambiguous clinical findings that were not in full agreement with the diagnostic imaging studies. At final follow-up, all still complained of neck pain (VAS 1 to 6) and all patients had been treated for extended periods by physiotherapists or chiropractors. One patient had severe neck pain that necessitated treatment with epidural steroids. All nine patients with radiating pain at 6 weeks also had radiating symptoms, pain, and sensory disturbances at follow-up. One patient who had declined surgery had radiating and neck intensity of VAS 5. Most patients in this group were off work repeatedly and for extended periods of time and one patient was still on sick leave after 5 years. The posteriorly fused patients had resumed unrestricted work and leisure activities, yet both reported residual neck pain of VAS grades 3 to 5 that required occasional analgesic medication. Of four patients with longstanding radiating pain preoperatively, three had numbness of their fingertips that resolved after 1 year.

Radiographic Evaluation and Outcome

All posterior fusions had healed in good anatomic position, and the discs above and below the fused segments had maintained normal height over 5 years. From the initial postinjury radiographs to the 5-year follow-up radiographs, no progression of degenerative changes was seen in any of the 50 patients. The three segments with unequivocal instability on the early flexion/extension radiographs were less unstable at follow-up. In the five segments with non-operated MRI disc protrusions, including the two grade 3 protrusions in the patients who declined surgery, and in the 13 segments rendering persisting segmental or radicular symptoms over 5 years, an average of 20% decrease in mobility was found on the flexion/extension films. The discs adjacent to the fusions had maintained normal height. Radiographs are notoriously negative in whiplash-type injuries and a suspicion of a soft-tissue lesion can only be inferred by indirect signs such as vertebral malalignment, ligament or muscle insertion site avulsions, or signs of segmental instability (21,31). This especially holds for emergency and bedside radiographs. The inability to detect even the most common and gross soft-tissue disruptions on plain radiographs does not preclude conventional radiography as being still the prime imaging modality in distortion accidents involving the cervical spine. In late stages, occult soft-tissue injuries are even more difficult to diagnose radiographically (1). Flexion/extension radiographs correctly showed segmental instability in patients with persistent neck pain and posterior soft-tissue ruptures (19). During posterior plating, we found hemarthrosis and ruptures of the neck muscles in the vicinity of the facet joints.

Surgical Findings

All nine surgically excised discs were severely ruptured: four herniations were midline or paramedian, and five were lateral. The midline herniations completely obliterated the combined anterior epidural and subarachnoid spaces (13) and were all in continuity with the disc space and easily extracted. By contrast, the lateral herniations were invariably sequestrated fragments that were trapped in the triangular space between the uncinate process, the traversing root bundle and ganglion, and the vertebral artery, explaining the incessant radiating pain and the instantaneous and complete pain relief after surgery in these patients. In our unselected, consecutive series of acutely injured patients, there was a surprisingly high incidence of positive clinical symptoms and signs corroborated by diagnostic imaging, and there was also unequivocal surgical confirmation of disc injuries and ruptures of the ligaments and joint capsules. Although the results of this surgical intervention in fresh or subacute injuries were very gratifying, our data should not be compared with those in inveterated and chronic conditions.

Traumatic Changes in Adolescents

Hyperextension or axial distraction injuries in adolescents differ from those in adults because the nonassimilated ring apophysis–endplate complex is more susceptible to injury than the disc itself (3,24,27,32). Traumatic cartilaginous endplate separations may explain why our two young patients with extensive posterior soft-tissue injuries had normal disc signals on MRI. Because the discs are structurally intact in these avulsion injuries, they may generate normal signals on MRI. In Table 1, the patients with persistent symptoms are listed by age in ascending order. It is noteworthy that patients with abnormal posterior gaping on the flexion/extension films all were young women who had neck pain without radicular symptoms. At follow-up, the two surgically treated patients complained of residual pain, although of lesser intensity. Among the patients who had only neck pain immediately after the accident and who developed radicular symptoms within 6 weeks, most who were nonsurgically treated (although improving over time) had residual symptoms, whereas those who were surgically treated made an immediate, complete, and lasting recovery. It is conceivable that disc herniations develop gradually over time by migration of nucleus material through traumatic annular fissures or annular detachment from the ring apophysis.

The source of pain following whiplash remains largely unknown. Pain can conceivably originate both from the ganglion and the richly innervated annulus fibrosus, as well as from the zygapophyseal (facet) joints (8,9), causing both local and referred pain. In some of our patients, the seemingly poor correlation between radiating pain and MRI abnormalities in several adjacent discs probably reflects multiple-level injuries. In a few patients with radiating pain, MRI showed grade 1 or 2 disc protrusions above the symptomatic level. The multiple disc injuries found in traffic accident victims strikingly resemble the disc abnormalities on MRI. Inconsistent radiating pain following whiplash-type trauma may well constitute pain referred via the sinuvertebral nerves from injured discs above the level of clinical symptoms. Perineural hematomas in nondiagnosed comminuted transverse process fractures may also cause radicular symptoms because of perineural scarring of the brachial plexus. Despite the fact that no studies thus far confirm these concepts, patients with neck symptoms after traffic accidents should probably be mobilized early and gently within the limits of pain to prevent hematoma-to-scar transformation, adhesions, and obliteration of the synovial recesses (37).

Degenerative Changes

Although surgical treatment for whiplash-type injuries has not been widely recommended except for patients with chronic pain (23), discectomy and fusion strikingly alleviated pain in our patients with disc herniations. Our patients were more than 10 years younger than the typical whiplash populations reported in the literature. This may in part be a result of the high proportion of students in our Uppsala population. Only acutely injured patients were admitted to our study. Patients with sequelae after whiplash-type neck distortions typically exhibit a plethora of diffuse and bizarre symptoms and signs from seemingly nonrelated organ systems. It has also been stated that patients with hidden soft-tissue lesions can develop abnormal mobility or degenerative changes such as spondylosis, subchondral endplate changes, and uncinate process osteophytosis (1,42). Our 5-year radiographic follow-up revealed no such acceleration of spondylotic changes in our nonsurgically treated patients with suspected discoligamentous injuries; to the contrary, the affected segments had, in fact, become increasingly stiffer over time, probably reflecting healing of unrecognized soft-tissue injuries (35).

"Exposed and Affected" Patients

A certain positive selection may well be inherent in the Swedish socioeconomic and insurance system that discourages patients' claims for costly settlements, compensations, litigations, and exorbitant lawyers' fees that are being reported from countries with a different medicolegal structure (18,23,29,51). All of our patients complained of neck pain (some also of radiating pain) immediately after the accident. In a controlled 6-year follow-up study of patients involved in rear-end car collisions, Nygren emphasized that 38% of the "exposed and affected" patients had constant or frequent neck pain, whereas only 15% of patients without immediate neck problems after the accident ("exposed, unaffected") or a control group that never had been exposed to any traffic accident had neck pain (Nygren, personal communication). Most of our patients had been "exposed and affected."

"Whiplash Injury"

The term *whiplash injury* sometimes leads to confusing an assumed mechanism with a structural injury. The trajectories of forces and the acceleration/deceleration moments can only rarely be inferred from the police reports, the damage to the vehicle, and impact marks in the patient. High-speed recordings in deceleration crashes in dummies, cadavers, and experimental animals have shown that the movements of the head and the site of the impact are highly complex and multidirectional. Nonengineer laymen (physicians, lawyers, insurance providers) can rarely appreciate the complex physics and biomechanics of an automobile collision. All of our patients reported that they wore seat belts at the time of the accident. This statement may be biased, because both front and rear seat belts are compulsory in Sweden. In our series, the traumatic events during the accident were not sufficiently clear to warrant a correlation of the impact forces with the pathoanatomic lesions. Both hyperextension and hyperflexion of the head in combination with frontal impact shearing forces are known to cause foramen magnum ring fractures (45). All but two of our cases with face injuries also had fractures of the skull base. It would appear plausible that skull fractures absorb much of the impact energy and transmit less of the impact forces to the cervical spine (39,44).

ACKNOWLEDGMENTS

Financial support was received from The Swedish Medical Research Council (Project No. B90-17X-07474-05A), and Trygg Hansa Insurance Company Research Foundation, Stockholm.

REFERENCES

1. Abel MS. Moderately severe whiplash injuries of the cervical spine and their radiologic diagnosis. *Clin Orthop* 1958;12:189–208.
2. Alker GJ, Young SO, Leslie EV, Lehotay J, Panaro VA, Eschner EG. Postmortem radiology of head and neck injuries in fatal traffic accidents. *Radiology* 1975;114:611–617.
3. Aufdermauer M. Spinal injuries in juveniles. *J Bone Joint Surg Br* 1974;56:513–519.
4. Balla JI. The late whiplash syndrome. *Aust N Z J Surg* 1980;50:610–614.
5. Bayless P, Ray VG. Incidence of cervical spine injuries in association with blunt head trauma. *Am J Emerg Med* 1989;7:139–142.
6. Berns DH, Blaser SI, Modic MT. Magnetic resonance imaging of the spine. *Clin Orthop* 1989;244:78–100.
7. Boden SD, McCowin PR, Davis DO, Dina TS, Mark AS, Wiesel S. Abnormal magnetic resonance scans of the cervical spine in asymptomatic subjects. *J Bone Joint Surg Am* 1990;72:1178–1184.
8. Bogduk N, Inglis A. The innervation of the cervical intervertebral discs. *Spine* 1988;13:2–8.
9. Bogduk N, Marsland A. The cervical zygapophyseal joints as a source of neck pain. *Spine* 1988;13:610–617.

10. Bohlman HH. Complications and pitfalls in the treatment of acute cervical spinal cord injuries. In: Tator CH, ed. *Early management of acute spinal cord injury.* New York: Raven Press, 1982;373–391.

11. Braakman R, Penning L. The hyperflexion sprain of the cervical spine. *Radiol Clin Biol* 1968;37:309–320.

12. Bucholz RW, Burkhead WZ, Graham W, Petty C. Occult cervical spine injuries in fatal traffic accidents. *J Trauma* 1979;19:768–771.

13. Bucy PC, Heimburger RF, Oberhill HR. Compression of the cervical spinal cord by herniated intervertebral discs. *J Neurosurg* 1948;5:471–492.

14. Cain CMJ, Simpson DA, Ryan GA, Manock CH, James RA. Road crash cervical injuries. *J Forensic Med Path* 1989;10:193–195.

15. Clark CR, Igram CM, El-Khoury GY, Ehara S. Radiographic evaluation of cervical spine injuries. *Spine* 1988; 13:742–747.

16. Davis D, Bohlman HH, Walker E, Fisher R, Robinson R. The pathological findings in fatal craniospinal injuries. *J Neurosurg* 1971;34:603–613.

17. Davis SJ, Tersei LM, Bradley WG Jr, Ziemba MA, Bloze AE. Cervical spine hyperextension injuries: MR findings. *Radiology* 1991;180:245–251.

18. Deans GT, Magalliard JN, Kerr M, Rutherford WH. Neck sprain—a major cause of disability following car accidents. *Injury* 1987;18:10–12.

19. Dvořák J, Froehlich D, Penning L, Baumgartner H, Panjabi MM. Functional radiographic diagnosis of the cervical spine: flexion/extension. *Spine* 1988;13:748–755.

20. Emery SE, Pathria MN, Wilber RG, Masaryk T, Bohlman HH. Magnetic resonance imaging of posttraumatic spinal ligament injury. *J Spinal Disord* 1989;2:229–233.

21. Gay JR, Abbott KH. Common whiplash injuries of the neck. *JAMA* 1953;152:1698–1704.

22. Goff CW, Alden JO, Aldes JH. *Traumatic cervical syndrome and whiplash.* Philadelphia: JB Lippincott, 1964.

23. Gotten N. Survey of one hundred cases of whiplash injury after settlement of litigation. *JAMA* 1956;162: 865–867.

24. Harris WH, Hamblen DL, Ojeman RG. Traumatic disruption of cervical intervertebral disk from hyperextension injury. *Clin Orthop* 1968;60:163–167.

25. Hohl M. Soft-tissue injuries of the neck in automobile accidents. *J Bone Joint Surg Am* 1974;56:1675–1682.

26. Hossack DW. The pattern of injuries received by 500 drivers and passengers killed in road accidents. *Med J Aust* 1972;2:193–195.

27. Jónsson H Jr, Bring G, Rauschning W, Sahlstedt B. Hidden cervical spine injuries in traffic accident victims with skull fractures. *J Spinal Disord* 1991;4:251–263.

28. Jónsson H Jr, Cesarini K, Sahlstedt B, Rauschning W. Findings and outcome in whiplash-type neck distortions. *Spine* 1994;19:2733–2743.

29. Larder DR, Twiss MK, Mackay GM. Neck injury to car occupants using seat belts. *Proceedings of the 29th meeting of American Association of Automotive Medicine*, Denver, 1985;153–168.

30. Levine A, Edwards C. Traumatic lesions of the occipitoatlantoaxial complex. *Clin Orthop* 1989;239:54–68.

31. Macdonald RL, Schwartz ML, Mirich D, Sharkey PW, Nelson WR. Diagnosis of cervical spine injury in motor vehicle crash victims: how many x-rays are enough? *J Trauma* 1990;30:392–397.

32. Macnab I. Acceleration injuries of the cervical spine. *J Bone Joint Surg Am* 1964;46:1797–1799.

33. Macnab I. The "whiplash syndrome." *Orthop Clin North Am* 1971;2:389–403.

34. Maimaris C, Barnes MR, Allen MJ. Whiplash injuries of the neck: a retrospective study. *Injury* 1988;19: 393–396.

35. Mark BM. Cervicogenic headache differential diagnosis and clinical management: literature review. *Cranio* 1990;8:332–338.

36. McGalliard JN, Rutherford WH. Incidence and duration of neck pain among patients injured in car accidents. *Br Med J* 1986;292:94–95.

37. Mealey K, Brennan H, Fenelon GC. Early mobilization of acute whiplash injuries. *Br Med J* 1986;292:656–657.

38. Neifeld GL, Keene JG, Hevesy G, Leikin J, Proust A, Thisted A. Cervical injury in head trauma. *J Emerg Med* 1988;6:203–207.

39. O'Malley KF, Ross SE. The incidence of injury to the cervical spine in patients with craniocerebral injury. *J Trauma* 1988;28:1476–1478.

40. Rauschning W, Sahlstedt B, Wigren A. Irreponible Luxationsfraktur der unteren Halswirbelsäule. *Chirurg* 1980; 51:529–533.

41. Rauschning W. Anatomy of the normal and traumatized spine. In: Sances A, Thomas DJ, Ewing CL, Larson SJ, eds. *Mechanisms of head and spine trauma.* Deer Park, NY: Aloray, 1986;531–563.

42. Rauschning W, McAfee P, Jónsson H Jr. Pathoanatomical and surgical findings in cervical spinal injuries. *J Spinal Disord* 1989;2:213–222.

43. Saternus KS. Die Wirbelsäulenuntersuchung im rahmen der forensischen obduktion. *Beitr Gerichtl Med* 1988; 46:489–495.

44. Sinclair D, Schwartz M, Gruss J, McLellan B. A retrospective review of the relationship between facial fractures, head injuries and cervical spine injuries. *J Emerg Med* 1988;6:109–112.

45. Sköld G, Voigt GE. Spinal injuries in belt-wearing car occupants killed by head-on collisions. *Injury* 1977;9: 151–161.

46. Sumchai A, Eliastam M, Werner P. Seatbelt cervical injury in an intersection type vehicular collision. *J Trauma* 1988;28:1384–1388.
47. Taylor AR, Blackwood W. Paraplegia in hyperextension cervical injuries with normal radiographic appearances. *J Bone Joint Surg Br* 1948;30:245–248.
48. Taylor TK, Bannister JH. Seat belt fractures of the cervical spine. *J Bone Joint Surg Br* 1976;58:328–331.
49. Thiemeyer JS, Ducan GA, Hollins GG. Whiplash injuries of the cervical spine. *Va Med* 1958;85:171–174.
50. Webb JK, Broughton RB, McSweeney T, Park WM. Hidden flexion injury of the cervical spine. *J Bone Joint Surg Br* 1976;58:322–327.
51. Yarnell PR, Rossie GV. Minor whiplash head injury with major debilitation. *Brain Inj* 1988;2:255–258.

Whiplash Injuries: Current Concepts in
Prevention, Diagnosis, and Treatment
of the Cervical Whiplash Syndrome,
edited by Robert Gunzburg and Marek Szpalski.
Lippincott–Raven Publishers, Philadelphia © 1998.

5

Soft-Tissue Injuries of the Cervical Spine (Whiplash Injuries): Classification and Diagnosis

Jiři Dvořák

J. Dvořák: Spine Unit, Department of Neurology, Schulthess Clinic, Zürich, Switzerland.

Evaluation of patients with cervical spine injury, particularly those with only soft-tissue injury, is very difficult. No unified opinion exists for diagnostic assessment during the acute and chronic stages.

When analyzing patient symptoms and signs after the injury, it is relevant to acknowledge the prevalence of chronic neck pain in the general population. In a population-based Finish questionnaire-study among 8,000 adults (15), chronic neck syndrome was identified in 9.5% of the male and 13.5% of the female population. The prevalence of chronic neck pain in a random sample of 10,000 persons of both sexes in Norway found an overall frequency of troublesome neck pain of 34.4%. A total of 13.8% of the total study group reported complaints lasting for more than 6 months (i.e., chronic neck pain). Such chronic complaints were significantly more frequent among women than men (3). The authors point out in their study that a prevalence of neck pain for more than 6 months is similar to the reported prevalence of persisting neck pain after whiplash injuries. However, because of different assessment techniques and methodology, a firm conclusion could not be drawn from this study.

Schrader et al. (27) studied the natural evolution of late whiplash syndrome outside the medicolegal context. In a control cohort study, the association between rear impact collision and chronic neck complaints was estimated. In this study, done in a country where financial gain was an unlikely influence, 202 people who had experienced a rear-impact car accident 1 to 3 years previously were matched to 202 controls and all were sent a series of questionnaires to ascertain the presence and frequency of symptoms such as neck pain, headache, and back pain. There was no significant difference in chronic symptoms between the accident victims and the controls. A family history of neck pain was the most important risk factor for current neck pain. The authors concluded that late whiplash syndrome has little validity and that accident victims tend to attribute preexisting symptoms to the whiplash and are affected by the expectation of disability. The results from Schrader's group confirm the previous finding (3,15) that neck pain and headache are common complaints in the general population. Bovim et al. (3) state that final answers to the questions related to the possible causal relationship between injuries with whiplash mechanism and chronic neck pain may be difficult to obtain as long as one is dependent on evaluation of subjective symptoms that are prone to exaggeration in a medicolegal context. For this reason, they suggest further epidemiologic studies that should avoid important sources of error that are inherent to situations with expectation of monetary compensation.

HISTORY, INITIAL SYMPTOMS, AND FINDINGS

Almost half of the injured patients consult the physician within the first 12 hours, and another 40% within the first 3 days (Fig. 1). In the majority of cases, the first consultation is performed at the office of a general practitioner or local specialist, or the patient is referred to a regional hospital. Only a small group (9%) are initially referred to a medical center (Fig. 2). This fact stresses the importance of the general practitioner for this particular problem, as the first assessment concerns prognostic values of great importance. Keeping in mind the epidemiologic studies in Finland and Norway (3,15) and the cohort study (27), the very first contact with the physician after injury might reveal anamnestic data related to previous history of neck pain or headache, for example, which later on might be suppressed unconsciously in light of the new symptoms. Preexisting symptoms such as headache and radiologic degenerative changes are important predictors for unfavorable outcome (21).

The history of the injured patient before the accident as related to absence from work and necessity of treatment resulting from disturbances of the musculoskeletal system must be recorded into the medical history.

The accident should be described as precisely as possible and according to the injury type as suggested by Krämer (13,14):

• Indirect cervical spine, indirect head injury (classical whiplash injury)
• Indirect cervical spine, direct head injury (head rest!)
• Direct cervical spine, direct head injury.

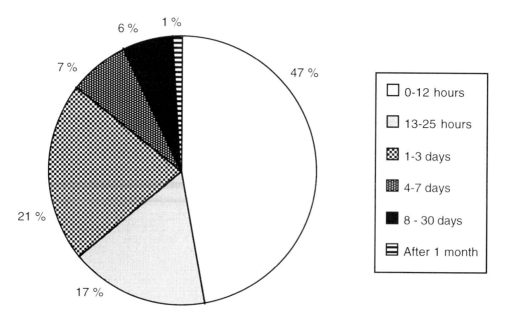

FIG. 1. Usual time interval before the first medical consultation after whiplash injury. From Dvořák, J, Valach L, Schmid S. Verletzungen der halswirbelsäule in der schwelz. *Orthopäde* 1987;16:2–12.

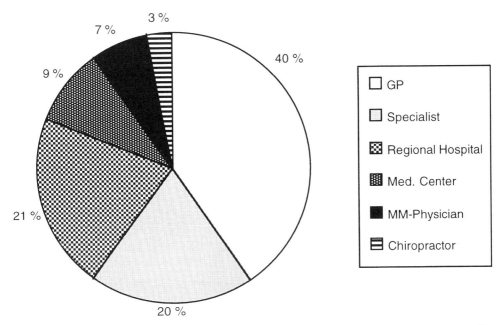

FIG. 2. Distribution of first referrals to medical institutions for whiplash patients. From Dvořák, J, Valach L, Schmid S. Verletzungen der halswirbelsäule in der schwelz. *Orthopäde* 1987;16:2–12.

Another significant point is whether the accident occurred unexpectedly or was expected. This information is important in determining the tone of the neck muscles (innervation, silent tone).

Concerning the biomechanics of the accident, not only is the speed important, but also the movement of the head, described as pure flexion/extension, bending (mainly in a side collision), and whether the head was rotated during the impact. Biomechanically, the last is probably the most vulnerable position of the head, as the alar ligaments are already stretched during rotation, and through additional flexion it is possible that the ligaments could be irreversibly overstretched or even ruptured (17).

Almost 70% of the injured patients report immediate occurrence of symptoms. The most frequent complaints were cervical spine pain and painful spine rotation. Shoulder pain and pain in the lumbar spine were also reported quite frequently. Disturbance of consciousness as well as dizziness were also common symptoms. Paresthesia and muscle weakness of the upper extremities, as well as radicular deficiency, found during clinical investigation are prognosed as unfavorable symptoms. In patient examinations, a painful rotation of the head and neck stiffness were observed most frequently.

Psychosocial symptoms or neuropsychological deficits were found in 79% of the patients who received later disability pensions, but the problems occurred in only 10% of other patients who suffered from pain. The neuropsychological deficits were present in 12% of the pensioned patients immediately after the accident, and in 30% several months later. The most common was a loss of general and occupational achievement ability, a depressive frame of mind, decreased vitality, lack of concentration, and sleep disturbances.

The Quebec Task Force (QTF) on Whiplash-Associated Disorders classifies the injuries symptoms and signs into four grades according to the clinical presentation (Table 1).

TABLE 1. *Proposed clinical classification of whiplash-associated disorders*

Grade	Clinical presentation[a]
0	No complaint about the neck No physical sign(s)
I	Neck complaint of pain, stiffness, or tenderness only No physical sign(s)
II	Neck complaint AND Musculoskeletal sign(s)[b]
III	Neck complaint AND Neurologic sign(s)[c]
IV	Neck complaint AND Fracture or dislocation

[a] Symptoms and disorders that can be manifest in all grades include deafness, dizziness, tinnitus, headache, memory loss, dysphagia, and temporomandibular joint pain.
[b] Musculoskeletal signs include decreased range of motion and point tenderness.
[c] Neurologic signs include decreased or absent deep tendon reflexes, weakness, and sensory deficits.
From ref. 27.

RELEVANT CLINICAL EXAMINATION AND ASSESSMENT

Based on the classification of the QTF (27), it is obvious that unrelated to the time axis, the clinical assessment is most relevant for the documentation of abnormal or pathologic signs. The functional examination of the cervical spine should include not only the measurements of the range of motion out of neutral position but also rotation out of flexion, and rotation out of extension to assess the function of the upper and lower cervical spine separately (4). The examination can be performed clinically (6–8), but also using electronic aids to document not only the main motion but also the coupled motion of the whole cervical spine (1,5). In the examination, it is important to compare the actively performed with the passively induced motion. The motion-induced pain is, however, the limiting factor for the interpretation of the results, especially for the total range of motion. The analysis of the motion pattern is difficult if the patients are suffering pain or are uncooperative. However, reduced mobility (compared with the age-related normal values) might be a sign of functional pathology (Fig. 3). The segmental manual examination of the cervical spine might be helpful to identify the most painful segment, or to determine whether the pain is attributable to the upper, middle, or lower cervical spine.

Neurologic deficit is known as an unfavorable predictor. For the sensory deficit, the dermatomal distribution and reproducibility is important.

The conventional radiographs in anteroposterior (AP) and lateral projection offer little information about soft-tissue injury, but they can offer information of the magnitude of preexisting degenerative changes (10,11).

Functional radiographs offer information about segmental instability. Using them, one can measure the range of motion consisting of segmental rotation and translation that might help to determine pathologic movement. Computer assisted measurement technique offers both the rotatory motion, the translation, and calculation of the center of rotation (7), and this is preferable to the simple superposition of radiographs which, however, is still a reliable and reproducible technique of measurement.

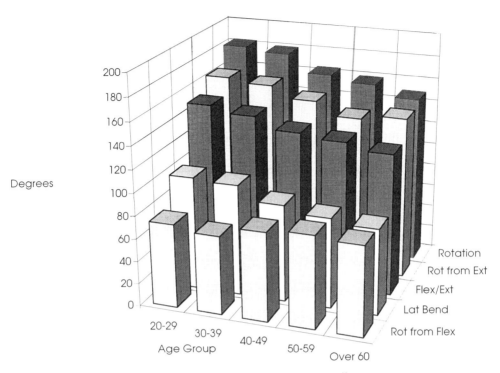

FIG. 3. Age related normal motion of cervical spine. From Dvořák J, Antinnes J, Panjabi M, Loustalot D, Bonamo M. Age and gender related normal motion of the cervical spine. *Spine* 1992;17:393–398.

Functional computer tomography (CT) (1,9) [and possibly in the future, functional magnetic resonance imaging (MRI)] can analyze segmental rotatory motion. The interpretation of the normal and pathologic findings is difficult and again dependent on the cooperation of the patient. Increased segmental rotation in atlanto-occipital and atlantoaxial joints might be a sign of suspected functional pathology of the upper cervical spine as a result of overstretching or rupture of the alar ligaments (25,26,29). The paradoxical rotation (1) within the upper cervical spine might be also considered as a pathologic sign underlying instability of the craniocervical junction.

CT AND MRI OF THE CERVICAL SPINE

Earlier examination (10,11,30) documented the high incidence of degenerative changes of the cervical spine as age related in a symptomatic population.

Boden and Wiesel (2) calculated the specificity (prevalence of false positive findings in healthy adults) of the MRI. Unrelated to patient age, 19% of asymptomatic subjects presented pathologic changes in the MRI of the cervical spine; when looked at by age, 14% of those were younger than 40, and 28% were older than 40. Among the younger subjects, 10% presented with a disc herniation and 4% with foraminal narrowing. The older patients presented with disc herniation in 5%, with disc protrusion in 3%, and with foraminal narrowing in 20%. Knowledge of the prevalence of false positive findings is important to understand and analyze posttraumatic intraspinal pathology (12).

NEURORADIOLOGIC EXAMINATION OF THE BRAIN

Several techniques for the examination of the brain are available: CT, MRI, single photon emission computed tomography (SPECT), and positron emission tomography (PET). Little information offered by CT and MRI scans can verify neuropsychological symptoms and signs. Occasionally, cortex atrophy or local demyelinization as result of a cerebrovascular blood-supply deficiency might be observed as underlying pathology in elderly patients, but those findings should not be misinterpreted as being result of an injury.

New results of the SPECT examination have been presented for discussion. Otte et al. (18) identified parieto-occipital hypoperfusion in 24 out of 28 patients after soft-tissue injury of the cervical spine with SPECT, whereas in 15 control subjects not a single abnormal perfusion was verified. Naturally, this finding could indicate a high sensitivity, but in this patient population, 6 of 7 patients with nontraumatic chronic neck pain also presented with parieto-occipital hypoperfusion. In another quantitative SPECT examination (19,20), 11 injured patients without preexisting neck pain or headache also presented with lower perfusion rate in the parieto-occipital region. This paper indicates that SPECT might be an alternative, important examination technique to analyze discrete regional hypoperfusion, which might be related to so-called minor injury of the brain.

Positron emission tomography has not been used yet in patients with so-called mild brain injury, but it has been utilized in patients after severe head and brain injuries. The observation by Otte et al. (20) is highly interesting and should be critically discussed. Generally, it can be said that SPECT and PET are functional examinations of the brain and therefore inadequate to analyze the brain structure, although little is known about the specificity and sensitivity of these nuclear tracer examinations as related to the influence of chronic intake of medication. In this respect, the fact that patients who have previously suffered injuries causing headaches are more likely to develop chronic neck pain after a soft-tissue injury has to be taken strongly into consideration (21,22).

We have studied neuropsychological testing by comparing sophisticated methods of cognitive testing, with advanced imaging techniques (MRI, PET, and SPECT) in patients suffering the so-called late whiplash syndrome who had strictly discontinued their medication before undergoing cognitive testing and neuroimaging studies. However, no significant correlation could be found between neuroimaging findings and patient performance in tests of divided attention and working memory. Neither was there a significant correlation between scores of both tests requiring working memory, and regional perfusion or metabolism in the areas of the brain that have been found to be the site of the working memory system (i.e., the dorsolateral prefrontal cortex), nor were there significant correlations between the test scores and regional perfusion or metabolism in any area of the brain. In contrast to morphologic or functional brain damage as a basis for cognitive impairment after whiplash injury, the present results support the previously suggested relationship between the two aspects of psychological functioning (i.e., the cognitive and emotional). Our findings support previous conclusions (16,23,24) that this position is not the principal factor influencing symptom development in whiplash patients, but pain experience is likely to trigger cognitive problems in these patients.

NEUROPHYSIOLOGIC EXAMINATION

Little is known about the sensitivity and specificity of neurophysiologic examination (electromyography, sensory and motor evoked potentials) in patients with soft-tissue injury suffering neck and arm pain. If there are clear signs of denervation observed, or if there is significant delay of central motor latency in the motor evoked potentials in concordance with the clinical symptoms, then these examinations are important to document the radicular origin of the pain.

REFERENCES

1. Antinnes JA, Dvořák J, Hayek J, Panjabi MM, Grob D. The value of functional computed tomography in the evaluation of soft-tissue injury in the upper cervical spine. *Eur Spine J* 1994;3:98–101.
2. Boden S, Wiesel S. Lumbrosacral segmental motion in normal individuals. *Spine* 1990;15(6):571–576.
3. Bovim G, Schrader H, Sand T. Neck pain in the general population. *Spine* 1994;19(12):1307–1309.
4. Dvořák J, Dvořák V, Schneider W, Tritschler, Spring H, eds. *Manuelle medizin: diagnostik.* Stuttgart: Thieme Verlag, 1997.
5. Dvořák J, Ettlin T, Jenzer G, Mürner J, Radanov BP, Walz F. Standortbestimmung zum Zustand nach Beschleunigungsmechanismus an der Halswirbelsäule. *Z Unfallchirur Versicherungsmed* 1994;87(2):86–90.
6. Dvořák J, Fröhlich D, Penning L, Baumgartner H, Panjabi MM. Functional radiographic diagnosis of the cervical spine: flexion/extension. *Spine* 1988;13(13):748–755.
7. Dvořák J, Panjabi M, Grob D, Novotny J, Antinnes J. Clinical validation of functional flexion/extension radiographs of the cervical spine. *Spine* 1993;18:120–127.
8. Dvořák J, Panjabi MM, Novotny JE, Antinnes JA. In vivo flexion/extension of the normal cervical spine. *J Orthop Res* 1991;9:828–834.
9. Dvořák J. Valach L, Schmid S. Verletzungen der halswirbelsäule in der schwelz. *Orthopäde* 1987;16:2–12.
10. Gore DR, Sepic S, Gardner G. Roentgenographic findings of the cervical spine in asymptomatic people. *Spine* 1986;11(6):521–524.
11. Gore DR, Sepic S, Gardner G, Murray P. Neck pain: a long-term follow-up of 205 patients. *Spine* 1987;12(1): 1–5.
12. Jonsson H, Bring G, Rauschning W, Sahlstedt B. Hidden cervical spine injuries in traffic accident victims with skull fractures. *J Spinal Disord* 1991;4(3):251–263.
13. Krämer G. Diagnostik neurologischer störungen nach schleudertraumen der halswirbelsäule. *Dtsch Med Wochensr* 1983;108:386–588.
14. Krämer G. HWS-Schleudertraumen. Zur Pathogenese der zerebralen beteiligung und persistierender posttraumatischer störungen. *Med Welt* 1983;34:1134–1140.
15. Mäkelä M, Heliövaara M, Sievers K, Impivaara O, Knekt P, Aromaa A. Prevalence, determinants and concequences of chronic neck pain in Finland. *Am J Epidemiol* 1991;134:1356–1367.
16. Mayou R, Bryant B, Duthie R. Psychiatric consequences of road traffic accidents. *Br Med J* 1993;307:647–651.
17. Ommaya AR. The head: kinematics and brain injury mechanisms. In: Aldman B, Chapon A, eds. *The biomechanics of impact trauma.* Amsterdam: Elsevier, 1984;117–138.
18. Otte A, Ettlin T, Fierz L, Mueller-Brand J. Parieto-occipital hypoperfusion in late whiplash syndrome: first quantitative SPECT study using technetium-99m bicisate (ECD). *Eur J Nucl Med* 1995;23:71–74.
19. Otte A, Ettlin TM, Mueller-Brand J. Comparison of 99m Tc-ECD with 99m Tc-HMPAO brain-SPECT in late whiplash syndrome. *J Vasc Invest* 1995;158–163.
20. Otte A, Mueller-Brand J, Fierz L. Brain SPECT findings in late whiplash syndrome. *Lancet* 1995;345: 1513–1514.
21. Radanov B, Sturzenegger M, Di Stefano G, Schnidrig A, Aljinovic M. Factors influencing recovery from headache after common whiplash *Br Med J* 1993;307:652–655.
22. Radanov B, Sturzenegger M, DiStefano G, Schnidrig A, Mumenthaler M. Ergebnisse der einjährigen verlaufsstudie nach HWS Schleudertrauma. *Schweiz Med Wochenschr* 1993;123:1545–1552.
23. Radanov BP, Di Stefano G, Schnidrig A, Sturzenegger M, Augustiny KF. Cognitive functioning after common whiplash: a controlled follow-up study. *Arch Neurol* 1993;50:87–91.
24. Radanov BP, Dvořák J, Di Stefano G. Attentional processing in common whiplash syndrome before and with immobilisation of the cervical spine. *Eur Spine J* 1993;2:72–75.
25. Saternus K. Verletzungen von halswirbelsäule und von halsweichteilen. In: Saternus K, ed. *Die wirbelsäule in forschung und praxis.* Stuttgart: Hippokrates, 1979.
26. Saternus KS. Dynamikversuch morphologie der HWS: bedeutung und wertigkeit von röntgenologischen veränderungen; pathologische bewegungsmuster: versteifung, hypermobilität, kneifzangenmechanismus. In: Hohmann D, Kügelgen B, Liebig K, Schirmer M, eds. *Neuroorthopädie 1.* Berlin: Springer-Verlag, 1983; 119–126.

27. Schrader H, Obelieniene D, Bovim G, et al. Natural evolution of late whiplash syndrome outside the medicolegal context. *Lancet* 1996;347:1207–1211.
28. Spitzer W, Skovron M, Salmi R, et al. Scientific monograph of the Quebec Task Force on whiplash-associated disorders: redefining "whiplash" and its management, section 3. Consensus findings. *Spine* 1995;20:21s–23s.
29. Taylor J, Tworney L. Acute injuries to cervical joints: an autopsy study of neck sprain. *Spine* 1993;18: 1115–1122.
30. Tepe HJ. Die Häufigkeit osteochondrotischer röntgenbefunde der halswirbelsäule bei 400 symptomfreien erwachsenen. *Röfo* 1985;6:659–663.

*Whiplash Injuries: Current Concepts in
Prevention, Diagnosis, and Treatment
of the Cervical Whiplash Syndrome,*
edited by Robert Gunzburg and Marek Szpalski.
Lippincott–Raven Publishers, Philadelphia © 1998.

6

Epidemiology of Whiplash

Mary Louise Skovron

M. L. Skovron: Genentech, Incorporated, South San Francisco, California 94080.

This chapter presents an overview of current understanding of the epidemiology and prognosis of whiplash, highlighting some risk factors that have been established and some whose role has not been clearly elucidated. Besides a brief presentation of the frequency and risk factors for whiplash injuries, this chapter will also present the clinical manifestations and prognosis of whiplash-associated disorders.

The term *whiplash* was first coined by Crowe (4) in 1928. Although there is a great deal of belief regarding its epidemiology, describing the epidemiology of whiplash based on sound evidence is difficult. The difficulty arises in part from variability of the meaning of the term *whiplash,* in part from difficulties in ascertainment, in part from variability in classification and diagnostic conventions among health professionals, and in part from the paucity of high-quality published studies.

The first point of variability is in the very use of the word *whiplash.* The word can signify a mechanism of injury, it can refer to injury resulting from that mechanism, and it can refer to the clinical manifestations of injury. Because the mechanism may or may not result in injury, and the injury may or may not have clinically detectable manifestations, this multiplicity of uses of the term can lead to apparent inconsistency in estimates of the frequency of whiplash. Recognizing the necessity for clarification of the uses of the term *whiplash*, the Québec Task Force on Whiplash-Associated Disorders adapted and modified the work of others (7,9) and proposed the following definitions:

> Whiplash is an acceleration–deceleration mechanism of energy transfer to the neck. It may result from rear-end or side-impact motor-vehicle collisions, but can also occur during diving or other mishaps. The impact may result in bony or soft-tissue injuries (whiplash injury), which in turn may lead to a variety of clinical manifestations (whiplash-associated disorders). (17)

Although the whiplash mechanism can result in both bony and soft-tissue injuries, and it may occur in diving or shaken-baby events, this chapter is focused primarily on soft-tissue injuries resulting from motor vehicle collisions.

FREQUENCY OF WHIPLASH INJURIES

Population rates of whiplash injury, determined from automobile insurance claims, vary from country to country and region to region. Table 1 shows that, applying the same definition of whiplash injury (namely, compensated claims), annual rates in three jurisdictions varied from 16 to 70 per 100,000 (8,20). Some explanations offered for this vari-

TABLE 1. Annual rates of compensated claims for whiplash injury

Jurisdiction	Years	Rate[a]
Québec Province[b]	1987	70
New Zealand[c]	1982–1983	16
Victoria, Australia[c]	1982–1983	39

[a] Rates are per 100,000 population.
[b] From Suissa S, Veilleux M. The Québec Whiplash-Associated Disorders cohort study. *Spine* 1995;20(8S):12S–20S.
[c] From Mills H, Horne G. Whiplash—manmade disease? *N Z Med J* 1986;99:373–374.

ability in rates include variability in actual incidence due to variability in accident rates, population and automobile density, and distances driven. Additionally, differences may be caused by variability of the automobile insurance structures and administrative rules governing claims and compensation. The high rate in Québec Province may be because universal single-payer automobile insurance through the Société assurance automobile du Québec allows virtually complete ascertainment. Still higher rates, however, are found in other Canadian provinces with universal single-payer automobile insurance. For example, in Saskatchewan, with a lower population density than Québec, the number of compensated whiplash injury claims in 1987 (16) leads to an estimated incidence rate of 700 per 100,000.

It has been hypothesized that the Saskatchewan tort system, which requires filing an auto insurance claim to support filing a lawsuit to be compensated for pain and suffering, encourages the filing of claims for whiplash injury, which are difficult to substantiate or disprove. This hypothesis has not yet been formally tested. However, Saskatchewan recently converted to a no-fault insurance system. Cassidy and colleagues, in cooperation with the Saskatchewan insurance agency, are currently collecting data to test the hypothesis.

Studies that rely on case ascertainment through emergency departments generally underrepresent the incidence of whiplash injury for several reasons. One is that people with whiplash injury may not develop whiplash-associated disorders for some time after the event. Indeed, in the Québec study, Suissa and colleagues (20) found that 22% of people with compensated claims did not appear injured at the scene. In an earlier study, Deans et al. (5) found that 22% of symptomatic whiplash patients had not developed symptoms until at least 12 hours after the event. Such patients are not likely to come for treatment to emergency departments. Underestimation of injury rates would result.

Another problem inherent in estimating whiplash injury rates from emergency department visits is that people come to the emergency department if they are injured while driving in the area. If the area is a major through route for long-distance travel, injuries in the area are not all attributable to the area population and therefore overestimate the population incidence rate. For instance, in a study in Suffolk County, New York, Barancik estimated the incidence of cervical strains caused by motor vehicle collisions, based on emergency room visits, as 3.60 per 1000, that is, 360 per 100,000 in a 1-year period before seat-belt laws went into effect (1). Suffolk County is a mixed small town, suburban, rural, and seaside resort area whose population density is multiplied by vacationers from May through October annually. The number of transients is not counted in the population census. These conditions suggest that the emergency-room-based incidence rates for this area are probably overestimates.

PERSONAL RISK FACTORS

Personal risk factors for whiplash injury include age and gender. Population-based studies in both northern Sweden (2) and Québec Province (20) have found that the 20s are the age decade of highest risk of whiplash injury. This partially but not entirely reflects overall collision injury rates, which are highest, for example, in the age group 15 to 19, followed by age group 20 to 24, in Québec.

Studies have repeatedly found that, except for children, women have higher incidence rates of whiplash injury than men. Barancik et al. in Suffolk County, New York, found the female-to-male ratio in emergency department whiplash injuries to be approximately 1.5 in 1984 (1); Suissa and colleagues found that women had 60% higher rates of compensated whiplash claims than men (20). A number of possible explanations have been offered for this frequently found difference, including that for a given head size, men have more neck musculature than women, and consequently they have lower actual injury rates. One may also speculate that women with whiplash injury are more likely to seek medical attention or file a compensation claim than men. To date, neither of these hypotheses has been tested satisfactorily.

SAFETY ENGINEERING

The role of safety engineering features of automobiles in whiplash injury prevention has been addressed in a number of studies. Several of these have examined the use of seat belts to prevent whiplash injuries. Barancik's study found a small increase in rate of cervical strain in the year following implementation of compulsory seat-belt laws in New York State (1985), compared to the year before those laws were in effect (1984) (1). Although this study overestimates the population rate of whiplash injuries, it can fairly be used to compare year-to-year trends in incidence. Unfortunately, the time periods compared were relatively brief. Consequently, the stability of the differences in rates has not been established. A study of longer duration by Tunbridge in Scotland found roughly a doubling of cervical sprain rates in the 3 years after the introduction of compulsory seat-belt use (21). In contrast, Salmi and colleagues found no significant change in the incidence of mild cervical spine injuries (MAIS 1) in Lyon, France, after the introduction of seat-belt laws (14).

Although the research is not entirely consistent, the preponderance of evidence suggests a slight increase in rate of whiplash injuries accompanying the implementation of seat-belt laws. However, suspension of these laws could not be an acceptable strategy for reducing whiplash injuries because of the increase in serious injuries that would ensue.

Another automobile safety engineering intervention has been the introduction of adjustable and fixed headrests. A number of investigations have demonstrated that fixed headrests are associated with reduced rates of whiplash injury. Stewart, in a study for the U.S. National Highway Transportation Safety Administration, found that the rate of whiplash injuries in front-seat occupants of towed vehicles with headrests was 10% lower than that in vehicles without head restraints. When fixed and adjustable headrests were evaluated separately, fixed headrests conveyed a 20% reduction in risk, whereas adjustable headrests were associated with a slightly but not significantly lower whiplash injury rate. Within the adjustable headrest group, properly adjusted headrests were associated with slightly but not significantly lower whiplash injury rates than improperly adjusted headrests (18). Additionally, Nygren and colleagues (10) found that the introduction of both fixed and adjustable headrests was associated with a reduction in claims of neck pain caused by rear-end collisions in two different car models, and that the fixed headrests had greater associated reductions than did the adjustable ones. However, the magnitude of the reductions was not similar in the two car models, indicating that more work was needed to elucidate the most effective type of head restraint.

CLINICAL MANIFESTATIONS

Table 2 shows the findings of the studies by Norris and Watt (9), Hildingsson and Toolanen (6), and Radanov and colleagues (13), that the most common manifestation of soft-tissue whiplash-associated disorder is neck pain (not unexpectedly, as it is part of the definition of the disorder). Headache is also very common, followed by shoulder pain and paresthesias. Dizziness and visual and auditory signs and symptoms are considerably less common, although they may be quite difficult to manage.

Several groups have attempted to classify the manifestations of whiplash-associated disorders according to their severity. The Québec Task Force (17), building on the work of others including Hirsch and colleagues (7) and Norris and Watt (9), developed the Québec Classification of Whiplash-Associated Disorders. In this classification, persons who have experienced a whiplash mechanism of energy transfer but have no complaints about the neck are grade 0. Patients with neck complaint of pain, stiffness, or tenderness only but no physical signs are grade I. Patients with neck complaints and musculoskeletal signs are grade II; patients with neck complaints and neurologic signs are grade III; and patients with neck complaints and cervical spine fractures or dislocations are grade IV. Patients in several studies were roughly classifiable in these categories. Of patients studied by Norris and Watt (9), 43% corresponded to Québec grade I, 29% were grade II, 12% grade III, and 6% had bony-tissue injury (grade IV). In a study by Burke et al. (3), 41% of patients corresponded to Québec grade I, 56% grade II and 3% grade IV.

PROGNOSIS

Recovery from whiplash-associated disorder has been, at least until recently, slower than would be expected based on our understanding of soft-tissue healing. Suissa and colleagues (20), for example, found that 22% of patients with paid whiplash claims returned

TABLE 2. *Presenting symptoms in whiplash-associated disorders*

Symptom	Patients (%)
Neck pain	88–100
Headache	54–66
Shoulder pain	40–42
Paresthesias	13–62
Visual disturbance	8–21
Auditory disturbance	4–18
Dizziness	17–25

Adapted from Spitzer WO, Skovron ML, Salmi LR, et al. Scientific monograph of the Québec Task Force on Whiplash-Associated Disorders: redefining whiplash and its management. *Spine* 1995;20(8 Suppl):1S–73S.

TABLE 3. *Recovery data of patients with compensated whiplash claims, Québec Province, 1987*

Time from collision	Percent returned to activity
≤ 1 week	22
≤ 4 weeks	47
≤ 1 year	98

Adapted from Suissa S, Veilleux M. The Québec Whiplash-Associated Disorders cohort study. *Spine* 1995;20(8S):12S–20S.

to usual activities within 1 week, 47% within 4 weeks, and 98% within 1 year (Table 3). Norris and Watt reported in their study (9) that all symptoms had declined somewhat by the 6-month follow-up, although it was not possible to estimate what proportion of their subjects had fully recovered. Radanov and colleagues (13) found that 27% of patients with whiplash-associated disorder in their series were still symptomatic after 1 year. However, the longer-term chronic whiplash syndrome may in fact not be attributable to whiplash injury. There is some suggestion that in the longer term, neck symptoms do not occur in any higher proportion in whiplash patients than in the general population. Notably, Schrader and colleagues (15) in a recent paper compared whiplash patients 1 to 3 years after collision to age- and sex-matched controls and found no differences in the prevalence of neck pain (33% to 35%) or headache (50% to 53%) in the two groups. These results are similar to those in earlier reports.

PROGNOSTIC FACTORS

Few potential prognostic factors have consistently been demonstrated in methodologically sound studies (Table 4). In a number of studies, female sex, besides conferring an increased risk of injury, has been found to confer a risk of delayed recovery from whiplash-associated disorder. Increasing age, particularly age over 50 years, is also a negative prognostic factor. The severity of symptoms as indicated by Québec grade or other severity classification such as the multiple symptom rating, is consistently predictive of time to recovery.

Results with regard to psychological factors have been mixed. In part, the mixed results may be attributed to differences in the way the psychological factors were measured, with the strongest evidence coming from the series of publications by Radanov and colleagues. This group has found that among a variety of psychosocial factors, including childhood factors, current psychosocial stress, and lifetime psychosocial stress, only cognitive disturbance after whiplash injury was prognostic of failure to recover within 6 months (11,12).

TABLE 4. *Prognostic factors in whiplash-associated disorders*

Factor	Association
Increasing age	+
Female sex	+
Severity of symptoms	+
Psychological factors	±
Severity of collision	±
Direction of impact	±

Evaluations of collision-related factors have also provided inconclusive results. Suissa and colleagues found, for example, that collision factors such as severity, presence of multiple injuries, non-rear-end direction, and vehicle other than car or taxi were associated with delayed recovery. Radanov and colleagues found that rotated or inclined head position was the strongest accident-related predictor of symptom persistence beyond 1 year (13).

SUMMARY

The epidemiology of whiplash, with the exception of a few risk factors, has not been well elucidated by sound research. Indeed, even the true frequencies of whiplash injury and whiplash-associated disorders are difficult to estimate. The reasons for the variability in estimates remain to be studied, as do the potentially causal roles of demonstrated risk factors (19).

With the exception of fixed headrests, few effective preventive measures beyond overall motor vehicle collision have been identified.

Recovery from whiplash-associated disorder appears to lag behind expectations; a few risk factors for delayed recovery have been identified and may point to ways of improving prognosis in subgroups at risk of delayed recovery.

To develop a better understanding of the epidemiology of whiplash injury and of whiplash-associated disorders, good population-based studies are needed, both for incidence rates and risk factors and for clinical presentation and prognosis. The good news is that such studies are currently ongoing. Two of note are the studies by Cassidy and colleagues in Saskatchewan, and by Nygren and colleagues in Sweden. The results of these and similar studies undertaken elsewhere are eagerly awaited.

REFERENCES

1. Barancik JL, Kramer CF, Thode HC. *Epidemiology of motor vehicle injuries in Suffolk County, New York before enactment of the New York State seatbelt use law.* Washington, DC: U.S. Department of Transportation, National Highway Traffic Safety Administration. June 1989; DOT HS 807 638.
2. Bjornstig U, Hildingsson C, Toolanen G. Soft-tissue injury of the neck in a hospital-based material. *Scand J Soc Med* 1990;18:263–267.
3. Burke JP, Orton HP, West J, Strachan IM, Hockey MS, Ferguson DG. Whiplash and its effects on the visual system. *Graefes Arch Clin Exp Ophthalmol* 1992;230:335–339.
4. Crowe H. Injuries to the cervical spine. *Presentation to the annual meeting of the Western Orthopedic Association.* San Francisco, 1928.
5. Deans GT, Magalliard JN, Kerr M, Rutherford WH. Neck sprain—A major cause of disability following car events. *Injury* 1987;18:10–12.
6. Hildingsson C, Toolanen G. Outcome after soft-tissue injury of the cervical spine. A prospective study of 93 car-accident victims. *Acta Orthop Scand* 1990;61:357–359.
7. Hirsch SA, Hirsch PJ, Hiramoto H, Weiss A. Whiplash syndrome. Fact or fiction? *Orthop Clin North Am* 1988;19:791–795.
8. Mills H, Horne G. Whiplash—manmade disease? *N Z Med J* 1986;99:373–374.
9. Norris SH, Watt I. The prognosis of neck injuries resulting from rear-end vehicle collisions. *J Bone Joint Surg Br* 1983;605:608–611.
10. Nygren Å, Gustaffson H, Tingvall C. Effects of different types of headrests in rear-end collisions. In: *Proceedings of the Tenth International Technical Conference on Experimental Safety Vehicles.* Oxford, Washington DC: U.S. Department of Transportation, National Highway Traffic Safety Administration, July 1–4, 1985;85–90.
11. Radanov BP, Di Stefano G, Schnidrig A, Ballinari P. Role of psychosocial stress in recovery from common whiplash. *Lancet* 1991;338:712–715.
12. Radanov BP, Hirlinger I, Di Stefano G, Vallach L. Attentional processing in cervical spine syndromes. *Acta Neurol Scand* 1992;85:358–362.
13. Radanov BP, Sturzenegger M, Di Stefano G, Schnidrig A. Relationship between early somatic, radiological, cog-

nitive and psychosocial findings and outcome during one-year follow-up in 117 patients suffering from common whiplash. *Br J Rheumatol* 1994;33:442–448.

14. Salmi LR, Thomas H, Fabry JJ, Girard R. The effect of the 1979 French seat-belt law on the nature and severity of injuries to front-seat occupants. *Accid Anal Prev* 1989;21:589–594.

15. Schrader H, Obelieniene D, Bovim G, et al. Natural evolution of the late whiplash syndrome outside of the medicolegal context. *Lancet* 1996;327:1207–1211.

16. Sobeco, Ernst, Young. *Saskatchewan Government Insurance automobile injury study.* Report to the Saskatchewan Government Insurance Office, March 1989.

17. Spitzer WO, Skovron ML, Salmi LR, et al. Scientific monograph of the Québec Task Force on Whiplash-Associated Disorders: redefining whiplash and its management. *Spine* 1995;20(8 suppl):1S–73S.

18. Stewart JR. *Statistical evaluation of the effectiveness of FMVSS 202: head restraints.* Chapel Hill, NC: Highway Research Center, University of North Carolina, 1980. Task 3 report 2:1-1-A-10. DOT HS 8 02014.

19. Stovner LJ. The nosological status of the whiplash syndrome: a critical review based on a methodological approach. *Spine* 1996;21:2735–2746.

20. Suissa S, Veilleux M. The Québec Whiplash-Associated Disorders cohort study. *Spine* 1995;20(8S):12S–20S.

21. Tunbridge RJ. *The long-term effect of seat belt legislation on road user injury patterns.* Crowthorne, UK: Transport and Road Research Laboratory, 1989. Research report No. 239.

Whiplash Injuries: Current Concepts in
Prevention, Diagnosis, and Treatment
of the Cervical Whiplash Syndrome,
edited by Robert Gunzburg and Marek Szpalski.
Lippincott–Raven Publishers, Philadelphia © 1998.

7

Injury Biomechanics

Mats Y. Svensson

M. Y. Svensson: Department of Injury Prevention, Chalmers University of Technology,
Göteborg, Sweden.

The symptoms of injury after neck trauma from rear-end collisions include pain, weakness, and abnormal responses in the parts of the body (mainly the neck, shoulders, and upper back) that are connected to the central nervous system via the cervical nerve roots. Vision disorders, dizziness, headaches, unconsciousness, and neurologic symptoms in the upper extremities are other symptoms that have been reported (5,10,16,19,23). The symptoms associated with soft-tissue neck injuries in frontal and side collisions appear to be very similar to those of rear-end collisions (10).

Rear-end car collisions typically occur in dense traffic situations. Sudden decreases in traffic tempo may cause a driver to start braking a little too late and, because of residual speed, bump into the vehicle in front. During the collision, the struck vehicle is subjected to a forceful forward acceleration and the car occupants are pushed forward by the seat backs. The head lags behind because of its inertia, forcing the neck into a swift extension (rearward bending) motion. This head motion continues until the neck reaches the end of its motion range or, if applicable, hits a head restraint or some other structure behind the head. Thereafter, the head moves forward relative to the torso and may stop in a somewhat flexed (forward bent) neck posture. This body motion has been described by McConnell et al. (13) and Ono and Kanno (17), among others, and is commonly called whiplash motion. The term *whiplash* has also been used in the literature for the neck motion in frontal and side collisions.

According to Svensson (21), a synthesis of findings by Mertz and Patrick (14,15) and by McConnell et al. (13) indicates that abbreviated injury scale (AIS) 1 neck injuries are prevented in a rear-end impact if the displacement between the head and the torso is avoided. The injury can, on the other hand, occur without exceeding the natural range of rearward angular head motion.

In frontal and side collisions, the neck usually experiences the same type of inertial loading from the head as in rear-end collisions. During the initial phase of these neck loading situations, the head normally undergoes a horizontal translational displacement relative to the torso. This is particularly evident in frontal (24) and rear-end collisions (7,9). This translational motion is called protraction for forward motion (Fig. 1) and retraction for rearward motion (Fig. 2). The neck is exposed to very significant mechanical loads when the end of the normal range of protraction or retraction of the neck is reached (see Figs. 1B,2B), and neck injuries may well occur at this point (6). This may be one explanation for the fact that modern head restraints do not provide better protec-

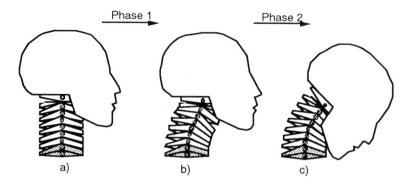

FIG. 1. Schematic drawing of the head–neck motion during a frontal collision. Phase 1: Protraction motion. Phase 2: Flexion motion.

tion. They may simply come into play too late, after the neck has exceeded the maximum range of retraction motion and gone into extension. Another possible explanation, involving transient pressure gradients in the central nervous system (CNS) causing cervical nerve root ganglion injuries at the point of maximum retraction or protraction, will be presented later in this chapter.

The aim of the neck injury project at Chalmers University of Technology, Göteborg, has been to find the phenomenon that could explain the various long-lasting symptoms that result from soft-tissue neck injuries and to establish how the risk of injury correlates to kinematic and kinetic parameters of the head–neck motion relative to the torso. The focus was on rear-end collisions at low impact velocities ($\Delta v < 20$ km/h). The work originated from a hypothesis by Aldman (1) postulating that injuries could be induced in the cervical spinal nerve root region as a result of transient pressure gradients during swift extension/flexion motion of the cervical spine. This chapter describes the further development of Aldman's hypothesis and the experimental set-up that was used to verify the hypothesis.

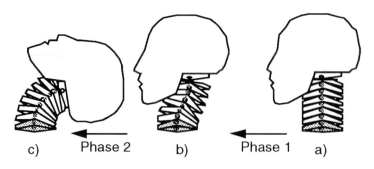

FIG. 2. Schematic drawing of the head–neck motion during a rear-end collision. Phase 1: Retraction motion. Phase 2: Extension motion.

THEORETICAL MODEL

The length of the cervical spinal canal increases at flexion and decreases at extension (4). A decrease of the cross-sectional area of the cervical spinal canal during neck extension is caused by the ligamenta flava protruding into the canal (4). This means that the inner volume of the spinal canal decreases during neck extension and increases during flexion of the neck. However, all the tissues and fluids inside the spinal canal are incompressible (8). This means that fluid transportation, to and from the cervical spinal canal, must take place during the flexion/extension motion of the cervical spine. The fluid could be either blood in the venous plexus of the epidural space or cerebrospinal fluid (CSF). Because of the relatively high flow resistance in the subarachnoid space, flow of CSF was thought to be of minor importance compared to vein blood flow in this type of volume compensation (22).

According to Batson (2), both the internal and external vertebral venous plexa that communicate via vein bridges through the intervertebral foramina have a capacity that exceeds that of the arteries supplying the tissues of the same region. Because these vein plexa do not have any valves, the blood can easily move in any direction within the plexa, and also back and forth between the inner and outer plexa. This means that blood volumes can move easily to compensate for the change in inner volume in the spinal canal during the flexion/extension motion (22).

During the extension/flexion motion, pressure gradients along the spinal canal and across the intervertebral foramina can occur. Because of flow resistance and the acceleration effect on fluid mass, the pressure gradients mentioned above may generate injurious stresses and strains to the exposed tissues.

A one-dimensional mathematical model of the flow and pressure phenomena in the spinal canal was developed (3). The model is based on the Navier Stokes equations and is built on the assumption that the flow along the cervical spinal canal is the most significant component in the process. The model predicts the risk of injury according to equation 1, where NIC stands for neck injury criterion, a_{rel} is the relative horizontal acceleration between T1 and the occipital joint, and v_{rel} is the relative horizontal velocity between T1 and the occipital joint:

$$NIC = 0.2a_{rel} + v_{rel}^2 \qquad [1]$$

A preliminary estimation yielded an NIC value that should not exceed 15 m^2/s^2 if injuries are to be avoided. The estimation is based on scaling of the pig anatomy to that of the human and comparisons with results from tests on volunteers (3).

EXPERIMENTAL NECK TRAUMA

Anesthetized pigs, males and females (28 animals in total) with body weights of 20 to 25 kg, were used in this work (3,18,22). The study was approved by the local animal experimentation and ethics committee. The first group of animals was used to measure pressure in the CNS during simulated rapid neck extension motion or neck flexion motion, and the second group was used for histopathologic examination. In the second group, some animals were exposed to simulated rapid neck motion and others served as sham-exposed controls. A schematic view of the test set-up for the experimental neck extension/flexion trauma is shown in Figure 3.

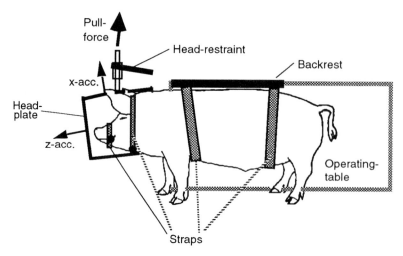

FIG. 3. The test set-up seen from above. The anesthetized animal is lying side-down on the operating table, strapped to the backrest. The head is strapped to the bolts in the horizontally movable head-plate. During the experiment, a pre-tensed rubber strap pulls the head-plate (in a posterior or an anterior direction) by the pull rod. The pull force is active until the pull rod is disconnected, and thereafter the head moves in the sagittal plane as a result of its inertia. In some tests, a head restraint was introduced to limit the maximal rearward displacement of the head.

The head was pulled either in the posterior or the anterior direction. In some extension-motion test runs, a head restraint was introduced. Gaps of 100 to 130 mm were used between head and head-restraint. A gap of 100 mm prevented the neck from reaching full retraction, and a gap of 130 mm allowed the neck to pass the point of full retraction but prevented it from reaching the maximum physiologic extension angle.

The animals used for the pressure measurement experiments had three pressure transducers introduced into the CNS (Fig. 4). Pressure measurements were taken under various loading conditions. The pull force (see Fig. 3) was varied from 150 newtons to 900 N.

The animals in the group that underwent histopathologic examination were given an intravenous injection of Evans blue dye conjugated to albumin (EBA) before the test. All animals in this group that underwent experimental neck trauma were exposed to a 600-N pull force. After the test, each animal remained anesthetized for an additional 2 hours and was thereafter sacrificed by transcardial perfusion with buffered formalin solution for fixation of the body. The brain and the spinal cord to about the T4 level were dissected. The spinal ganglia and proximal parts of corresponding nerves were identified and isolated (18). Cryostate microtome sections were prepared and examined in a fluorescence microscope according to a procedure described by Suneson et al. (20).

The function of EBA is to indicate the damage sustained to the blood–brain barrier in the CNS. If at microscopic examination EBA can be detected outside the blood system, the blood vessels have been damaged. Because of the fenestration of the capillaries in the spinal ganglia, however, EBA will normally pass into the intercellular space, but not into the nerve cells. Thus, EBA inside the nerve cells indicates damage to the nerve cell membranes and to satellite cells.

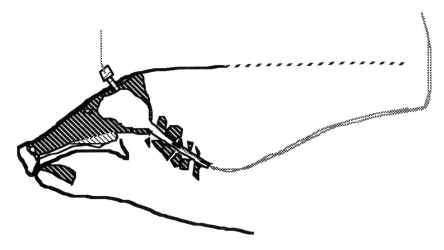

FIG. 4. Schematic sagittal cross-section of the pig head and cervical spine displaying the positions of the three pressure transducers, one in the frontal skull bone and two in the cervical spinal canal.

RESULTS

Pressure measurement results from one whiplash extension run are shown in Figure 5. The pull-force was 600 N, which is the same as that for the animals in the histopathologic examination group. The angular displacements and linear x-displacements of the head, the x- and z-accelerations of the head plate, and the readings from the three pressure transducers in the CNS are shown (see Fig. 5). The onset of the angular motion of the head is delayed about 30 ms compared to the linear x-displacement, indicating that the head moves mainly translationally during the first 30 ms. The general pattern of the pressure pulse in the spinal canal is the same for all degrees of pulling force, but the duration of the pulse becomes shorter and its magnitude higher with increasing pulling force (22). The maximum angular head displacement occurs earlier and increases in magnitude with increasing pulling force (22). According to the mathematical model by Boström et al. (3), the two distinct pressure dips at 25 ms and 60 ms in Figure 5 are caused by a water-hammer effect. The dips occur as the flow of vein blood along the spinal canal swiftly alters direction when the cervical spine changes its bending mode (3).

A comparison of the pressure readings in the spinal canal at C4 level between a test without a head restraint (PW 03.04) and a test with a head restraint positioned 100 mm behind the head (PW 03.03) are shown in Figure 6. The pressure pulse is drastically reduced after head to head-restraint contact at about 60 ms in test PW 03.03 (see Fig. 6). With a 130-mm head-restraint gap, the contact would occur at about 80 ms, which means that the deep pressure dip at about 70 ms would not be avoided.

The pressure readings from an experimental neck flexion trauma test are shown in Figure 7. The pull force was 300 N and the magnitude of the pressure dip is in the same order as for an experimental neck extension trauma at the same pull force level (22).

Macroscopic inspection during the autopsies of the animals exposed to trauma revealed no bleeding or fractures of vertebral structures, or ruptures of ligaments (18).

However, fluorescence microscopic examination of the satellite cells and nerve cells in the spinal ganglia of the animals exposed to neck extension trauma (without head

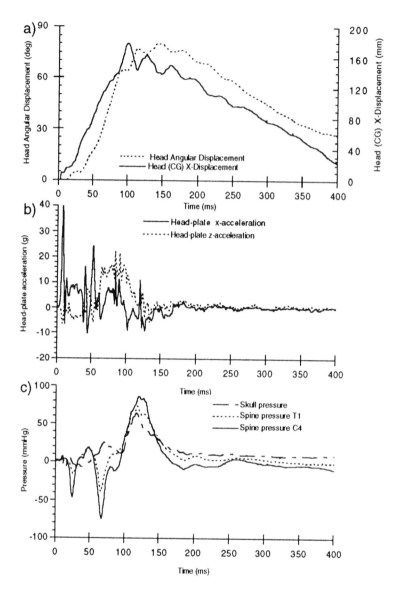

FIG. 5. The results from one whiplash extension run with pressure measurements. The applied pull force on the head-plate was 600 N. **A:** Angular displacement and the linear x-displacement of the head CG (center of gravity) versus time. **B:** Accelerations of the head-plate versus time. **C:** The pressure versus time in the CNS at three levels: skull, C4, and T1.

restraint) disclosed red fluorescent material, indicating EBA leakage and thus membrane dysfunction. These findings were most obvious at the C6 to C8 levels. There were no signs of such leakage into the satellite cells or the nerve cells in the spinal ganglia from the sham-exposed animals (18).

In the tests with a head restraint in place, there were no signs of EBA leakage at a 100-mm head-restraint gap, but for tests with 130-mm head-restraint gap the frequency of leakage was the same as in the animals where no head restraint was used (3). Preliminary

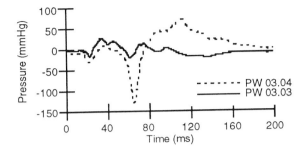

FIG. 6. The pressures inside the spinal canal at the C4 level during swift extension motion at a pull force of 600 N (3). PW 03.03 was carried out with a head-restraint gap of 100 mm and PW 03.04 was carried out without a head restraint.

results indicate that the animals exposed to neck-flexion trauma had a frequency of EBA leakage similar to that of the animals exposed to neck-extension trauma without a head restraint (Svensson et al., 1997, manuscript in preparation).

Static loading of the cervical spine under loading conditions resembling those caused by a posterior pull force of 600 N did not result in any pressure gradients or any histopathologic findings (3).

DISCUSSION

The overall anatomy of the cervical spine of the pig is similar to that of humans even though the dimensions and the detailed shapes of different tissues differ somewhat between the two species. The spine and head of the pig serve as a qualitative substitute of the corresponding parts of the human body and have served as guidance in terms of what kinematic and kinetic parameters are related to the risk of injury. Identical experiments using anesthetized sheep resulted in virtually identical pressure readings, which indicates that this type of pressure will probably occur in all mammals during this type of swift extension/flexion motion of the neck (Svensson et al., 1997, manuscript in preparation). Repeatability and reproducibility was found to be adequate in the test set-up, and the loading conditions and time history of the neck trauma experiments were considered relevant (21).

Symptoms similar to those incurred during rear-end collisions also occur in patients who have been involved in frontal impacts (10–12), although the relative incidence appears to be smaller in the latter circumstance. Pressure measurements in the CNS during swift experimental flexion motion of the neck revealed only negative pressures (see

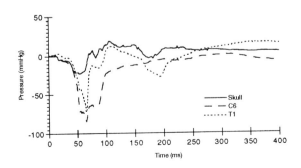

FIG. 7. The pressures inside the skull and in the spinal canal at the C6 and T1 levels during swift flexion motion at a pull force of 300 N (22).

Fig. 7), but these were of magnitudes similar to those in the extension motion experiments (22). The positive histopathologic findings from swift experimental flexion motion indicate that the negative portion of the pressure readings corresponds to the occurrence of nerve cell membrane dysfunction.

In the neck extension trauma experiments, the negative part of the pressure readings was avoided only with the head restraint at the closest distance, 100 mm behind the head, and only at this narrow head-restraint gap were the injuries to the spinal ganglia avoided. This is another indication that the negative part of the pressure readings is responsible for the nerve-cell membrane dysfunction. The findings also indicate that a head restraint, to be effective, must intervene with the head motion early, before the point of maximal neck retraction has been reached.

ACKNOWLEDGMENTS

This work was a joint project involving Chalmers University of Technology, the University of Gothenburg, The National Defense Research Establishment, and Autoliv AB. I want to thank my co-workers Bertil Aldman, Ola Boström, Hans-Arne Hansson, Yngve Håland, Per Lövsund, Tore Örtengren, Torsten Seeman, Anders Suneson, and Anett Säljö. This work was supported by the Swedish Transport and Communications Research Board (KFB) and the Swedish National Road Administration (VV).

REFERENCES

1. Aldman B. An analytical approach to the impact biomechanics of head and neck. *Proceedings of the 30th annual Association for the Advancement of Automotive Medicine (AAAM) conference*, LC 64-1965, 1986;439–454.
2. Batson OV. The vertebral vein system, Caldwell Lecture, 1956. *Am J Roentgenol* 1957;48:195–212.
3. Boström O, Svensson MY, Aldman B, et al. A new neck injury criterion candidate-based on injury findings in the cervical spinal ganglia after experimental sagittal whiplash. *Proceedings of the International Research Council on the Biokinetics of Impacts (IRCOBI) conference*. Dublin, Ireland, 1996;123–136.
4. Breig A. *Adverse mechanical tension in the central nervous system*. Stockholm: Almqvist & Wiksell, 1978.
5. Deans GT, Magalliard JN, Kerr M, Rutherford WH. Neck sprain—a major cause of disability following car accidents. *Injury* 1987;18:10–12.
6. Deng Y-C. Anthropomorphic dummy neck modelling and injury considerations. *Accid Anal Prev* 1989;21:85–100.
7. Eichberger A. Comparison of different car seats regarding head-neck kinematics of volunteers during rear-end impact. *Proceedings of the international IRCOBI conference*, Dublin, Ireland, 1996:153–164.
8. Estes MS, McElhaney JH. Response of brain tissue to compressive loading. American Society for Mechanical Engineers, paper no. 70-BHF-13,1970.
9. Geigl BC, Steffan H, Dippel C, Muser MH, Walz F, Svensson MY. Comparison of head-neck kinematics during rear end impact between standard hybrid III, RID neck, volunteers and PMTO's. *Proceedings of the international IRCOBI conference*, Brunnen, Switzerland, 1995:261–270.
10. Hildingsson C. *Soft tissue injury of the cervical spine*. Umeå University medical dissertations, new series no. 296, ISSN 0346-6612, 1991.
11. Larder DR, Twiss MK, Mackay GM. Neck injury to car occupants using seat belts. *Proceedings of the 29th annual AAAM conference*, Washington D.C, LC 64-1965, 1985:153–168.
12. Maimaris C, Barnes MR, Allen MJ. "Whiplash injuries" of the neck: a retrospective study. *Injury* 1988;19:393–396.
13. McConnell WE, Howard RP, Guzman HM, et al. Analysis of human test subject responses to low velocity rear end impacts. SP-975, Society of Automotive Engineers paper no. 930889, 1993:21–30.
14. Mertz HJ, Patrick LM. Investigation of the kinematics and kinetics of whiplash. *Proceedings of the 11th STAPP car crash conference*, Anaheim, CA. New York: Society of Automotive Engineers, LC 67-22372, 1967:267–317.
15. Mertz HJ, Patrick LM. Strength and response of the human neck. *Proceedings of the 15th STAPP car crash conference*. New York: Society of Automotive Engineers, LC 67-22372, 1971:207–255.
16. Nygren Å, Gustafsson H, Tingvall C. Effects of different types of headrests in rear-end collisions. *Proceedings of the 10th international conference on experimental safety vehicles*, National Highway Traffic Safety Administration (NHTSA), 1985:85–90.

17. Ono K, Kanno M. Influences of the physical parameters on the risk to neck injuries in low impact speed rear-end collisions. *Proceedings of the international IRCOBI conference*, Eindhoven, The Netherlands, 1993: 201–212.
18. Örtengren T, Hansson H-A, Lövsund P, Svensson MY, Suneson A, Säljö A. Membreáne leakage in spinal ganglion nerve cells induced by experimental whiplash extension motion: a study in pigs. *J Neurotrauma* 1996;13: 171–180.
19. Spitzer WO, Skovron ML, Salmi LR, et al. Scientific monograph of the Québec Task force on whiplash-associated disorders: redifining "whiplash" and its management. *Spine* 1995(Suppl);20:1S–73S.
20. Suneson A, Hansson H-A, Seeman T. Peripheral high-energy missile hits cause pressure changes and damage to the nervous system: experimental studies on pigs. *J Trauma* 1987;27:782–789.
21. Svensson MY. *Neck injuries in rear-end car collisions—sites and biomechanical causes of the injuries, test methods and preventive measures.* Department of Injury Prevention, Chalmers University of Technology, S-412 96 Göteborg, Sweden, 1993.
22. Svensson MY, Aldman B, Lövsund P, Hansson HA, Seeman T, Suneson A, Örtengren T. Pressure effects in the spinal canal during whiplash extension motion—a possible cause of injury to the cervical spinal ganglia. *Proceedings of the interational IRCOBI conference*, Eindhoven, The Netherlands. Society of Automotive Engineers paper no. 1993-13-0013, 1993:189–200.
23. Watkinson A, Gargan MF, Bannister GC. Prognostic factors in soft tissue injuries of the cervical spine. *Injury* 1991;22:307–309.
24. Wismans J, Spenny CH. Head-neck response in frontal flexion. *Proceedings of the 28th STAPP car crash conference.* Society of Automotive Engineers paper no. 841666, SAE/P-84/152, 1984:161–172.

*Whiplash Injuries: Current Concepts in
Prevention, Diagnosis, and Treatment
of the Cervical Whiplash Syndrome,*
edited by Robert Gunzburg and Marek Szpalski.
Lippincott–Raven Publishers, Philadelphia © 1998.

8

Whiplash Trauma Injury Mechanism: A Biomechanical Viewpoint

Manohar M. Panjabi, Jonathan N. Grauer, Jacek Cholewicki, Kimio Nibu, Lawrence Brett Babat, and Jiři Dvořák

*M. M. Panjabi, J. N. Grauer, and J. Cholewicki: Biomechanics Laboratory,
Department of Orthopaedics and Rehabilitation, Yale University School of Medicine,
New Haven, Connecticut 06520-8071.
K. Nibu: Department of Orthopaedics, Yamaguchi University School of Medicine,
Ube City Yamaguchi Pref. 755, Japan.
L. B. Babat: Department of Orthopaedic Surgery, Brown University, Providence,
Rhode Island 02912.
J. Dvořák: Spine Unit, Department of Neurology, Schulthess Clinic, Zürich, Switzerland.*

Whiplash has been loosely defined as an acceleration injury, and it most commonly involves an unaware victim in a stationary vehicle being struck from behind. Cervical spine injuries are an important, but poorly understood, resulting problem.

Fifty percent of car-to-car traffic accidents in Japan result in neck injuries (19). Reports from several European countries indicate an alarming increase in the annual number of neck injuries in recent years because of the increased traffic density (27). Resulting symptoms, including neck pain, dizziness, and headaches, are nonspecific and are reported up to months or years after accidents (1,2,7).

The National Highway Traffic Safety Administration in the United States estimates that 84% of all neck injuries are classified as AIS1, or soft tissue injuries (3). Such injuries are most commonly not a complete failure of particular anatomic structures, but are subfailure injuries. Although the presently available imaging methods such as magnetic resonance imaging (MRI) often do not have sufficient resolution to identify these injuries, the decreased function and pain associated with whiplash trauma may be explained by these subfailure injuries.

Whiplash investigations have ranged from reviews of clinical data to a number of different laboratory approaches. Nevertheless, a solid understanding of whiplash injuries requires knowledge of intervertebral kinematics, which is not yet available. The relatively recent Québec Task Force on Whiplash-Associated Disorders found a need for further biomechanical information about whiplash (26).

Several attempts have been made to define the mechanism of whiplash injuries. Mac-Nab, realizing the difficulties of clinical studies, turned to experimental trauma of anesthetized monkeys (12–14). He found a predominance of anterior element injuries, which he ascribed to hyperextension of the entire cervical spine.

Penning postulated that the primary mechanism of whiplash injury is hypertranslation of the head as opposed to the more conventional view of hyperextension (23,24). Penning studied lateral radiographs of "chin-in and chin-out" subjects as representative of back-ward and forward head translations. He then compared associated intervertebral sagittal plane rotations with those of actively flexed and extended functional radiographs. He found that the rotations of the craniovertebral junction (C0-C2) were greater with simple head translations than with head flexion or extension. This was not the case for the lower cervical intervertebral joints. He thus concluded that upper level rotational injuries should predominate.

Svenson et al. studied a neck dummy model and noted that the cervical spine initially forms an S-shaped curve and then complete extension (28). However, they focused on the effects of such behavior on cerebrospinal fluid pressure in a pig whiplash model rather than overall osteoligamentous injuries.

Other experiments have used various human volunteer models to study head and neck motions during whiplash (8–10,15,16,25). By the nature of human investigations, instrumentation is limited, accelerations are predominantly below injury thresholds, and the subjects are aware of impending collisions. Whole cadavers, anthropomorphic dummies, and mathematical models have also been used to study whiplash injuries (5,6,17,18,27,29).

Our laboratory has developed a benchtop model of whiplash to approach the question of what mechanism is most directly responsible for cervical spine trauma in rear-end car collisions (21). We have studied human cervical spines in a highly controlled and instrumented system. Intervertebral motions were tracked with high speed cinematography (11). Physiologic intervertebral rotations were studied before and after experimental trauma to determine specific physiologic derangements (22). Such measurements have never been made before.

WHIPLASH TRAUMA MODEL

Eight fresh-frozen human cadaveric cervical spine specimens were studied. Occiput to C7 or T1 osteoligamentous specimens were mounted in resin molds in neutral position. The mechanical properties of the intact cervical spines were determined with flexibility testing as has been previously described (Fig. 1) (20,22). This was accomplished by applying pure flexion and extension moments in a stepwise fashion to the occiput while monitoring intervertebral motions with sets of infrared-emitting diodes mounted on each vertebra. One newton-meter (Nm) was defined as the physiologic limit of loading that did not result in injury by experiments of repeatability. Two flexibility parameters were studied: range of motion (ROM) and neutral zone (NZ).

The whiplash trauma was produced with a specially developed trauma apparatus (Fig. 2) (21). A trauma sled was mounted on horizontal linear bearings and was accelerated by a pneumatic piston, power springs, and an electromagnet release. The lower end of each spine specimen was attached to the sled, and the upper end carried a steel head surrogate designed to represent a 50th-percentile human head (18). The weight of the surrogate head was fully balanced by a pneumatic suspension system, but the inertial components of the head were effective. The suspension of the head was such that the head was completely free to move within its three degrees of freedom in the sagittal plane. A head rest was empirically set at a 45-degree angle so that the natural extension of the head led to a perpendicular contact of the head and head rest. Additionally, each vertebra was fitted with a motion-monitoring flag completely visible from a lateral perspective to allow sagittal plane vertebral motions to be recorded with a movie camera during the trauma.

Once a specimen was mounted on the sled, the springs were compressed with the piston. At time zero, magnets were released, the sled was struck from the rear, and it accel-

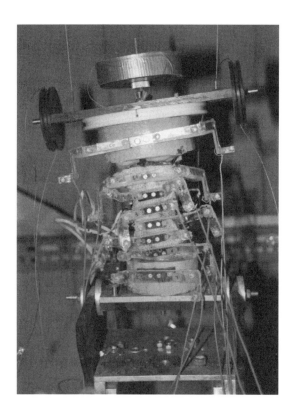

FIG. 1. Cervical spine specimen in flexibility testing machine. Pure moments were applied to a headpiece, and individual intervertebral motions were tracked with infrared-emitting diodes attached to detection flags using an optoelectronic three-dimensional motion measurement system.

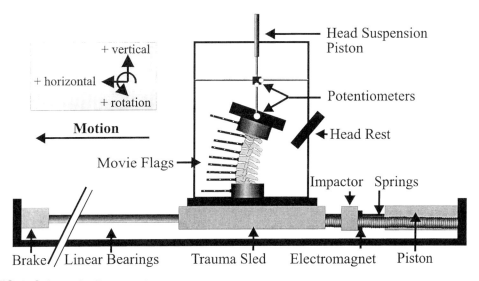

FIG. 2. Schematic diagram of the benchtop whiplash apparatus. Trauma sled was drawn to the negative horizontal direction with the pneumatic piston and released in the positive horizontal direction. Flexion was defined as positive rotation and extension as negative rotation.

erated, reached maximum velocity, decelerated as it hit breaks, and finally came to rest. The traumas were recorded with high speed filming at 500 frames per second. Movie flags were later digitized and the data converted to intervertebral rotations (11).

The maximum sled acceleration for the initial trauma for each specimen was 2g. After this trauma, flexibility testing was repeated to determine any mechanical changes of the cervical spine. Trauma was then increased in increments of 2g, until specimen failure. Flexibility testing was repeated after each trauma.

INJURY-CAUSING MOTIONS DURING WHIPLASH

Analysis of the high speed films revealed a distinctive kinematic response of the cervical spine to whiplash trauma. Digitized intervertebral data from one specimen is shown in Figure 3 and is represented schematically in Figure 4. The 50- to 75-ms time period illustrates an initial phase with development of S-shaped curvature of the cervical spine with extension at the lower levels and flexion at the upper levels. The 100- to 125-ms time period represents the final phase with extension of the entire cervical spine. This was seen in all trauma classes with an average time difference of 25±48 ms.

The intervertebral motions of trauma were then contrasted to the physiologic limits of the cervical spines by comparing maximum intervertebral flexion and extension as determined from the digitized films to that determined from the flexibility testing of the intact cervical spines. As an example, the 6g trauma class is graphically contrasted to the phys-

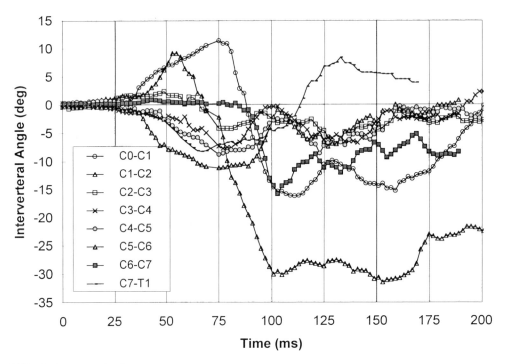

FIG. 3. Intervertebral rotation data obtained from high speed cinematography of an 8.4*g* whiplash trauma. Time zero was defined at the magnet release. Negative values indicate extension, positive values flexion.

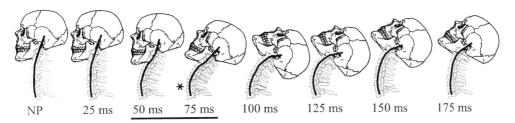

NP   25 ms   50 ms   75 ms   100 ms   125 ms   150 ms   175 ms

FIG. 4. Schematic of a head and neck demonstrating time points during the whiplash represented in Figure 3. A line is drawn through the vertebrae to highlight the curvature of the spine. A skull is shown for illustration only (surrogate head used in studies). NP, neutral posture.

iologic limits in Figure 5. As represented in this figure, intervertebral rotations of C6-C7 and C7-T1 significantly exceeded the maximum physiologic rotations of extension for all trauma classes. The maximum extension of these lower levels occurred during the initial stage of trauma, significantly before full neck extension. Hyperflexion of the upper cervical spine was previously proposed (23,24), but significant hyperflexion was observed only in the 4g trauma class.

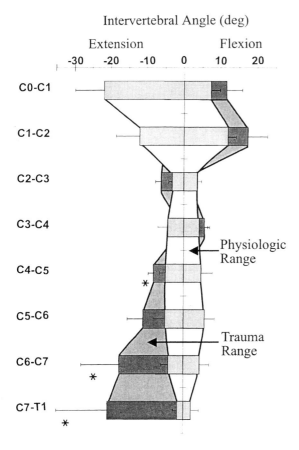

FIG. 5. Physiologic and 6g trauma class intervertebral rotations. Physiologic range outlines the flexion/extension ranges of motion for each intervertebral joint as determined from flexibility testing of the intact spines *(lightly shaded bars/regions)*. The trauma ranges demonstrate where average film rotational data exceeded physiologic limits *(darkly shaded bars/regions)*. The *asterisks* denote significant difference between physiologic and trauma rotations.

Flexibility testing revealed general increased net flexion/extension ROM and NZ, with incrementally increasing trauma as would be expected. To visualize the changes in the flexibility parameters of ROM and NZ caused by trauma, averages at each trauma class and spinal level were computed as percentage increases from intact values.

Range-of-motion analysis demonstrated significant ($p<0.005$) increase in the extension at the C5-C6 levels after 4g trauma (Fig. 6). Flexion ROM significantly increased only at the C2-C3 level after 10g trauma. NZ analysis also demonstrated significant increase in extension at the C5-C6 level after 4g trauma. Extension NZ was also observed to increase at C0-C1 and C6-C7 after 6g trauma but was not statistically significant ($p < .1$) (Fig. 7).

CURRENT CONCEPTS OF WHIPLASH TRAUMA MECHANISM

The mechanism of whiplash has remained unclear over the past 70 years since the term was first coined in 1928 by Crowe (4). Our laboratory has approached the question of whiplash injury mechanism in two stages. First, to establish which mechanism produces such trauma, the intervertebral rotations of the cervical spine were studied with high speed cinematography. Second, to quantify the injuries, the changes in mechanical properties of the cervical spine at each intervertebral level after whiplash trauma were measured with flexibility testing.

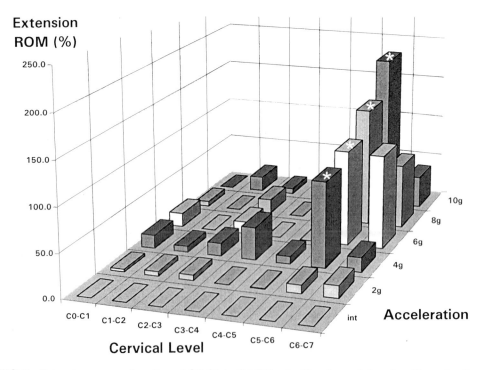

FIG. 6. Extension range of motion at C0-C1 to C6-C7 spinal levels as determined from the flexibility test after 2g to 10g whiplash traumas. The increases are percentage increases above the corresponding intact values. *Asterisks* denote significant change from intact values ($p < .05$).

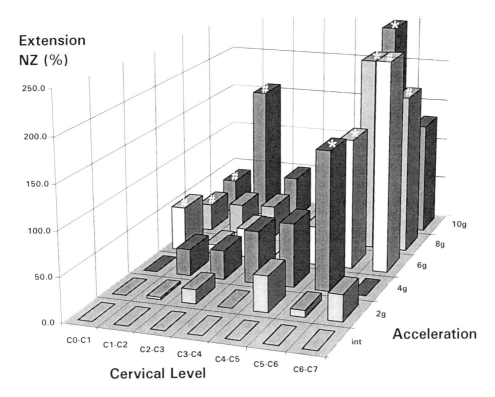

FIG. 7. Extension neutral zone at C0-C1 to C6-C7 spinal levels as determined from the flexibility test after 2*g* to 10*g* whiplash traumas. As in Figure 6, the increases are percentage increases above the corresponding intact values. *Asterisks* denote significant change from intact values ($p < .05$); pound symbols *(#)* denote trends ($p < .1$).

We started from the assumption that intervertebral motions beyond physiologic limits have the potential to cause soft-tissue injury. Furthermore, we define the physiologic limits as the rotations that are reproducible under the application, in this case, of 1 Nm pure moment.

Based on high speed filming of the experimental whiplash trauma, we propose that whiplash is a two-staged response of the neck to a forward acceleration of the thoracic spine. The first stage of whiplash involves the development of S-shaped curvature of the cervical spine with lower level extension and upper level flexion. This S-shaped cervical curvature was noted in a dummy preparation by Svenson, but it was not related to spinal column injury (28). This curvature was also an assumption on which Penning's theory of injury mechanism is based (23,24). However, Penning hypothesized that the cranioverte-bral junction is the principal site of cervical trauma in whiplash. In contrast, our experimental findings show that the lower cervical levels more consistently exceeded their physiologic motion limits.

The second stage of whiplash involves the change to extension of the entire cervical spine. This is associated with a lesser degree of lower level extension and thus less potential for soft-tissue injury. Many of the early whiplash studies that attributed injuries to this full neck extension may have missed the potentially more damaging initial S-shaped trauma stage because of lack of accurate methods to continuously monitor individual intervertebral rotations during the trauma.

It is of further note that the simulated whiplash did not produce occiput extension beyond the physiologic limits. The average peak head extension was, in fact, significantly less than the physiologic head extension. This means that injury could not have been caused by simple neck extension. This directly contradicts the concepts put forth by such authors as MacNab (12,13). Other whiplash studies have also observed the lack of head hyperextension (15,16).

The concept of lower cervical extension trauma is reinforced by the repeated flexibility testing, which found significant increases of ROM and NZ mostly in the lower levels (i.e., C5-C6), although there was a tendency to increase at the upper level (C0-C1) at higher trauma intensities. As would be expected, the magnitude of these increases was related to the magnitude of the peak accelerations imparted to the base of the cervical spine.

There are limitations to our studies. Namely, there are no muscles that in accident victims would serve several roles. First, muscles stabilize the neck and thus help carry the weight of the head. This function has been simulated in our model by suspending the head with a well-developed suspension system that negates gravitational forces without compromising inertial effects. Second, muscles can act in response to trauma to produce forces to limit the motions. However, the reaction time for an unwarned victim to develop sufficient muscle force to brace the spine is approximately 200 ms (30). This is longer than the time to peak trauma, which we observed to be less than 125 ms. Finally, muscles may assist in passively tethering the spine; this was not simulated in our model.

We now see the mechanism of cervical spine whiplash injury to revolve around an initial S-shaped curvature stage that primarily produces hyperextension at lower levels. This suggests the stretching of anterior elements of the lower cervical spine beyond their normal yield limits consistent with AIS1 type injuries. This theory is substantiated by flexibility testing, which has demonstrated corresponding functional changes. Additionally, hyperextension also implies that the corresponding facet joints will be traumatized.

This further understanding of the whiplash mechanism will help in the interpretation of ongoing biomechanical and clinical studies. As the understanding of whiplash continues to improve, the associated prevention, clinical diagnosis, and treatment will be facilitated.

REFERENCES

1. Balla JI. The last whiplash syndrome. *Aust N Z J Surg* 1980;50:610.
2. Braaf MM, Rosner S. Trauma of the cervical spine as cause of chronic headache. *J Trauma* 1975;15:441–446.
3. Compton C. The use of public crash data in biomechanics research. In: Nahum A, Melvin J, eds. *Accident injury biomechanics and prevention.* New York: Springer-Verlag, 1993;49–66.
4. Crowe HE. Injuries of the cervical spine. Presented at the meeting of the Western Orthopaedic Association, San Francisco, 1928.
5. Deng Y-C, Goldsmith W. Response of a human head/neck/upper-torso replica to dynamic loading: I. Physical model. *J Biomech* 1987;20:471–486.
6. Deng Y-C, Goldsmith W. Response of a human head/neck/upper-torso replica to dynamic loading: II. Analytical/numerical model. *J Biomech* 1987;20:487–497.
7. Dvořák J, Valach L, Schmid ST. Cervical spine injuries in Switzerland. *J Manual Med* 1989;16:7–16.
8. Ewing CL, Thomas DJ, Lustick L, Becker E, Willems G, Muzzy WH III. The effect of the initial position of the head and neck on the dynamic response of the human head and neck to -Gx impact acceleration. *Proceedings of the 19th STAPP car crash conference.* Warrendale, PA: Society of Automotive Engineers, 1975: paper no. 751157.
9. Ewing CL, Thomas DJ, Lustick L, Muzzy WH, Willems G, Majewski PL. The effect of duration, rate of onset, and peak sled acceleration on the dynamic response of the human head and neck. *Proceedings of the 20th STAPP car crash conference.* Warrendale, PA: Society of Automotive Engineers, 1976: paper no. 760800.
10. Ewing CS, Thomas DJ, Patrick LM, Beeler GW, Smith MJ. Living human dynamic response to -Gx impact acceleration. II. Accelerations measured on the head and neck. *Proceedings of the 13th STAPP car crash conference.* Warrendale, PA: Society of Automotive Engineers, 1969: paper no. 690817.

11. Grauer JN, Panjabi MM, Cholewicki J, Nibu K, Dvořák J. Whiplash produces bi-phasic curvature of the neck with hyper-extension at lower levels. *Spine* 1997; (in press).
12. MacNab I. Acceleration injuries of the cervical spine. *J Bone Joint Surg* 1964;46A:1797–1799.
13. Macnab I. Whiplash injuries of the neck. *Manit Med Rev* 1966;46(3):172–174.
14. MacNab I. Acceleration extension injuries of the cervical spine. In: Rothman RH, Simeone FA, eds. *The spine.* Philadelphia: WB Saunders, 1982.
15. Matsushita T, Sato TB, Hirabayashi K, Fujimura S, Asazuma T, Takatori T. X-ray study of the human neck motion due to head inertia loading. *Proceedings of the 38th STAPP car crash conference.* Warrendale, PA: Society of Automotive Engineers, 1994: paper no. 942208.
16. McConnell WE, Howard RP, Guzman HM, et al. Analysis of human test subject responses to low velocity rear end impacts. *Proceedings of the 37th STAPP car crash conference.* Warrendale, PA: Society of Automotive Engineers, 1993: paper no. 930889.
17. McKenzie JA, Williams JF. The dynamic behaviour of the head and cervical spine during whiplash. *J Biomech* 1971;4:477–490.
18. Mertz HJ, Patrick LM. Strength and response of the human neck. *Proceedings of the 15th STAPP car crash conference.* Warrendale, PA: Society of Automotive Engineers, 1971: paper no. 710855.
19. Ono K, Kanno M. Influences of the physical parameters on the risk to neck injuries in low impact speed rear-end collisions. International Research Council on Biokenetics of Impacts (IRCOBI) conference on the biomechanics of impacts, Sept 8-10, Eindhoven, The Netherlands, 1993.
20. Panjabi MM, Abumi K, Duranceau J, Crisco JJ. Biomechanical evaluation of spinal fixation devices: II. Stability provided by eight internal fixation devices. *Spine* 1988;13:1135–1140.
21. Panjabi MM, Cholewicki J, Babat LB, Nibu K, Dvořák J. Whiplash trauma can be stimulated using whole cervical spine specimens. *Spine* 1997 (in press).
22. Panjabi MM, Nibu K, Cholewicki J. Whiplash injuries and potential for mechanical instability. *J Spinal disorders* (in press).
23. Penning L. Acceleration injury of the cervical spine by hypertranslation of the head: Part 1. Effect of normal translation of the head on the cervical spine motion: a radiological study. *Eur Spine J* 1992;1:7–12.
24. Penning L. Acceleration injury of the cervical spine by hypertranslation of the head: Part 2. Effect of hypertranslation of the head on the cervical spine motion: discussion of literature data. *Eur Spine J* 1992;1:13–19.
25. Severy DM, Mathewson JH, Bechtol CO. Controlled automobile rear-end collisions, and investigation of related engineering and medical phenomena. *Can Serv Med J* 1955;11:727–759.
26. Spitzer WO, Skovron ML, Salmi LR, Cassidy JD, Duranceau J, Suissa S, Zeiss E. Scientific monograph of the Quebec Task Force on whiplash-associated disorders: redefining "whiplash" and its management. *Spine* 1995; 20(suppl):10S–73S.
27. Svensson M. *Neck-injuries in rear-end car collisions—sites and biomechanical causes of the injuries, test methods and preventive measures.* Chalmers University of Technology, Department of Injury Prevention, 1993.
28. Svensson MY, Aldman B, Hansson HA, Lovsund P, Seeman T, Suneson A, Ortengren T. Pressure effects in the spinal canal during whiplash extension motion: a possible cause of injury to the cervical spinal ganglia. *Proceedings of the 1993 international IRCOBI conference on the biomechanics of impacts,* Eindhoven, The Netherlands, 1993:189–200.
29. Svensson MY, Haland Y, Larsson S. Rear-end collisions—a study of the influence of backrest properties on head-neck motion using a new dummy neck. *Proceedings of the 37th STAPP car crash conference.* Warrendale, PA: Society of Automotive Engineers, 1993: paper no. 930343.
30. Tennyson SA, Mital NK, King AI. Electromyographic signals of the spinal musculature during +Gz impact acceleration. *Orthop Clin North Am* 1977;8:97–119.

Whiplash Injuries: Current Concepts in Prevention, Diagnosis, and Treatment of the Cervical Whiplash Syndrome, edited by Robert Gunzburg and Marek Szpalski. Lippincott–Raven Publishers, Philadelphia © 1998.

9

Neurophysiologic Mechanisms of Low-Velocity Non-Head-Contact Cervical Acceleration

Malcolm H. Pope, Assen Aleksiev, Leif Hasselquist, Marianne L. Magnusson, Kevin Spratt, and Marek Szpalski

M. H. Pope, A. Aleksiev, L. Hasselquist, M. Magnusson, K. Spratt: Iowa Spine Research Center, Department of Orthopaedics, University of Iowa, Iowa City, Iowa 52242. M. Szpalski: Department of Orthopaedic Surgery, Centre Hospitalier Molière Longchamp, Brussels, Belgium.

Whiplash syndrome has become surrounded by both legal and medical controversy. The rate has increased dramatically in the last decade and now reaches 70 per 100,000 in Quebec [Québec Task Force on Whiplash-Associated Disorders (QTF)](4). The rate is greatest in females and those in the 20- to 24-year-old age group. The neurophysiologic aspects of the whiplash injury are not well understood. Our study questions the old assumption that the cervical muscles do not have a significant effect in the mechanism of whiplash-associated disorders, and it tests a simple protective maneuver for its efficacy during sudden acceleration. None of the available biomechanical models include the cervical muscles. The idea that the human subject is a helpless victim of whiplash-associated disorders during collision may not be completely true. The sickness absence resulting from whiplash appears to increase if no seat belt was used and with the severity of impact (QTF). There is consensus that a whiplash occurs with no warning, no bracing, trunk acceleration followed by deceleration, and head hyperextension followed by hyperflexion. What appears to be important is the temporal nature of the events. Severy et al. (3), in controlled rear-end collisions, found peak head accelerations at 235 ms. The first purpose of the present study was to establish how quickly the neck musculature of a subject could respond to a controlled impact. The second purpose was to determine if a program based on motor control principles may have preventative potential in subjects, allowing them to cope better with sudden cervical accelerations.

HYPOTHESES

The hypotheses were as follows:

1. The cervical muscles do have a significant influence in the mechanism of whiplash injury.

2. A simple protective maneuver (shoulder elevation) prior or during sudden cervical acceleration may have preventative potential.

TABLE 1. *Experimental design*

- A $2 \times 2 \times 2 \times 2 \times 2 \times 2 \times$ within subjects factorial experiment.
- 2wTraining $\times$ 2wDirection $\times$ 2wExpectancy $\times$ 2wRecoil $\times$ 2wSpeed $\times$ 2wMuscle group.
- Ten subjects in each of 32 conditions with two muscle groups assessed within each condition.
- A total of $10 \times 32 \times 2 = 640$ observations.

3. There is an interaction between expectation, velocity, direction, recoil, and training effect on the cervical muscle electromyogram (EMG) responses and the head acceleration.

METHODS

Ten healthy men (ages, 18 to 25) were tested after approved consent. Each subject was positioned in a bucket seat from a standard compact automobile with an adjustable head rest. The seat was mounted to a movable sled with four wheels. Spring mechanisms were attached to the base of the sled. A standard tension to the springs was applied so that minimal acceleration (much below any discomfort limit) to the cervical spine was experienced. Surface EMG activity was recorded laterally, 3 cm from the midline at C4, and at the upper part of the sternocleidomastoideus muscle. One accelerometer recorded the head acceleration, and a second one the sled acceleration. A video camera recorded the movement of the head, neck, and seat. The subjects were tested during expected and unexpected acceleration, and before and after safety instructions containing a brief explanation of the quick shoulder elevation protective maneuver. The subjects were instructed to elevate their shoulders just before the sudden acceleration for the expected case, and as soon as possible for the unexpected case.

The experimental design is summarized in Tables 1 and 2.

The influence of the neck muscles depends on how fast they can respond (reaction time), how strongly they can respond (magnitude), and how long they maintain their activity (duration). These characteristics were calculated using wavelet transformation (WT) of the EMG signals with automatic detection (1,2). The short latency (reflexive) responses and long latency (anticipatory) responses were calculated as time lags [in milliseconds (ms)] between the first acceleration increment and the corresponding burst of EMG activity. The magnitude of the response was calculated in millivolts (mV) and the duration in milliseconds. The video analysis was performed using Primer 4.2 and Photo 3.0 to calculate velocity, and linear and angular displacement.

TABLE 2. *Experimental Design: 2wTraining $\times$ 2wDirection $\times$ 2wExpectancy $\times$ 2wRecoil $\times$ 2wSpeed $\times$ 2wMuscle group*

Outcomes	Definition	Units of measurement
Response amplitude	Muscle response	mv
Response duration	Muscle response	ms
Number of responses	Muscle response	Frequency
Lag time 1: sled	Onset to first EMG	ms
Lag time 1: head	Onset to first EMG	ms
Lag time max: sled	Onset to max EMG	ms
Lag time max: head	Onset to max EMG	ms

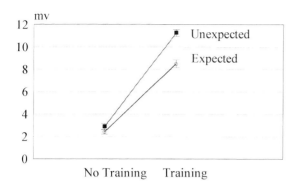

FIG. 1. Training × expectancy effects for response amplitude.

RESULTS

The response amplitude is greater after training, and after training it is greater when the impact is unexpected (Fig. 1). The response duration, relative to the sled impact, is shown in Figure 2. Training appears to improve the response duration. Figure 3 summarizes the training and expectancy effects. The pattern of results is consistent for reaction times assessed from the sled and the head. Of importance is the temporal ordering of the sled relative to the head reaction times. The response time is fast enough to affect the response of the head, because it appears to be initiated by the initial sled impact. Training in the expected condition demonstrated much shorter anticipatory reactions. Significant interaction effects for reduced models are shown in Figure 4. Figure 5 shows training × speed × muscle group (flexor versus extensor) for interaction for response duration.

DISCUSSION

The hypothesis that the cervical muscles cannot react fast enough for protection during sudden acceleration was not supported from these results. Thus, the assumption that humans are helpless during collision is premature. The muscle reaction appears to be initiated by the initial impact, and it will affect the biomechanics and could even be a secondary source of injury. The shoulder elevation has a great protective potential. Increased magnitude and duration of the muscle activity, decreased duration of the head acceleration, and decreased angular displacement during this maneuver showed more efficient

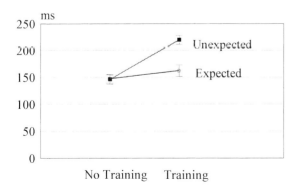

FIG. 2. Training × expectancy effects for response duration.

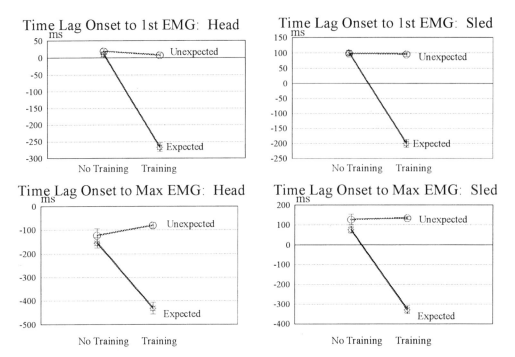

FIG. 3. Summary of training × expectancy effects.

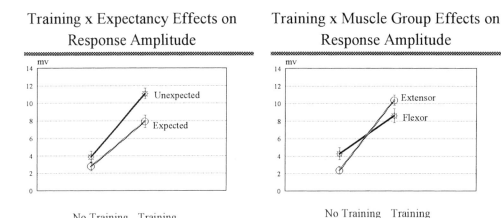

FIG. 4. Significant interaction effects for reduced models.

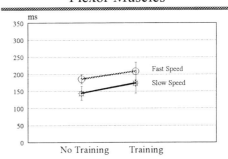

FIG. 5. Training × speed × muscle group interaction for response duration. For both the flexor and extensor muscles, there is a significant difference between the fast and slow speeds in the *No Training* condition, but no significant difference between the fast and slow speeds in the *Training* condition.

self-bracing. The decreased bursts of EMG activity suggests that the cervical muscles have been pre-tuned by the co-contraction of the shoulder muscles to become better dampers of sudden acceleration. If this simple maneuver proves to be practically applicable as well, an inexpensive alarm device, indicating unusually short distances between two cars, may be a small investment to the safety and health of passengers.

CONCLUSIONS

The results from the study would be helpful in preventing or reducing the severity of the whiplash-associated disorders as a result of sudden cervical accelerations by a simple safety instruction for quick shoulder elevation before or during sudden accelerations. Further studies testing the feasibility of an alarm device, and this maneuver in a driving simulator with distraction of the subject's attention, are needed to verify the value of these findings.

ACKNOWLEDGMENTS

Supported by Injury Prevention Research Center (IPRC) (CCR 703640-06), The University of Iowa (P 1 0542), and National Institutes of Health (NIH) grant 1 R01 AR43652-01.

REFERENCES

1. Bruce A, Donoho D, Gao H. Wavelet analysis. *IEEE Spectrum* 1996;0018-9235:26–35.
2. Chui CK. Wavelet transforms. *An introduction to wavelets*. San Diego: Academic Press, 1992;49–80.
3. Severy DM, Mathewson JH, Bechtol CP. Controlled automobile rear-end collisions: an investigation of related engineering and mechanical phenomenon. *Can Services Med J* 1955;11:727.
4. Spitzer W, Skovron ML, Salmi R, Cassidy D, Duranceau J, Suissa S, Zeiss E. Scientific monograph of the Quebec Task Force on whiplash-associated disorders: redefining whiplash and its management. *Spine* 1995;20: 8S–11S,27S–30S.

*Whiplash Injuries: Current Concepts in
Prevention, Diagnosis, and Treatment
of the Cervical Whiplash Syndrome,*
edited by Robert Gunzburg and Marek Szpalski.
Lippincott–Raven Publishers, Philadelphia © 1998.

10

The Minimal Collision Velocity for Whiplash

Stefan Meyer, Michael Weber, William Castro, Markus Schilgen,
and Christoph Peuker

S. Meyer and M. Weber: Ingenieurbüro Schimmelpfennig und Becke, Münster, Germany.
W. Castro and M. Schilgen: Academy for Manual Medicine,
University of Münster, Germany.
C. Peuker: Department of Radiology, Clemens-Hospital, Münster, Germany.

Since the 1970s, an increasing number of whiplash injuries have been observed in Germany. At present, enormous sums of money, exceeding DM 1 billion each year, are being paid by the insurance companies alone for injury damages after whiplash traumas. In 1990, a comprehensive evaluation called Fahrzeugsiclerheit 90 (FS90) was carried out on 15% of all car–car accidents involving injury to occupants. It was found that half of these accidents were rear-end impacts, and in 94% of these impacts at least one of the occupants claimed to have suffered whiplash injury (4). Fig. 1 shows the statistical distribution of rear-end impacts in terms of the level of damage. Only accidents with injury victims are counted. Damage is classified into five classes, as detailed schematically in Figure 2. An interesting point to note is that in 65% of all rear-end impacts, the vehicles show only slight to moderate damage. An example of slight damage is shown in Figure 3; vehicles were placed in this class only when they suffered scratches and slight dents. An example of moderate damage can be seen in Figure 4; only vehicles with deformations up to a depth of about 10 cm were classified in this category.

The study also evaluated what percentage of the occupants claimed whiplash injury in accidents with the various levels of vehicle damage. This evaluation produced the astonishing result that rising severity of damage did not produce an increase in injuries, but a decrease instead. The highest level of injury claims was in vehicles with the slightest levels of damage.

Various studies showed that the biodynamic stresses arising in the cases of slight to moderate vehicle damage cannot be sufficient to cause injuries to the cervical spine (6,7,10,1,8,9,11). Higher stresses occur in normal, everyday movements, and especially in sports, and there is no question that these are tolerated by the cervical spine. Therefore, from a biomechanical point of view, it is not possible to explain the very high percentage of whiplash trauma with slight to moderate levels of vehicle damage. The insurance companies in Germany, Austria, and Switzerland are responding increasingly critically towards whiplash claims in the event of nonsevere rear-end impacts; more and more cases are being brought before the courts, and consequently the courts themselves have also become aware of the problems involved. In 1994, the issue of whiplash trauma was dealt with at a judges' conference, which adopted a recommendation that in cases of

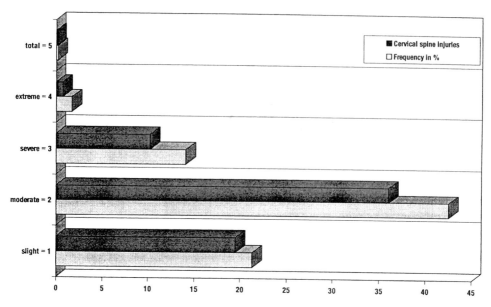

FIG. 1. Statistical evaluation of whiplash in Germany.

disputes, interdisciplinary technical and medical expertise should be obtained on the actual biomechanical stresses involved (2). In 1996, the subject was raised again in connection with claims for indemnification; the judges recommended that no damages should be paid for slight injuries, whereas the damages for severe injuries should be increased instead, and also that fraudulent exploitation of damages law should be combated more energetically (3).

As technical experts in the field of traffic accidents, we are being increasingly asked in court proceedings whether the stresses occurring in a vehicle were sufficient to cause injury to the cervical spine. As a matter of principle, the level of stress can be reconstructed by evaluating the vehicle damage. However, the question of what forces are exerted on the vehicle occupants for the various levels of vehicle deformation was poorly investigated. Therefore, since 1988, we have been carrying out crash tests with live test subjects at our crash test facility. The first systematic study was carried out in 1993 (6), and we are currently engaged in a second study in interdisciplinary cooperation with the Academy for Manual Medicine at the University of Münster.

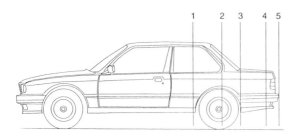

FIG. 2. Classification of rear-end deformation in FS 90 (*y*-axis in Fig. 1).

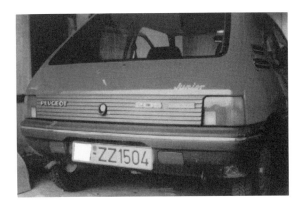

FIG. 3. Slight deformation in FS 90.

The results of the first study and the current status of the second study will be detailed here. To provide a general understanding of the technical and biomechanical factors involved, some explanations will first be given.

INTERDEPENDENCE BETWEEN VEHICLE DEFORMATION AND BIOMECHANICAL STRESS

It is fundamentally possible to infer the velocity of impact from the deformation of the vehicles. As the deformation intensity increases with the square of the impact velocity, this velocity can be stated with precision by evaluating the deformation. By now, a large number of crash tests have been carried out, which in normal cases allow impact velocities to be reliably determined from the deformation found. However, it is not only the impact velocities that determine the stresses exerted on the occupants. Other factors must also be taken into consideration:

The *weights of the vehicles* are very important. An extreme example of this is shown in Figure 5. If a heavy truck crashes into a normal car, the occupants of the target vehicle will be subject to high forces, even at a low impact velocity. Conversely, if a normal car crashes into a heavy truck, the force in the truck exerted by the same impact velocity will be slight.

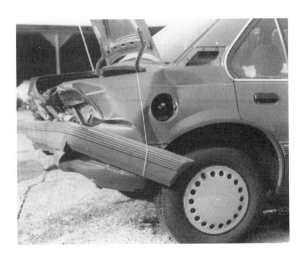

FIG. 4. Moderate deformation in FS 90.

Heavy vehicle against light vehicle = high force

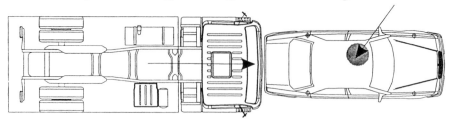

Light vehicle against heavy vehicle = low force

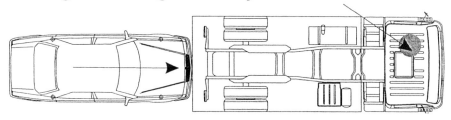

FIG. 5. Influencing factor: vehicle weights.

The level of stresses in the target vehicle is also influenced by the *degree of overlap.* The greater the degree of overlap, the higher the force (Fig. 6).

Another important factor is the *impact height.* In the case of rear-end collisions, the driver of the bullet vehicle usually has enough time to apply the brakes before impact occurs. This causes the vehicle to nose-dive (Fig. 7).As the bumpers of the two vehicles are at the same height when the vehicles are unbraked, nose-diving inevitably results in submarining of the bullet vehicle under the bumper of the target vehicle. According to measurements performed by us, the nose-dive depth is 10 to 15 cm (12). As a result, the direct contact, and therefore the exchange of forces, is between the headlamp plane and the rear bumper, and not, as in the case of unbraked impact, between the hard zones of the bumpers. In our view, most studies into the stress tolerance of the cervical spine (whiplash) do not take sufficient account of this factor. It is usually the case in rear-end collisions that the vehicles impact at different heights because of the nose-diving effect, and therefore tests that simulate bumper–bumper collisions are of little relevance to practical reality.

In principle, there are various possibilities for describing the forces occurring in vehicles. In practical terms, however, only a description of the acceleration phases over time and the change in velocity are useful. The acceleration phases over time is the more

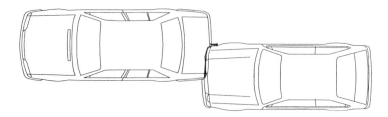

FIG. 6. Influencing factor: overlap.

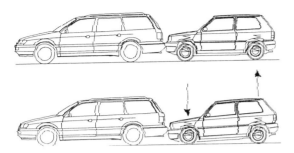

FIG. 7. Influencing factor: impact heights (**top**: unbraked impact; **bottom**, braked impact).

meaningful method, but it has the disadvantage of being abstract to people who are not technical experts. The change in velocity is much easier to imagine, but it does not take the duration of impact into account. In the case of longer-lasting collisions, the stresses are lower because of the longer impact duration in which the velocity change is produced; in the case of short impact duration, the velocity change is produced very quickly. Long and soft impacts occur when there is nose-diving and/or a small degree of overlap. Short and hard impacts occur in bumper–bumper contact with a greater degree of overlap. For practical purposes, a description using the velocity change ΔV (Fig. 8) is normally sufficient. Before impact, the bullet vehicle B is travelling at velocity V_B faster than the target vehicle T. During impact, about half of V_B is transmitted to T. This is only the case, however, if both vehicles are of approximately the same weight and the collision is not elastic. For a general consideration, though, this statement is adequate. After the collision, T continues to move with the velocity change ΔV. In the collision, this vehicle has undergone velocity change ΔV within a time of 1/10 to 2/10 s; the higher this velocity change is, the higher also is the biomechanical stress.

In the case of greater differences between the weights of the vehicles, the velocity change can be calculated according to the following formula (plastic impact):

Before collision:

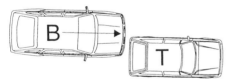

During collision:

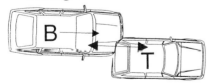

After collision:

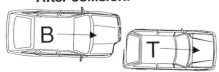

FIG. 8. Definition for change in velocity ΔV.

TABLE 1. *The same stress as produced by different velocity combinations*

Bullet vehicle (kph)	Target vehicle (kph)	Relative impact velocity (= biomechanical stress) (kph)
120	100	20
70	50	20
20	0	20
10 (forwards)	−10 (backwards)	20

$$\Delta V = [m_B/(m_T + m_B)]v_B$$

The foregoing applies when both vehicles are in motion. In this case, the relative impact speed must be used for calculation. For example, the velocity combinations shown in Table 1 produce the same stresses.

Furthermore, the level of stress in the target vehicle is not significantly influenced by whether either of the drivers or both of them brake before, during, and after impact. It is not the case that higher velocity changes occur with an unbraked target vehicle; rather, the effect of the braking forces is negligible as compared to the impact forces.

The only significant influence of braking is the change in impact height. An uphill or downhill gradient at the site of the accident also has no significant influence.

As practice shows, most impacts are not plastic but partially elastic. This means that in the target vehicle slightly higher velocity changes occur in a magnitude of 60% of the relative impact velocity. Further details on this can be taken from the evaluation of the trials presented later, particularly in Figure 11.

METHODOLOGY

In the 1993 study (6), a total of 22 rear-end impacts were carried out at a ΔV of 6 kph to 12 kph. In 14 of the tests, live test subjects were located in the target vehicles; in the remaining tests, dummies were used. Recordings were made of the vehicle acceleration, the chest acceleration, and the head acceleration. Additionally, the muscle tone was recorded synchronously with the other data by means of surface electromyograms (EMGs).

Analysis of the kinematics was done by markers applied to the passenger compartment, the seat, and the body of the occupant. To prevent anticipation, some of the test persons were screened off acoustically. Additionally, the 1993 study also performed practical measurements at a bumper-car ride.

In the 1996 study (which is still continuing), the same basic instrumentation layout has been retained, but with significant improvements. The velocity change in the target vehicle has been considerably increased to a ΔV of 10 kph to 15 kph. It should be emphasized, however, that, as will be shown below, even at 15 kph the forces that occur are still comparable to those measured in bumper cars. Before the trials, all the test persons were informed of the possible risks. Most of them were technical or medical experts who also had a personal interest in the results of the trials. Comprehensive medical examinations took place 6 days before, 24 hours after, and 4 weeks after the trials. The test persons were subject to orthopedic/manual medical/neurologic examinations. On the same dates, a computer-controlled ultrasound examination of the motility of the cervical spine and spin tomography of the cervical spine with and without gadolinium-diethylene-triamine penta-acetic acid (DTPA) were performed.

All the crash tests were performed at the facility of Ingenieurbüro Schimmelpfennig + Becke. The medical examinations were carried out at the Academy for Manual Medicine and at Clemens Hospital in Münster. The Institute for Sports Medicine at the University of Münster was responsible for recording and evaluating the movement markers.

VEHICLES USED

In the 1993 study, no systematic selection of the test vehicles was made. All were fitted with normal European bumper systems, without energy-absorbing components. In the 1996 study, a systematic selection was made. The trials included five modern compact cars (Volkswagen Golf), five station wagons (Opel Kadett), and five limousines (Opel Rekord). Additionally, crash tests were carried out with two bumper cars of the type found at funfairs.

OCCUPANTS AND INSTRUMENTATION SETUP

In the 1993 study, only two different test subjects were used. These were both men, aged about 30, and neither complained of injury after the collisions. The trials were not subject to medical monitoring. The 1996 study includes women, and the trials are medically monitored. All volunteers are subject to only one rear-end collision. The test persons are chosen with a wide spread in terms of age, preexisting degenerative conditions, and physical constitution.

To prevent anticipation by the test persons, they are all completely screened off visually (by blindfold) and acoustically (Walkman with loud rock music). Most of the test subjects stated after the trials that they had been able to discern nothing of the further trial preparations, which took between 5 and 15 minutes. The EMG recordings of all the test subjects show typical rest potentials before the trials with no anticipation of the neck muscles.

The instrumentation applied to the test persons is shown in Figure 9. The test subject is already completely screened off at the time of recording. Accelerometers are installed

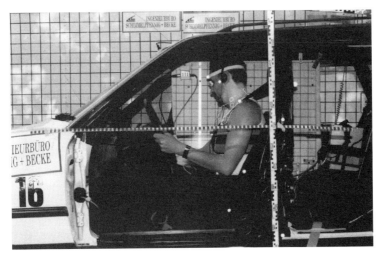

FIG. 9. Instrumentation of the occupant.

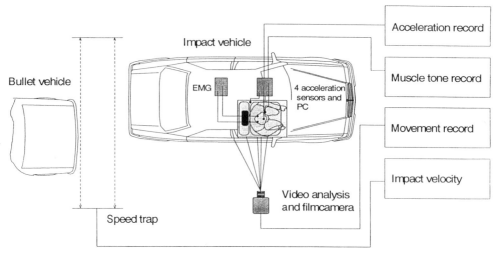

FIG. 10. Instrumentation layout for all tests.

in the vehicle's passenger compartment and on the chest and the head of the occupant. Additionally, movement markers are fitted at the shoulder, the center of gravity of the head, the forehead, and the hip of the test person. Other movement markers are located on the seat, the head restraint, and the "B" pillar. EMG signals are obtained from various neck muscles.

Figure 10 shows the schematic setup for the 1993 and 1996 studies. Besides passenger compartment acceleration, the kinematics of the occupant were also recorded in these rear-end impacts. The movement data were recorded by a video evaluation system and by additional biomechanical acceleration data. In addition to the kinematic data, the activity of the neck muscles was also recorded using surface EMGs.

For the 1996 study, the instrumentation setup was developed further, with accident data recorders (manufactured by Mannesmann-Kienzle, Villingen, Germany) being installed in both the bullet and the target vehicle. This enabled the acceleration effects to be recorded for the passenger compartment not only of the target vehicle but also of the bullet vehicle. For kinematic analysis, the screening frequency was increased from 50 to a good 700 Hz. Additionally, EMG signals were obtained from several neck muscles. The contact phase of the vehicle structures and the kinematics of the occupants were recorded using high-speed cameras.

VEHICLE MOVEMENTS

Table 2 lists the data of all persons and the most important data of all tests in the ongoing 1996 study. Figure 11 shows the impact velocity (V_I) and ΔV for all trials so far carried out in both studies. For the impact velocities of the vehicles, which in some cases differed significantly in weight, the weight influence has been eliminated. This allows a better comparison of the impact velocities. The x-axis shows the weight-adjusted impact velocities in the trials, the y-axis the velocity change ΔV. The line k = 0 stands for plastic collisions, whereby the velocity change ΔV is precisely half of the weight-adjusted impact velocity. The second line, k = 1, stands for elastic collisions. A virtually elastic impact takes place when, for example, two billiard balls strike each other. In vehicle col-

TABLE 2. *Data from all tests in the ongoing 1996 study*

Trial no.(yr)	Subject age	Height (m)	Weight (kg)	Sex	Overlap (%)	Time (s)	V_1 (kph)	ΔV_2 (kph)
I	36	1.84	76	M	75 l.	0.119	17.5	8.7
II	37	1.77	61	F	100	0.107	21	13.6
III	33	1.8	72	M	50 r.	0.108	18.5	9
IV	32	1.84	84	M	50 l.	0.105	18.5	9.4
V	48	1.74	82	M	100	0.106	19.5	11.4
VI	33	1.8	70	M	100	0.132	20.5	12.8
VII	30	1.85	78	M	100	0.13	19	12.7
VIII	30	1.89	80	M	85 r.	0.12	22.5	14.2
IX	28	1.75	63	M	50 l.	0.137	20	12.7
X	26	1.74	71	F	50 r.	0.128	22	13.3
XI	30	1.85	90	M	50 l.	0.119	25	12.6
XII	32	1.7	68	F	100	0.121	20.5	9.5
XIII	34	1.8	95	M	100	0.117	21	9.7
XIV	35	1.75	65	M	100	0.131	19.5	9.4
XV	36	1.81	72	F	50 r.	0.105	25	11
XVI	37	1.82	82	M	30 l.	0.169	27.5	13.3

V_1, impact velocity of bullet vehicle; ΔV_2, velocity change of the target vehicle.

lisions, however, elastic impacts are not observed. Figure 12 also shows that with rising collision velocity, the character of the impact becomes increasingly plastic.

The relevant impact times are stated in Figure 12. These are around 0.1 s; with greater intrusions, impact times of up to 0.16 s have also been observed. All the impacts are generally between 0.075 s and 0.16 s.

BUMPER CAR MOVEMENTS

In funfair bumper car tests, a total of about 70 impact events were recorded and evaluated. Figure 13 shows that for bumper cars, the collision times for all individual impacts

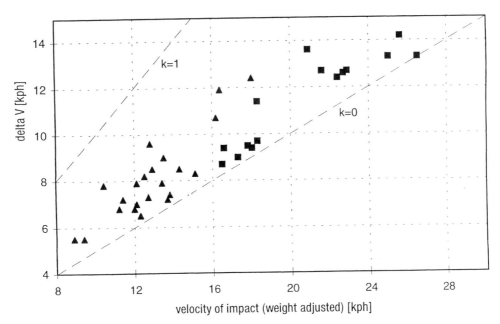

FIG. 11. Crash velocities (weight adjusted) and ΔV for all tests in the 1993 study (▲) and ongoing 1996 study (■).

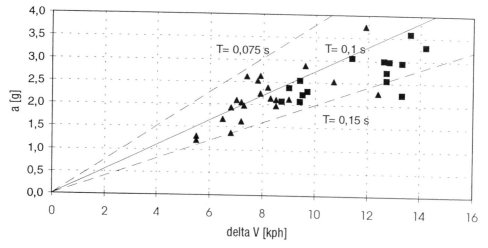

FIG. 12. Rear-end collision impact times, Δ V, and average acceleration in the 1993 study (▲) and ongoing 1996 study (■).

are in a range between 0.075 s and 0.15 s. Most of the values are grouped very densely around the mean impact time of 0.1 s (1/10 s). For bumper cars, Δ V values of approximately 4 kph to a maximum of 15 kph were found. This corresponds to mean vehicle passenger compartment accelerations of about 1g to 4g.

Figure 14 gives a direct comparison between vehicle and bumper car impacts. The vehicle acceleration shows typical high-frequency oscillations *(right)*. Because of the

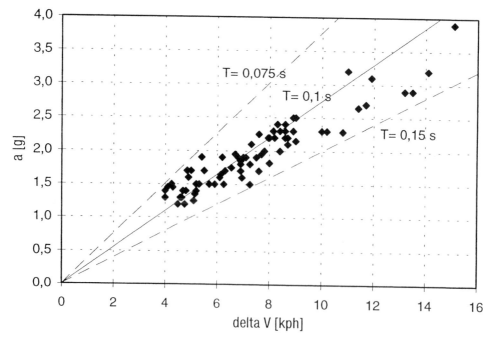

FIG. 13. Bumper car collision impact times, Δ V, and average acceleration for 70 impacts at a funfair.

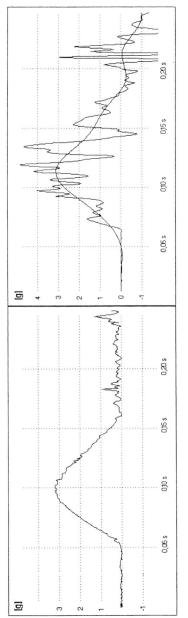

FIG. 14. Comparison of acceleration between bumper car collision (*left*) and vehicle collision (*right*).

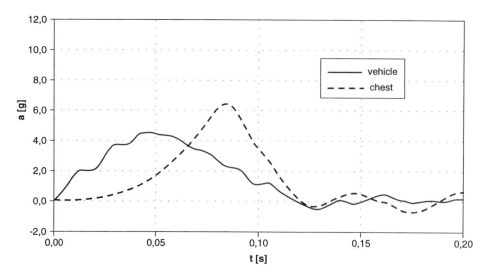

FIG. 15. Bumper car collision acceleration curves for car and chest in a trial.

mechanical inertia of the torso and body of the occupant, these oscillations are of no relevance for the biomechanical stress on the occupant. The digitally filtered signal that is also shown demonstrates that impacts between vehicles are highly comparable with impacts between bumper cars in respect to the time sequence of passenger compartment acceleration.

In the 1996 study, a test subject was used in the test vehicles at similar ΔV values in a bumper car collision and a car impact. The acceleration curves of the bumper car, motor car, and occupant's chest are very similar, whereas the head acceleration in the car is substantially higher. The explanation for this is that the head impacts on the head restraint in the car. In the bumper car, the head is not stopped; instead, its relative rearward movement is unrestrained. This results in a comparatively large angle between torso and head of the occupant. As an example, in Figure 15 the acceleration curves for car and chest of a rather hard bumper-car impact with a ΔV of 11 kph is shown. The peak acceleration of the bumper car went up to 4g. In this trial, we observed hyperextension of the cervical spine with a head–torso angle up to 80°! The volunteer in this test complained of no trouble.

OCCUPANT INJURIES AND SUBJECTIVE IMPRESSIONS

The test subjects in the 1993 did not complain of any trouble immediately after the crash or indeed at any time since then. It should further be noted in this context that because of the small number of test persons, each one was subjected to numerous impacts in the bumper car collisions and up to 50 impacts in the car crashes. As the test subjects were involved in both the bumper car and the motor vehicle impacts, they were able to give a subjective assessment of both types of impact. They stated unanimously that because of the unfavorable seat geometry and the absence of head restraints they found the bumper car impacts to be more unpleasant than the car collisions.

In the trials performed in the 1996 study to date, most of the occupants did not complain of pain after the test. Some test subjects stated immediately after the collision that they felt pain through contact of the head restraint with the back of the head. Two test subjects reported slight tension of the neck muscles in conjunction with slight restriction of movement, which, however, disappeared within the next few days.

OCCUPANT MOTION

In the following section, we take a closer look at the phases of motion of the vehicle occupants, produced by rear-end impacts. The aim is to obtain more detailed information on the injury mechanism. On the basis of motion analysis from the video recordings in the 1993 study, it was possible to determine the absolute and relative movements of the vehicle, of the seat and head restraint, and also of the occupant from the movement of the markers. In the example, impact velocity was 13.5 kph and ΔV was 7.5 kph. Figure 16 shows ten positions evaluated during the first 180 ms of a collision. The absolute movements of the passenger compartment, of the seat back and head restraint, and of the occupant were documented. Two markers each were attached to the head and chest. The motions shown for the head and chest could be calculated from the paths of movement. The absolute movements of the head restraint and seat back were also determined in the same way. Using this depiction, it was then possible to break occupant movement down into four constantly recurring movement phases in the case of rear-end impacts.

These movement phases are described in Figure 17. On the right, the lines of movement are shown in isolation (i.e., detached from the body of the test subject). If these individual pictures are superimposed on each other and the end points of the lines are joined, the result are the paths of movement as recorded by the video camera. The occupant movement can be split into four phases:

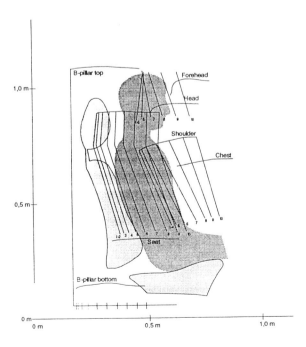

FIG. 16. Evaluation of the marker-movements.

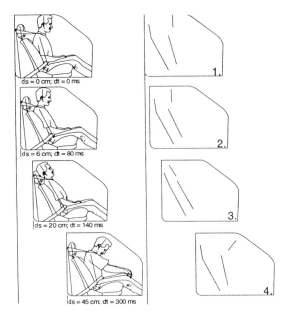

FIG. 17. Four phases of movement.

Phase 1

The characteristic of this phase is that the passenger compartment and the car seat move towards the occupant's torso, which is at rest. In this phase, therefore, there is as yet no movement of the occupant. The start of this phase is identical with the start of the impact, or the time of first contact between the two vehicles.

Phase 2

The second phase begins with the contact between the torso and the seat back. As the deformation margin of the seat back is consumed, the occupant's torso is more and more included in the general forward movement. Up to this time, the head has not moved at all. With the start of forward movement of the torso, the relative movement between the head and torso begins. At the start of the second phase, the passenger compartment has already moved forwards about 6 cm, without the body of the occupant participating in this movement at all. The second phase begins about 80 ms after first contact between the vehicles.

Phase 3

When the passenger compartment has already moved forwards a distance of about 20 cm, and a time of about 140 ms from the start of the impact has elapsed, the approaching head restraint contacts with the back of the head. The start of this third phase is thus determined by the contact between the head restraint and the head. From this point on, the head follows the general forward movement, whereby, provided it is correctly positioned, the head restraint ensures that after the start of the third phase the relative angle between the torso and the head of the test subject cannot increase further.

Phase 4

The three primary movement phases are followed by the fourth phase, in which the low-energy secondary movement of the occupant in the form of a forward motion takes place (rebound). Because of the fact that the occupant follows the movement of the passenger compartment with his own time lag, he also reaches ΔV with only this time lag. He consequently moves forward relative to the passenger compartment and is finally restrained by the seat belt. In contrast to the primary movement (phases 1 to 3), however, this secondary movement is very low in energy and therefore certainly not liable to induce injuries.

For example, Figure 18 shows the acceleration curves recorded during an impact trial together with the EMG signal. In this figure, the first three of the four collision phases can be clearly seen. The acceleration of the passenger compartment, the chest, and the head were marked. The start of chest acceleration indicates the start of contact between the torso and the seat back, and the start of head acceleration marks the contact with the head restraint. In the periods between the start of the various accelerations, there is in each case the phase of relative movement between the passenger compartment and the torso, and the torso and head of the occupant. After passing the start point of head acceleration, which is shown as a broken line, the fourth and final phase of movement then begins, in which the test person moves forwards. In this context, it should be noted that for determining the relative movement between the head and the torso, only the time sequence of head acceleration is of interest. The maximal acceleration value, on the other hand, is only an indication for the strength of head impact with the head restraint. This impact therefore occurs during the phase of contact with the head restraint and is therefore not suitable for characterizing the relative movement between the head and torso.

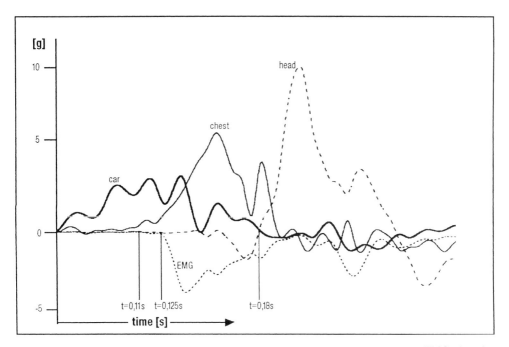

FIG. 18. Acceleration curves recorded during an impact trial together with the EMG signal.

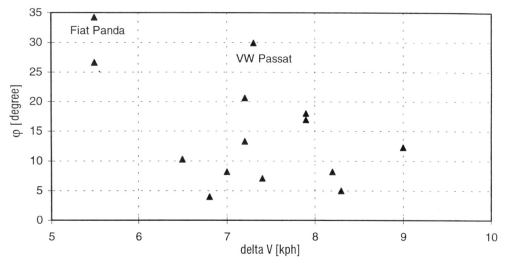

FIG. 19. Maximal angle of torso–head and change in velocity Δ *V* (1993 study only).

Figure 19 shows the maximal angle of movement between the head and body, as determined from motion analysis, in relation to Δ *V*. A uniform trend to the effect that the maximal angle increases with increasing Δ *V* cannot be found. Analysis of the occupant movement shows that the maximal relative angle is rather determined by the geometric factors of the seat construction. The greatest head–torso angle was found in impacts in the lower velocity range, with the test person located in a Fiat Panda. In this vehicle, the angle of the seat back could not be adjusted. A relatively large angle to the vertical was therefore predetermined. The so-called head restraint in this vehicle was integrated into the seat back and could not be adjusted in height, so it would be more accurate to speak of a neck roll than of a head restraint. The head is not supported at all; instead, rear hyperextension

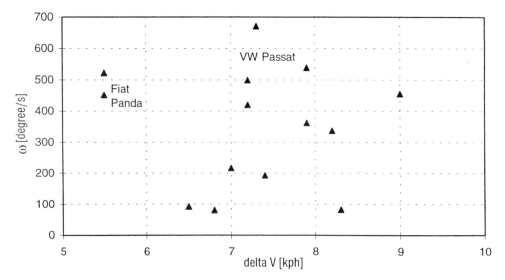

FIG. 20. Relative angle velocity over Δ *V* (1993 study only).

over the top of the head restraint is reinforced. Seat geometry of this type must be considered as promoting injury.

Irrespective of this, the maximum relative angle in all the trials was in a range that can also easily be reached with a slow, conscious movement. As the geometric arrangement of the seat in the area of head contact is independent of the speed of travel, an injury mechanism in the form of mechanical hyperextension through the extent of head displacement appears unlikely even for higher-impact velocities.

Figure 20 shows the maximal relative angle velocities measured between head and torso over ΔV. The maximal value is reached shortly before contact between the head and the head restraint (i.e., during the phase when movement between the head and torso is still unrestricted by external factors). What is conspicuous is that the rotation angle velocity of the head, in contrast to the relative angles, can achieve a considerable magnitude even at low impact velocities. The trials therefore indicate that with a correct geometric seat arrangement in the area of head contact, the injury-relevant parameter can lie only in the velocity of the relative movement between the head and torso.

BIOMECHANICAL ACCELERATION AND EMG SIGNAL

Figure 21 shows the time lag between the biomechanical signals in relation to the ΔV of the target vehicle. In this graph, the start of acceleration of the passenger compartment is defined as the zero point. It is evident here that with a normal seating position, the acceleration of the chest begins immediately after acceleration of the passenger compartment (irregularities begin to appear in the signals about 10 ms after the start of the impact), whereas acceleration of the head shows a time lag of about 110 ms relative to the acceleration of the passenger compartment. Within this period of time between the start of acceleration of the passenger compartment and the start of acceleration of the head, the head restraint travels a distance of about 20 cm. This distance also approxi-

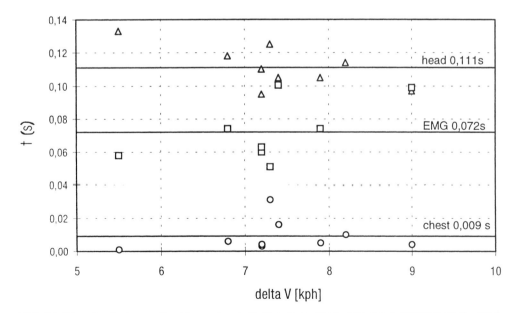

FIG. 21. Time lag between the biomechanical signals in relation to the ΔV (1993 study only).

mately corresponds to the distance between the head and the head restraint in normal circumstances. On the basis of this movement, a decreasing time lag between the acceleration of the passenger compartment and that of the head might be inferred at higher ΔV values. The measurement data, however, do not indicate such a relationship. The reaction time found for the neck muscles starts approximately 72 ms after the start of acceleration of the passenger compartment and 63 ms after the start of chest acceleration. Muscle activity therefore does not start until after the relative movement between the torso and head of the occupant, but on average almost 40 ms before the start of head acceleration. In view of the fact that in about half of the trials carried out in 1993 the test subject's attention was screened off, it can be concluded, despite the small number of trials, that this reaction must be a kind of reflex. As even in the case of conscious activity, the minimal reaction time to individual signals is 200 ms, the reaction time value we obtained of about 60 ms is plausible only for an unconscious reflex, and it is also in line with the reflex times for the neck muscles found by Foust (5).

EXAMPLE OF A TRIAL IMPACT

Figure 22 gives comparative pictures for the damage occurring in a real accident and that in a crash test carried out in the 1996 study. The aim was to determine the stresses on the occupant during the real accident, because the driver of the impacted Mercedes station wagon *(B)* claimed to have been severely injured. As the bottom pictures show, impact at a velocity of just under 28 kph produced comparable or somewhat more severe damage. ΔV in the impacted vehicle could therefore be determined at under about 13 kph.

Finally, Figure 23 documents the effect of nose-diving in this trial. The rigid structural parts in the area of the front bumper of the bullet Mercedes were subject to only little stress, whereas the higher body work sections were substantially deformed. The volunteer test person complained of no trouble after the trial, nor were any injuries found in the various medical examinations that were subsequently carried out.

For the same trial, Figure 24 shows the accelerations of the vehicle, chest, and head. The time lag between these accelerations is typical for rear-end collisions, for the increase of accelerations between vehicle, chest, and head, which depends on the distance between body and seat back and also on the seat construction. The lowest biomechanical stress occurs when there is no distance between seat and body and when the seat is rather stiff. After this test, we can say that the force level is similar to a slight bumper collision. We find no explanation for a severe whiplash.

RESULTS AND DISCUSSION

The question of whether a direct cause-and-effect relationship exists between an accident and an injury to the cervical spine can be answered only on the basis of a known ΔV of the vehicle concerned. In determining ΔV, the technical expert must, using the available photographs of damage, take into account the degree of overlap, and the differences in heights and the structural rigidity of the vehicle parts involved. Additionally, information on the vehicle weights is necessary.

To make statements with a high degree of statistical reliability, it is helpful to compare bumper car impacts at funfairs, whose forces are tolerated by the occupants without injury, with car–car collisions at ΔV values of the same magnitude. The occupants of bumper cars have very poor support, as the seats are of inadequate height and there are

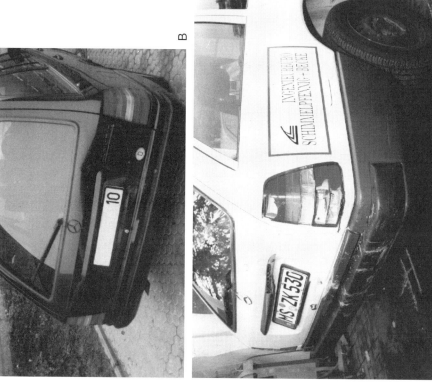

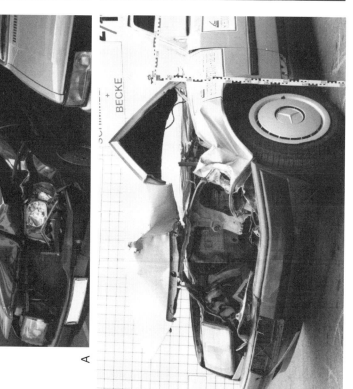

FIG. 22. A,B: A rear-end accident between two station wagons. **C,D:** The trial we made to determine the impact speed.

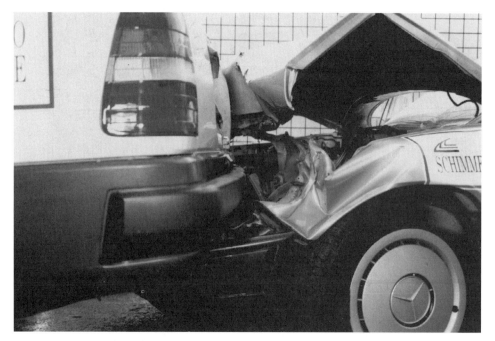

FIG. 23. The result of nose-diving in a rear-end impact.

no head restraints to prevent hyperextension of the cervical spine. Additionally, all possible directions of impact, body postures, and levels of muscle tension are observed in bumper car collisions (Fig. 25). We observed also that many older men and women, mostly with children but also alone, use bumper cars. Moreover, the occupants are in many cases taken completely by surprise by the impact and can therefore not adopt a protective posture.

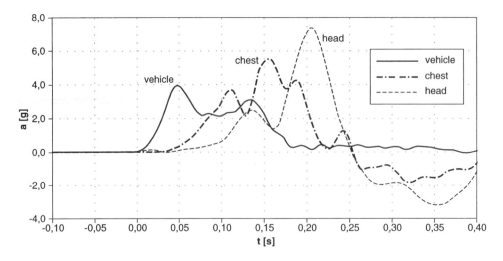

FIG. 24. Acceleration curves for car, chest, and head for the test shown in Figures 23 and 24.

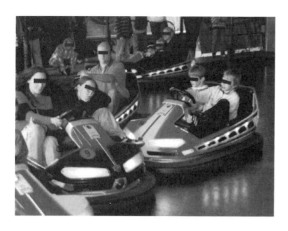

FIG. 25. All kinds of impact directions and seating positions occur in bumper cars.

Despite these unfavorable circumstances, millions of bumper car collisions occur at funfairs every year, with symptoms being reported in only a statistically negligible number of cases, and indeed no such case being known to us in Germany. From this, it can be deduced that the forces occurring in bumper cars are tolerated by the cervical spine, even in the case of preexisting pathologic damages and major interpersonal differences. The assessment of injury causality requires an interdisciplinary (technical and medical) approach. On the basis of the knowledge acquired in the 1993 study, such interdisciplinary cooperation is essential at a ΔV greater than 10 kph, as, in addition to the technical collision parameters, factors related to the individual people involved must be taken into account.

However, on the basis of our 1993 study and our knowledge today, it can be stated that the limit of harmlessness for stresses arising from rear-end impacts lies around a ΔV of 10 kph. Taking the results of the initial part of the 1996 study into account, it appears probable that the injury threshold is much higher than a ΔV of 10 kph.

REFERENCES

1. Deutscher C. *Bewegungsablauf von Fahrzeuginsassen beim Heckaufprall.* Eurotax (International) AG, CH-8807 Freienbach, 1994.
2. *Deutscher Verkehrsgerichtstag.* Deutsche Akademie für Verkehrswissenschaft Hamburg, 1994.
3. *Deutscher Verkehrsgerichtstag.* Deutsche Akademie für Verkehrswissenschaft Hamburg, 1996.
4. *Fahrzeugsicherheit 90, Analyse von Pkw-Unfällen, Grundlagen für künftige Forschungsarbeiten.* München: Büro für Kfz-Technik, 1994.
5. Foust D, Chaffin D, Snyder R, Baum J. Cervical range of motion and dynamic response and strength of cervical muscles. Warrendale, PA: Society of Automotive Engineers, paper 7309756, *Biomech Impact Inj* 1993;43.
6. Meyer S, Hugemann W, Weber M. Zur Belastung der Halswirbelsäule durch Auffahrkollisionen. *Verkehrsunfall und Fahrzeugtechnik* 1994;32:15–21, 187–199
7. Schuller E, Eisenmenger W. Die verletzungsmechanische Begutachtung des HWS-Schleudertraumas. *Unfall- und Sicherheitsforschung Strassenverkehr* 1993;89:193–196.
8. Steffan H, Geigl B. Zur Problematik von HWS-Verletzungen. *Verkehrsunfall und Fahrzeugtechnik* 1996;34: 35–39.
9. Szabo TJ, Welcher JB. *Human subject kinematics and elektromyographic activity during low speed rear end impacts.* Warrendale, PA: Society of Automotive Engineers, paper 962432, 1996.
10. Szabo TJ, Welcher JB, Anderson RD, Rice MM, Ward JA, Paulo LR, Carpenter NJ. *Human occupant kinematic response to low speed rear-end-impacts.* Warrendale, PA: Society of Automotive Engineers, paper 940532, 1994.
11. Weber M. *Die Aufklärung des Kfz-Versicherungsbetruges—Grundlagen der Kompatibilitätsanalyse und Plausibilitätsprüfung.* 1. Auflage, Schriftenreihe Unfallrekonstruktion, Münster, 1995.
12. Weber M, Dieling W. Die Zuordnung von Beschädigungszonen bei Berücksichtigung von Beladung, Verzögerung und Querbeschleunigung. *Verkehrsunfall und Fahrzeugtechnik* 1990;28:179–182.

*Whiplash Injuries: Current Concepts in
Prevention, Diagnosis, and Treatment
of the Cervical Whiplash Syndrome,*
edited by Robert Gunzburg and Marek Szpalski.
Lippincott–Raven Publishers, Philadelphia © 1998.

11

Natural Evolution and Resolution of the Cervical Whiplash Syndrome

Michel Benoist

*M. Benoist: Department of Orthopaedic Surgery, Section of Rheumatology, Hôpital
Beaujon, University of Paris VII, Paris, France.*

Despite numerous investigations, the evolution and resolution of the whiplash syndrome are still a matter of controversy. Most studies indicate that a substantial proportion of patients still complain of neck pain and/or headache in the months or years after their acceleration–deceleration injury, which was usually caused by a rear-end car collision. The number of patients who develop chronic symptoms varies according to the studies. The factors predicting persistent chronic complaints are another source of debate. Litigation neurosis for financial gain has been proposed as the cause by a few authors (17,31). In contrast, other studies conclude that chronicity of symptoms is principally a consequence of initial severe and evolutive organic lesions (9,10,22,23,41,43). This chapter is an attempt to estimate the outcome of the syndrome and the proportions of patients who develop chronic complaints. Attributing persistent symptoms to psychological factors or malingering versus somatic lesions will also be discussed.

Estimates will be based on published series in the literature according to the definition proposed by the Quebec task force (37). Only grades 1, 2, and 3 will be discussed, excluding grade 4 with fractures and dislocations. However, it should be pointed out that grade 4 is sometimes difficult to recognize because of occult, or hidden, bone or soft-tissue lesions not readily detectable by early radiographic evaluation (9).

Studies on the prognosis of whiplash syndrome are numerous. Many of them are difficult to compare because of multiple methodologic differences such as selection criteria of patients, study designs, number of patients reviewed, length of follow-up, and therapy used. Moreover, a good number of these studies should be discarded because of their lack of meeting acceptable criteria of validity. For example, among the 10,382 abstracts and titles collected by the Quebec Task Force, only 1204 met the criteria for the preliminary screening. Of those, 294 were selected by the scientific secretariat for independent review. Among these selected studies, only 16.7% were considered as relevant in the domain of evolution and resolution (38). Finally, scientifically valid studies of prognosis are rare. Most of these studies are hospital based and concern patients identified by a clinician immediately after the accident, or by insurance claims with medical examination performed rapidly after the injury. These studies include samples of good size with a low attrition rate and an inception cohort correctly evaluated and assembled at the outset. This chapter, devoted to evolution and resolution of the whiplash syndrome after a whiplash injury, is based on estimates identified by these studies. Evolution of the lesions and of the clinical symptoms will be briefly discussed. Symptoms and pathology of whiplash have been reviewed in detail (2).

EVOLUTION OF THE LESIONS

By definition, all structures of the neck can be traumatized by a whiplash injury. These include discs, zygapophysial joints, muscles, and ligaments. Injuries to cervical vertebrae, with overt fractures corresponding to grade 4 of the Quebec Task Force definition, are excluded (37). The main difficulty at the initial examination is to appreciate which tissues are injured and the severity of the lesions. Clinically, little information can be obtained. Some patients complain of neck pain without physical signs; others experience neck pain with stiffness and decreased range of motion. In these two categories, the presumed pathology is related to a neck sprain indicating injury of the soft tissues (37). However, neither history taking nor physical examination is able to appreciate the site and the severity of the pathology. In patients with neck and radiating pain, neurologic signs, such as motor weakness, sensory deficits, and absent or decreased reflexes, the clinical picture is more suggestive of the presumed pathology. In this category of patients, the neurologic examination may lead to identification of lesions related to a mechanical injury of the neurologic system (37). A small proportion of these patients undergo surgery, enabling identification of the site and nature of the lesions, but early surgery is rarely indicated after a whiplash injury.

Initial imaging studies usually consist of plain radiographs with flexion and extension films. Cervical spondylosis, reduced height of the intervertebral discs, and abnormalities of the cervical curvature are frequent but not specific findings (19). Plain radiographs may be normal and cannot be used to detect abnormalities of the soft tissues of the zygapophysial joints, such as tears of the capsule, hemarthrosis, or damage of the articular cartilage. However, such lesions have been demonstrated at surgery in cadaver and animal experiments and in postmortem studies (6,22,24,26). Similarly, injuries to the intervertebral disc, such as tears of the annulus fibrosus, cannot be identified on plain radiographs, although such tears, as well as avulsion of the disc from the endplate, have been demonstrated at surgery, experimentally, and in cadaver studies (6,10,22,24,25). Muscle tears, avulsions, and hemorrhages are also beyond the scope of a standard radiologic examination, but in some instances, swelling and tenderness of the muscles can be disclosed during the physical examination. Lesions of the ligaments, often associated with disc injuries, cannot be detected radiologically. However, tears of the anterior longitudinal ligaments and other ligaments have been documented in several studies, as have lesions of the upper cervical ligaments (6,10,12,22,25).

In summary, at the individual level the initial lesions caused by a whiplash injury usually remain unknown. Magnetic resonance imaging (MRI) is rarely used immediately after the accident, except in patients with neurologic symptoms and signs leading to more sophisticated imaging studies, and in patients with a more severe injury. Autopsies of accident victims, and experimentally caused whiplash injuries in monkeys and in cadavers, have demonstrated that severe structural damage can be associated with whiplash injury. The above pathologies can be combined in various ways, and in cases with continuing chronic complaints the injury may have created lesions more severe than initially suspected. Theoretically, two main categories of patients can be distinguished: patients with a simple sprain of the cervical spine and patients with severe structural damage of the posterior joints, discs, or ligaments. In the first instance, the sprained neck may be compared to the sprained ankle, or to strains of other soft tissues (21). Muscles and ligaments as well as joint capsules are endowed with nerve endings and nociceptors. Healing of soft-tissue trauma is usually rapid. The initial inflammatory period of capillary hemorrhage, edema, synovial swelling, and release of chemicals subsides in a few days and is followed by a period of repair by new collagen, lasting a few weeks or months.

In contrast, more severe damage to the disc or to the posterior joint cartilage or to the ligaments may create irreversible lesions and the previously described model cannot be applied. These lesions can initiate degenerative and biomechanical abnormalities, with chronic instability, capable of stimulating the nociceptive system and of releasing inflammatory mediators. For example, secondary osteoarthritic changes have been described after whiplash injury (44). The problem with whiplash is that at presentation, differentiation between a simple sprain and more severe organic lesions is difficult even with the use of MRI, considering the relatively high proportion of false positive findings. For example, abnormal MRI scans of the cervical spine in asymptomatic subjects have disclosed abnormalities such as discal herniation or bulging or foraminal stenosis in 19% of 63 subjects and in 28% in individuals over 40 years old (4). Surveillance of the evolution of the lesions is as difficult as their appreciation at the initial examination. In those patients with chronic complaints, the use of computed tomography (CT) scans and MRI may disclose hidden bone lesions or serious discal or ligament abnormalities in patients initially considered as having a simple sprain (9,10). Difficulties in evaluating the anatomic lesions explain the difficulties in predicting the clinical outcome.

CLINICAL SYMPTOMS

The symptoms most commonly reported in the literature are listed in Table 1. Neck pain is present in almost all symptomatic subjects after a whiplash injury. Pure neck pain without any other musculoskeletal disorders defines grade I of the Quebec Task Force proposed clinical classification of whiplash-associated disorders (37). Neck pain may be associated with decreased range of motion and point tenderness, which defines grade 2 of the Quebec classification (37). It may be accompanied by neurologic signs including radiating pain, motor or sensory deficits, and decreased or absent reflexes, which defines grade 3 of the Quebec classification. After the accident, the onset of neck pain usually occurs within the first hours, but it is sometimes delayed within to 2 or 3 days (11,13). Neck pain may radiate to the shoulder or interscapular region, but patterns of referred pain do not give any indication of the exact source of the pain. Provocative discography and stimulation of the cervical zygapophysial joints in normal volunteers disclose the

TABLE 1. *Subjective complaints after whiplash injury, as commonly reported in the literature*

Neck pain
Headache
Back pain
Dizziness
Visual disturbances
Paresthesias
Fatigability
Concentration impairment
Sleep disturbances
Irritability
Anxiety–depression

same referred distribution. Moreover, the cause of neck pain after whiplash is probably multifactorial. Recent studies using diagnostic blocks seem to indicate that the posterior joints are a common source of pain (1,3,5). However the blocks do not give clear information on the pathology.

Headache is the second most frequent symptom. It is usually occipitally located, but it can be generalized and can radiate anteriorly in the orbital region. The origin of whiplash headache is usually cervical, although concussion has also been suggested (16). Several causes of cervical origin have been advocated, such as referred pain from muscle contraction or trauma of the greater occipital nerve (13). Diagnostic blocks of the C2-C3 posterior joints indicate that referred pain from these joints was the source of the headache in approximately half of the cases (2). Internal derangement of the temporomandibular joint can also be associated with referred headache (48).

Visual disturbances with blurred vision are present in approximately 10% of the patients (43). Abnormalities of the accommodation power and of oculomotor function have been demonstrated, but their mechanisms remain hypothetical (18).

Dizziness and auditory disturbance with sensitivity to noise and feeling of disequilibrium have been described in many studies in spite of normal neurologic examination (2,13,43). The mechanism of these auditory and vestibular dysfunctions is not clear, although abnormalities of electronystagmography have been identified (2,13,34).

Weakness of the upper limbs is reported in a small percentage of whiplash patients. The muscular fatigue occurring when lifting or carrying is similar to that described by fibromyalgia patients. It is not accompanied by objective signs or by neurologic abnormalities suggesting irritation of a nerve root. As in fibromyalgia, the sensation of muscular fatigue has no clear explanation. Weakness has been attributed to malingering by some authors. Others are in favor of a neurophysiologic mechanism induced by a reflex inhibition of the muscles acting in conjunction with the neck (2).

RESOLUTION OF THE CLINICAL SYMPTOMS

As mentioned earlier, sources of information come from the few scientifically relevant studies, and they include patients seeking medical care in a hospital-based emergency department and those consulting a physician immediately after the accident with a claim for indemnity. We will briefly review the studies falling in this category.

The study of Norris and Watt (33) comprised three groups of patients categorized according to their presenting symptoms, the groups being very similar to the Quebec Task Force grades 1, 2, and 3. All 61 accident victims were reviewed with a mean follow-up of 20 months. At final follow-up, 67% of the patients were still complaining of neck pain, which was statistically more frequent in group 3 than in group 1. In each group, 20% of patients found the pain severe enough to require time off work. In group 3, the neck pain was sufficiently severe in 70% of patients to interfere with recreational activities, whereas only 25% of the group 1 were affected. Similarly, headache was persistent in 70% of the patients in group 3, whereas only 37% of the patients in groups 1 and 2 were still complaining of headache.

In the study of Radanov et al. (43), the sample investigated consisted of 117 patients, all injured in automobile accidents and referred by primary care physicians. Patients with fractures and dislocations were excluded. The investigated group corresponded to the Quebec Task Force grades 1, 2, and 3. Symptoms at presentation were similar to those reported by Norris and Watt (33). All patients had neck pain and 57% had headache. The rate of recovery was as follows: 44% at 3 months, 30% at 6 months, 24% at 1 year, and 18% at 2 years were still complaining of symptoms related to the accident. Persistence of neck pain or other symptoms appears to be determined by the severity of the injury.

The prospective study of Hildingsson and Toolanen (19) included 93 consecutive patients. Neck pain and stiffness were the main initial symptoms. At the final follow-up, with an average of 2 years, symptomatic recovery occurred in 39 patients (42%). Thirteen patients (15%) reported some minor discomfort and 41 patients (43%) had severe persisting symptoms. Analysis of 17 factors including accident parameters, subjective parameters, objective parameters, and radiographic parameters did not disclose any factor of prognosis.

Pennie and Agambar (36) have conducted a prospective study of 144 consecutive patients who were followed with a mean duration of 5 months. The follow-up rate was 95%. The proportion of patients with neck pain at the end of the follow-up was 14%. The authors concluded that in their series, it was impossible to identify the possible pathologic basis of the symptoms and signs by clinical and radiologic examination alone.

Maimaris et al. (27) studied 120 consecutive patients who had sustained whiplash injuries of the neck in road traffic accidents during a 6-month period. The follow-up rate was 85%. One third of all patients were still symptomatic 2 years after the accident. Of those patients asymptomatic at the end of 2 years, 88% were symptom free within 2 months.

In the study of Deans et al. (11), 137 patients were contacted regarding pain in the neck 1 and 2 years after a road traffic accident. Eighty-five (62%) had suffered pain in the neck at some time after the accident. Thirty-one patients (22.6%) still felt occasional pain 1 year after the accident and five had continuous pain at 1 year.

Miles et al. (30) have followed prospectively 73 consecutive patients after a whiplash injury. The follow-up rate was 100%, and after 2 years, 29% were still complaining of neck pain. In 1990, Gargan and Bannister (15) were able to review the cohort described by Norris and Watt in 1983. Forty-three of the 61 patients initially studied could be traced. The mean follow-up period was 10.3 years. Of these 43 patients, only 12% had recovered completely, and 74% were still complaining of neck pain. Residual symptoms were intrusive in 28% and severe in 12%.

Barnsley et al. (2) have applied a worst-case analysis of these various studies, assuming that all those patients who were unable to be followed up recovered completely. Their conclusion was that between 14% and 42% of patients with whiplash injuries will develop chronic neck pain and that approximately 10% will have constant severe neck pain.

Only one study, by Schrader et al. (46), suggests that chronic symptoms were not caused by the car accident, and that expectation of disability, family history, and attribution of preexisting symptoms to the trauma may be more important for the evolution of the late whiplash syndrome. This study was a retrospectively based cohort study of 202 individuals, identified from the records of the traffic police department in Kaunas Lithuania. In this country, most drivers do not have personal insurance and the likelihood of disability compensation is remote. The group of injured patients was compared with an age-matched control group of uninjured individuals selected randomly from the same geographic area. No significant difference in the proportions of neck pain between accident victims and controls was found. The proportions of neck pain before versus 1 to 3 years after the accident were similar. However, this study raises a serious methodologic problem, as individuals were selected retrospectively from the police departments' records, and they were not examined by a physician, either private or hospital based.

Therefore, the authors were unable to identify the initial presenting symptoms and consequently their evolution.

According to most of the pertinent studies, 15% to 40% of the whiplash patients have symptoms persisting over 6 months. Among those, a small percentage become disabled. In the Quebec whiplash-associated disorders cohort study (39), disability was defined as the number of days between the date of the collision and the last date for which compensation to replace regular income was made by the Société d'Assurance Automobile de Québec (S.A.A.Q). This outcome corresponded to the time off work and off usual activities. In the study cohort of 2810 members 22% recovered within 1 week, and 53% took more than 4 weeks to recover from their injuries. After 1 year, 2.9% were still absent from usual activities or work. Recurrences, defined as symptoms after a symptom-free interval, occurred in 6.8% of the study subjects. In the prospective study of Radanov et al. (43) including 117 patients, disability was certified in five patients (4%) 2 years after injury. This is in keeping with the 3% disabled patients after 2 years in the study by Maimaris et al. (27) including 102 patients. It also corresponds roughly to the 6% of patients still absent from work after 1 year in the study by Pearce which included 100 patients (35).

In conclusion, although the majority of the whiplash-injured individuals become rapidly asymptomatic regardless of the treatment used, the reality is that some patients do not recover completely, with a small proportion (2% to 5%) being unable to resume work or usual activities.

Why do the illness and symptoms persist in various proportions according to the different studies? Whether the persistent symptoms are caused by organic lesions, by psychological factors, or by expectation of financial gain is still a matter of debate. The late whiplash syndrome has become a major controversial condition, not yet completely resolved (7). Chronic pain is not morphologic. It cannot be measured and includes three major components. First, severe organic lesions, not necessarily detected on radiographs or on MRI, can perpetuate the peripheral nociceptive input and create hyperexcitability of the nociceptors. Second, the excessive nociceptive input in the dorsal horn of the cord may sensitize the nociceptive neurons, which become in a state of permanent hyperexcitation (8). Finally, the brain processing may involve psychological factors including litigation neurosis (20). As mentioned earlier, in the case of whiplash, appreciation of the soft-tissue pathology is often limited, with the exception of the more severe injuries with neurologic complications. Thus, persistence of symptoms by perpetuation of the nociceptive peripheral input remains questionable when MRI and CT scans are normal or show discrete structural changes. On the other hand, it is well known that injuries of soft tissues elsewhere in the body undergo a rapid healing within a few weeks or months. Central sensitization of the nociceptive neurons cannot be demonstrated at the present time and it is not yet possible to evaluate the fluctuations of the neuromediators. In contrast, the influence of psychosocial factors and of litigation on the modulation of pain has been emphasized (20).

LITIGATION

Malingering for financial remuneration is considered by some authors to be the major determinant for why patients with no evident pathology fail to improve until settlement (17,31,32). However, many studies report that persistence of symptoms is independent of litigation. In the study of Norris and Watt (33), 41 of the 61 patients followed for 13 to 31 months were involved in litigation. In groups 1 and 2, patients who pursued claims were either improved after settlement or were no worse. In group 3, with more severe initial presentation, there were only two patients who felt improved after settlement. These findings suggest that litigation per se has little influence on symptoms. Maimaris et al. (27) evaluated the influence of insurance claims made by 20 out of 35 symptomatic patients. One half had their claims settled an average 9 months after the accident but still remained symptomatic. The remaining ten had not yet settled their claims. In the study of Pennie and Agambar (36), 81% of the 144 patients followed were claiming compensation. There was no significant difference in recovery between claimants and non-claimants. More recently, Schofferman and Wasserman (45) evaluated prospectively 39 consecutive patients with neck pain and low-back pain after a motor vehicle accident who had litigation pending. Pain and function were quantified by the McGill pain questionnaire and the Oswestry disability questionnaire. The authors observed a statistically significant improvement with treatment despite ongoing litigation. All together, these studies indicate that late whiplash symptoms "are usually not cured by verdict," as suggested by Mendelson (28).

In contrast, evidence to support the assertion that litigation is the main reason for prolonged chronic symptoms is not based on scientifically relevant studies. The report by Gotten (17) is often used to indicate that settlement of litigation is the key factor for recovery. The conclusions of that study indicated that financial compensation was the most important factor in evaluating whiplash patients and that settlement of the claim resulted in improvement of the residual symptoms. However, this study has numerous methodologic flaws, which casts a serious doubt on the conclusion of the author. For example, selection of patients was not made consecutively, but only if they were suitable for the study. Evaluation was made by a medical student on the basis of an unvalidated questionnaire. Moreover, the attrition rate was high, as only 100 of the 219 patients could be located and contacted, a response rate of 45%.

In summary, close analysis of the reports having studied the influence of litigation settlement on the natural evolution indicates that conscious malingering for financial gain has little influence on the evolution of symptoms and probably involves a minority of patients. In that case, chronicity of symptoms could be attributed to nonhealed organic lesions in genuine patients with minimal apparent abnormalities on the imaging studies. In these chronic patients, a complete clinical, functional, and neurologic assessment should be completed, as well as functional radiographs, MRI, and neurophysiologic examination including evaluation of the motor pathways looking for some kind of physical damage. However, these investigations often fail to discover major organic lesions. Alternatively, the role of psychological factors primary or secondary to the accident and not necessarily linked to financial settlement should be discussed.

PSYCHOLOGICAL FACTORS: THE WHIPLASH NEUROSIS

Some authors (14,20) have suggested that whiplash injury represents a psychophysiologic reaction to a particularly stressful situation. Accordingly, predisposing personality type has been suggested in persons developing chronic symptoms. The preexisting psychological characteristics, including strong elements of hostility and dependency, could lead to the development of psychosomatic symptoms determined by an external precipitating stress such as the whiplash injury (20). However, in the prospective study of Radanov et al. (43) involving 117 patients, a set of formal psychological and cognitive tests was performed to assess whether the psychosocial variables significantly influenced the outcome 2 years after the trauma. Interestingly, there were no significant differences between the symptomatic and nonsymptomatic groups with regard to psychosocial stress and virtually all psychological variables. However, the symptomatic group performed higher on the initial score of the well-being scale and worse on tests requiring a more complex level of attentional processing. These findings indicate that primary psychological factors do not predict the chronicity of symptoms. However, persistent pain, sleep disturbances, cognitive deficits, legal dispute, use of narcotics, and potential loss of job may create secondary psychological disturbances (20,40,42), including anxiety, depression, and emotional instability with a tendency to hostility and dependency (29). These accident-induced psychological disturbances may be exaggerated by the attitude of those physicians or lawyers who look upon these patients as consciously malingering for financial reasons. Taken together, the physical, mental, social, and legal consequences of the injury are a good example of the clinical model of illness presented by Waddel et al., including physical problems, nociception, distress, illness behavior, and sick role (47). In this context, it is obviously difficult to separate the effects of seeking compensation from other factors.

PROGNOSTIC VARIABLES

The statistical analysis performed in the study by Radanov et al. (43) indicates that older age of patients is prognostically significant in persistent symptoms. Other risk factors disclosed in the same study include the position of the head (inclined or rotated) at the time of the impact, the greater variety of the subjective complaints at the initial examination, higher pain rating for neck pain and headache, and radicular deficits. These features indicate the prognostic significance of the initial severity of the injury (41).

Features on plain radiographs seem to have a prognostic value, such as the existence of degenerative changes on initial radiographs (43). Abnormal curvature changes are associated with a poor prognosis in one study (33), but in another report, reversal of the cervical spine to a kyphotic position was not associated with prolonged disability (27). Similarly, one study reports that the presence of an angular deformity is not associated with a poor outcome (30). As mentioned earlier, the psychosocial factors of patients, the family history, or different aspects of stress at baseline do not have a prognosis significance (43).

CONCLUSION

Whiplash injuries usually result in neck pain and headache, sometimes associated with other symptoms such as visual or auditory disturbances, muscular weakness, concentration impairment, and sleep disturbances. Most patients recover within a few weeks to a few months. However, persistent neck pain and headaches after 1 or 2 years are reported by 15% to 40% of the patients. In some of these chronic cases, severe organic lesions such as discal herniations, anterior annular tears, occult vertebral endplate fractures, or segmental instability are sometimes demonstrated a few months after injury. This group of patients may require surgery. In the majority of the late whiplash syndrome patients, functional radiographs, CT, and MRI do not disclose serious abnormalities. However, tears of muscles or ligaments, and lesions of the annulus or the posterior joints including capsule and cartilage, are not readily detectable by the most sophisticated imaging. These lesions may form the basis of an ongoing nociceptive input. Most studies indicate that pure malingering for financial gain is rare and that most of these chronic patients are not cured by a verdict. However, the consequences of the injury, including persistent pain, sleep disturbances, and legal dispute, may induce secondary psychological factors that in turn participate in the chronicity of the symptoms and create distress and illness behavior. Most data available in the literature indicate that the late whiplash syndrome is a combination of organic lesions created by a severe injury and of secondary psychological factors. The therapeutic attitude should be structured accordingly, acting on both the physical problem and the psychological consequences of the injury.

REFERENCES

1. Aprill C, Bogduk N. The prevalence of cervical zygapophyseal joint pain: a first approximation. *Spine* 1992;17: 744–747.
2. Barnsley L, Lord S, Bogduk N. Whiplash injury, clinical review. *Pain* 1994;58:283–307.
3. Barnsley L, Lord S, Wallis BJ, Bogduk N. The prevalence of chronic cervical zygapophyseal joint pain after whiplash. *Spine* 1995;20:20–25.
4. Boden SD, Mccowin PR, Davis DO, et al. Abnormal magnetic resonance scans of the cervical spine in asymptomatic subjects. *J Bone Joint Surg* 1990;72:1178–1184.
5. Bogduk N, Aprill C. On the nature of neck pain, discography and cervical zygapophyseal joint blocks. *Pain* 1993; 54:213–217.
6. Buonocore E, Hartman JT, Nelson LL. Cineradiograms of cervical spine in diagnosis of soft tissue injuries. *JAMA* 1966;198:143–147.
7. Carette S. Whiplash injury and chronic neck pain. *Lancet* 1994;330:1083–1084.
8. Coderre TJ, Katz J, Vaccarino AL, Melzack R. Contribution of central neuroplasticity to pathological pain: review of clinical and experimental evidence. *Pain* 1993;52:259–285.
9. Davis JW, Phreaner DL, Hoyt DB, Mackersie RC. The etiology of missed cervical spine injuries. *J Trauma* 1993; 34:342–346.
10. Davis SJ, Teresi LM, Bradley WG, et al. Cervical spine hyperextension injuries: M.R. findings. *Radiology* 1991;180:245–251.
11. Deans GT, Magalliard JN, Kerr M, Rutherford WH. Neck sprain. A major cause of disability following car accidents. *Injury* 1987;18:10–12.
12. Dvořák J, Hayek J, Zehnder R. CT functional diagnostics of the rotatory instability of the upper cervical spine. 2. An evaluation of healthy adults and patients with suspected instability. *Spine* 1987;12:726–731.
13. Evans RW. Some observations on whiplash injuries. *Neurol Clin* 1992;10:975–997.
14. Farbman AA. Neck sprain. Associated factors. *JAMA* 1973;223:1010–1015.
15. Gargan MF, Bannister GC. Long term prognosis of soft time injuries of the neck. *J Bone Joint Surg* 1990;72: 901–903.
16. Gay JR, Abbott KH. Common whiplash injuries of the neck. *JAMA* 1953;152:1698–1704.
17. Gotten N. Survey of one hundred cases of whiplash injury after settlement of litigation. *JAMA* 1956;162: 865–867.
18. Hildingsson C, Wenngrenn BL, Bring G, Toolanen G. Oculomotor problems after cervical spine injury. *Acta Orthop Scand* 1989;60:513–516.
19. Hildingsson C, Toolanen G. Outcome after soft tissue injury of the cervical spine. A prospective study of 93 accident victims. *Acta Orthop Scand* 1990;61:357–359.
20. Hodge JR. The whiplash neurosis. *Psychosomatics* 1971;12:245–249.
21. Janes JM. Severe extension–flexion injuries of the cervical spine. *Mayo Clin Proc* 1965;40:353–369.
22. Jonsson H, Bring G, Rauschning W, Sahlsted B. Hidden cervical spine injuries in traffic accident victims with skull fractures. *J Spinal Disord* 1991;4:251–263.
23. Jonsson H, Cesarini K, Sahlstedt B, Rauschning W. Findings and outcome in whiplash type neck distorsions. *Spine* 1994;19.2733–2734.
24. La Rocca H. Acceleration injuries of the neck. *Clin Neurosurg* 1978;25:209–217.
25. MacNab I. Whiplash injuries of the neck. *Manit Med Rev* 1966;46:172–174.
26. MacNab I. The whiplash syndrome. *Orthop Clin North Am* 1971;2:389–403.
27. Maimaris C, Barnes MR, Allen MJ. Whiplash injuries of the neck: a retrospective study. *Injury* 1988;19: 393–396.
28. Mendelson G. Not cured by a verdict. Effect of legal settlement on compensation claimants. *Med J Aust* 1982;2: 132–134.
29. Merskey H. Psychological consequences of whiplash. *State of the Art Rev* 1993;7:471–480.
30. Miles KA, Maimaris C, Finlay D, Barnes MR. The incidence and prognostic significance of radiological abnormalities in soft tissue injuries to the cervical spine. *Skeletal Radiol* 1988;17:493–496.
31. Miller H. Accident neurosis. *Br Med J* 1961;1:992–998.

32. Mills H, Horne G. Whiplash, man-made disease. *N Z Med J* 1986;99:373–374.
33. Norris SH, Watt I. The prognosis of neck injuries resulting from rear-end vehicle collisions. *J Bone Joint Surg* 1983;65:608–611.
34. Oosterveld WJ, Kortschot HW, Kingma GG, et al. Electronystagmographic findings. *Acta Otolaryngol* 1991; 111:201–205.
35. Pearce JM. Whiplash injury: A reappraisal. *J Neurol Neurosurg Psychiatr* 1989;52:1329–1331.
36. Pennie BH, Agambar LJ. Patterns of injury and recovery in whiplash. *Injury* 1991;22:57–59.
37. Quebec classification of whiplash associated disorders. Section 3. Consensus findings. *Spine* 1995;20:21–23.
38. Quebec Task Force report on whiplash associated disorders. Section 4. Best evidence synthesis. *Spine* 1995;20: 24–33.
39. Quebec whiplash associated disorders cohort study. *Spine* 1995;20:12–20.
40. Radanov BP, Dvořák J, Valach L. Cognitive deficits in patients after soft tissue injury of the cervical spine. *Spine* 1992;17:127–131.
41. Radanov BP, Sturzenegger M, Di Stefano G, et al. Factors influencing recovery from headache after common whiplash. *Br Med J* 1993;307:652–655.
42. Radanov BP, Di Stefano G, Schnideig A, Sturzenegger M. Common whiplash psychomatic or somatopsychic ? *J Neurol Neurosurg Psychiatr* 1994;57:484–490.
43. Radanov BP, Sturzenegger M, Di Stefano G. Long term outcome after whiplash injury. A 2 year follow-up considering features of injury mechanism and somatic radiologic and psychosocial findings. *Medicine* 1995;74: 281–296.
44. Rauschning W, McAffe PC, Jonsson H. Pathoanatomical and surgical findings in cervical spine injuries. *J Spinal Dirsord* 1989;2:213–221.
45. Schofferman J, Wasserman S. Successful treatment of low-back pain and neck pain after a motor vehicle accident despite litigation. *Spine* 1994;19:1007–1010.
46. Schrader H, Obelieniene D, Bovim G, et al. Natural evolution of late whiplash syndrome outside the medicolegal context. *Lancet* 1996;347:1207–1211.
47. Waddel G, Main CJ, Morris EW, et al. Chronic low-back pain, psychological distress and illness behaviour. *Spine* 1984;9:209–213.
48. Weinberg S, Lapointe H. Cervical extension–flexion injury (whiplash) and internal derangement of the temporomandibular joint. *J Oral Maxillofac Surg* 1987;45:653–656.

Neurological and Psychological Consequences

Whiplash Injuries: Current Concepts in Prevention, Diagnosis, and Treatment of the Cervical Whiplash Syndrome, edited by Robert Gunzburg and Marek Szpalski. Lippincott–Raven Publishers, Philadelphia © 1998.

12

The Acute Traumatic Central Cord Syndrome

Didier H. Martin

D. Martin: Department of Neurosurgery, University Hospital, University of Liège, Liège, Belgium.

It is not uncommon for patients with cervical myelopathy to present with an acute traumatic degradation associating weakness or paralysis of the hands and arms, with relatively preserved lower extremity strength. This situation can be observed after cervical trauma even without any predisposing abnormality. Two clinical syndromes can fit this description: (a) cruciate paralysis (CP) and (b) acute traumatic central cord syndrome (ATCCS), depending on the localization of the central nervous system injury (9).

Cruciate paralysis was first described by Bell (2). The clinical characteristics of this syndrome are the paralysis of both arms without weakness in the legs . The majority of the patients had sustained an upper cervical spine fracture. The basis for the clinical presentation is thought to result from midline damage to the rostral portion of the pyramidal decussation, which would selectively ablate the fibers of the corticospinal tract (CST) that subserve the hand and arm function (9).

Acute traumatic central cord syndrome was first described by Schneider et al. (17). The clinical manifestations are characterized by disproportionate impairment of motor function of the arms compared to the legs, and predominant impairment of distal motor function, with complete or nearly complete paralysis of the hands. Bladder dysfunction and varying degrees of sensory deficit below the level of injury also characterize this syndrome. The etiologic mechanism of injury is thought to be hyperextension of the cervical spine and squeezing of the spinal cord in the anteroposterior plane by an inward bulging of the ligamentum flavum in an already narrowed spinal canal. The pathophysiology and histologic findings remain, for the most part, controversial.

NEUROLOGIC PRESENTATION

Acute traumatic central cord syndrome is a common clinical presentation observed after a cervical hyperextension injury. It is a complex spinal cord syndrome. The deficits are incomplete and usually associated with motor, sensory, and sphincter disturbances.

The motor deficits are disproportionate and the impairment predominates in the upper extremities (because the lower extremities can be moved), with usually a paralysis of both hands. Often the patients are even able to walk, but they are unable to use their hands because of extreme weakness. In some cases, the weakness is asymmetrical and may mimic a Brown-Séquard syndrome.

The sensory impairment associated with the central cord syndrome is quite variable and may not follow any definite anatomic pattern. Some patients complain of paresthesia in both upper limbs according to a radicular topography. Often, this was present before the spinal cord trauma. Most of the patients describe varying degrees of diffuse sensory loss below the level of the lesion. The sensory aspects of ATCCS have assumed added importance since the description by Maroon (10) in 1977 of the burning hands syndrome, characterized by burning dysesthesia in the hands and fingertips and occasionally in the feet. Typically, the burning sensation lasts for 18 to 24 hours before dissipating.

Most of the patients with an ATCCS exhibit bladder dysfunction (usually urinary retention). The bladder needs to be catheterized for several days.

The generally good prognosis is noted. The typical pattern of recovery, with return of lower extremity power, bladder function, upper extremity power, and intrinsic hand function, in that order, is also typically noted. The varied pattern of recovery of sensation is also noted. According to Penrod et al. (15), the prognosis for functional recovery depends partly on the patient's age. The prognosis is less optimistic in older patients and considerably more favorable in younger patients.

PATHOPHYSIOLOGY

The syndrome occurs most frequently in severe hyperextension injuries of the cervical spine. Often, facial abrasions, contusions, and lacerations, or a history of striking the forehead, suggest this hyperextension mechanism. This movement causes squeezing or pinching of the spinal cord both anteriorly and posteriorly. Usually, there is no traumatic bony damage, but spondylotic changes are observed, particularly in the older age group. The cervical spinal canal, often already congenitally narrow, is compromised in its anteroposterior diameter because of the presence of spurs developed posteriorly. Nevertheless, the syndrome may be associated with other causes of spinal injuries such as fracture dislocation, hyperflexion injury, and compression fractures or even spinal malformations [e.g., os odontoideum (13)].

The main biomechanical characteristic is that during a hyperextension movement the cord is compressed anteriorly and posteriorly, inducing a pinching between the spurs, with bulging of the ligamentum flavum. This produces an injury of the cord that has been considered, since the classic description by Schneider et al. (17), to be associated with a hemorrhage located at the center of the cord but also spreading to the medial part of the white matter funiculi. Thus, the name of central cord syndrome was used in the first description.

In the proposed pathophysiologic mechanism that resulted in ATCCS (17), the initial injury causes a hematomyelic necrosis to form within the central gray matter of the spinal cord. This area of central cord injury involves the medially placed fibers of the CST within the posterolateral funiculus. The medially placed corticospinal fibers were presumed by Foerster (6) to specifically represent those subserving arm and hand function. Thus, injury to these medially placed fibers could theoretically result in relatively greater upper extremity weakness. Foerster thought that the CST had a somatotopic organization, as did the fasciculi cuneatus and gracilis and the lateral spinothalamic tract. He presented no evidence for this somatotopic organization, however, and no neuroanatomic evidence has subsequently been presented to support these assertions. Later, detailed anatomic studies in primates and tracing procedures in monkeys demonstrated that the CST present a somatotopic organization in the motor cortex, the internal capsule, and the cerebral peduncles, but not caudal to the pons [i.e., with decussation of the pyramids or the spinal cord (9,14)]. According to Levi et al. (9), an alternative explanation may be that the function of the CST in the human is more important for hand and arm function than it is for lower extremity use. This would explain why diffuse injury of the CST (see later) could compromise predominantly the function of the hands rather than the function of the legs.

RADIOLOGIC AND PATHOLOGIC FINDINGS

Because ATCCS is usually associated with a good prognosis (the recovery often occurs within a few days or weeks), detailed pathologic studies are lacking. The presence of a hematomyelic necrosis with a pencil-shaped rostral and caudal extension and edema, as reported by Schneider et al. (17) in their seminal paper, remains controversial.

Using magnetic resonance imaging (MRI), several authors (5,12,16) tested the validity of this widely disseminated hypothesis. In all cases studied in the reports by Quencer et al. (16) and by Martin et al. (12), bony spine and canal exhibited pathologic

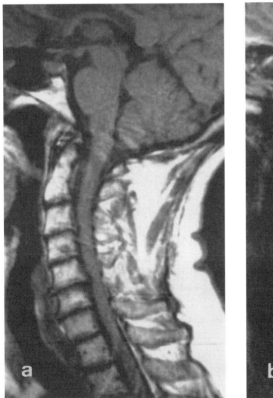
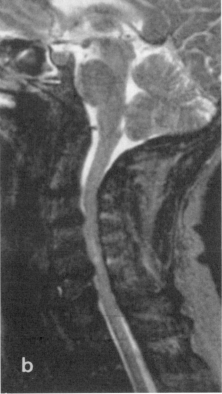

FIG. 1. MRI of the cervical spinal cord of a patient with a typical ATCCS. **A:** Sagittal T1-weighted images (500/20) obtained 2 days after injury show multilevel disc protrusions reducing the anteroposterior diameter of an already narrow canal, but no abnormal signal within the cord. **B:** Sagittal T2*-weighted images (2000/90) disclose a hyperintense signal occupying the whole section of the cord and centered on the C5 segment.

modifications. The most frequent were multilevel cervical spondylosis (after the sixth decade) or disc herniation and congenital canal stenosis (in young patients). Cervical spine fracture occurred in only one case.

Furthermore, there were no signal changes in the spinal cord to suggest the presence of intramedullary blood or blood products in the acute or subacute stages of hemorrhage. T2*-weighted gradient refocusing echo (GRE) images showed no areas of low signal indicating acute bleeding, and T1-weighted spin echo images showed no areas of high signal corresponding to subacute hemorrhage. Instead, high signal was seen in the cord on GRE images and was interpreted as focal edema. This intramedullary hypersignal was either very restricted (Fig. 1), or it could extend over several segments (Fig. 2).

In the five published cases (5,12) presenting an MRI–pathology correlation, no evidence of central cord hemorrhagic necrosis was disclosed. On gross anatomy, the cord appeared normal. After blocking the cord, either it appeared normal (5), or the anterior horns at the C4 and C5 segments were slightly brownish and softened (12). On microscopic examination, the most striking changes were in the white matter tracts of the lateral and, to a lesser extent, the dorsal funiculi. They consisted of marked axonal swelling and disruption with relative sparing of myelin sheaths. These axonal lesions

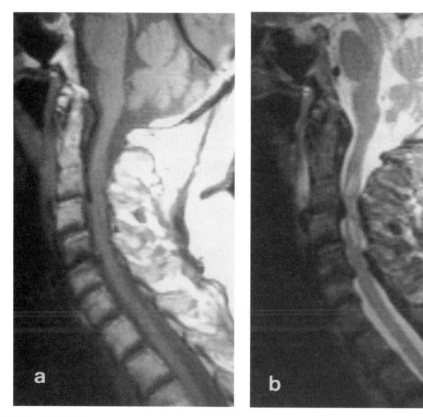

FIG. 2. MRI of the cervical spinal cord of a patient with a typical ATCCS. The MRI parameters are the same as those described in Figure 1. **A:** The sagittal T1-weighted images demonstrate the spinal cord compression at several levels without hyper- or hypointense intramedullary signal. **B:** A hyperintense signal is observed in the cord, extending from C3 to C5 segments on T2*-weighted images.

were predominantly in the central portions of the dorsolateral columns, including the totality of the CST. They were less pronounced, but obvious, in the dorsal columns, and mainly in the fasciculus cuneatus, whereas the ventral funiculi were preserved. Neuropathologic findings in the case described by Martin et al. (12) differ from the cases published by Quencer et al. (16) only in that there was a recent coagulative necrosis in the right C4 anterior horn of the gray matter at the injured level, a factor that could affect the motor impairment of the upper limbs.

Clearly, most of the cases of ATCCS do not present a hemorrhagic lesion and are characterized by white matter injury centered on the lateral columns, involving the CST completely. Nevertheless, hemorrhage and central necrotic lesions or delayed cavitation have been occasionally documented by MRI (7,11) and pathologic (1,3,8,17) studies, and this could explain the lack of functional recovery or even secondary neurologic deterioration that has been observed in some cases.

TREATMENT

Because the pathologic process was considered to be within the central spinal cord with varying degrees of edema and hematomyelia, Schneider et al. (17) recommended nonsurgical treatment for patients with ATCCS. Nevertheless, Brodkey et al. (4) reported a series of seven patients with ATCCS who were thought to benefit from operative intervention (either anterior cervical decompression and fusion, or laminectomy) during the subacute period of their evolution.

Our current therapeutic attitude for patients with ATCCS is based on neurologic and MRI findings as described by Maroon (11). Patients with fracture–dislocation of the cervical spine or traumatic disc herniation are rapidly operated on and the cervical spinal cord is decompressed. When spondylotic changes are the main features, the patient is allowed to recover. If the neurologic evolution is characterized by a plateauing or a deterioration, the spinal cord is decompressed by an anterior cervical decompression and fusion, or a laminectomy, depending on the location, and on the degree and extent of the spondylotic abnormalities.

REFERENCES

1. Barraquer-Bordas C, Vrendrell-Torne E, Peres Serra J. Le syndrome médullaire cervical central aigu par hyperextension. *Neurol Psychol* 1964;147:3–19.
2. Bell HS. Paralysis of both arms from injury of the upper portion of the pyramidal decussation: "cruciate paralysis." *J Neurosurg* 1970;33:376–380.
3. Bohlman HH. Acute fractures and dislocations of the cervical spine. An analysis of three hundred hospitalized patients and review of the litterature. *J Bone Joint Surg Am* 1979;61A(8):1119–1142.
4. Brodkey JS, Miller CF, Harmody RM. The syndrome of acute central cervical spinal cord injury revisited. *Surg Neurol* 1980;14:251–257.
5. Bunge RP, Puckett WR, Becerra JL, Marcillo A, Quencer RM. Observations on the pathology of human spinal cord injury. A review and classification of 22 new cases with details from a case of chronic cord compression with extensive focal demyelination. In: Seil JF, ed. *Advances in neurology.* New York: Raven Press, 1993:75–89.
6. Foerster O. Symptomatologie der Erkankpungen des Rusckenmarks und Zeiner Wurzeln. Bunke Foerster's Handbuch. *Neurology* 1936;5:1–403.
7. Fox JL, Wener L, Drennan DC, Manz HJ, Won DJ, Al-Mefty O. Central spinal cord injury: magnetic resonance imaging confirmation and operative considerations. *Neurosurgery* 1988;22:340–347.
8. Fuentes JM, Vlahovitch B, Nègre C. La diplégie brachiale d'origine traumatique consécutive aux atteintes de la moelle épinière. *Neurochirurgie* 1984;30:165–170.
9. Levi ADO, Tator CH, Bunge RP. Clinical syndromes associated with disproportionate weakness of the upper versus the lower extremities after cervical spinal cord injury. *Neurosurgery* 1996;38:179–185.
10. Maroon JC. "Burning hands" in football spinal cord injuries. *JAMA* 1977;238:2049–2051.

11. Maroon JC, Abla AA, Wilberger JI, Bailes JE, Sternau LL. Central cord syndrome. *Clin Neurosurg* 1991;37: 612–621.
12. Martin D, Schoenen J, Lenelle J, Reznik M, Moonen G. MRI/pathological correlations in acute traumatic central cord syndrome: case report. *Neuroradiology* 1992;34:262–266.
13. McGoldrick JM, Marx JA. Traumatic central cord syndrome in a patient with os odontoideum. *Ann Emerg Med* 1989;18:1358–1361.
14. Nathan PW, Smith MC, Deacon P. The corticospinal tracts in man. Course and location of fibres at different segmental levels. *Brain* 1990;113:303–324.
15. Penrod LE, Hegde SK, Ditunno JF Jr. Age effect on prognosis for functional recovery in acute, traumatic central cord syndrome. *Arch Phys Med Rehabil* 1990;71:963–968.
16. Quencer RM, Bunge RP, Egnor M, et al. MR/pathological correlations in acute traumatic central cord syndrome. *Neuroradiology* 1992;34:85–94.
17. Schneider RC, Sherry G, Pantek H. The syndrome acute central cervical spinal cord injury. *J Neurosurg* 1954; 11:546–577.

Whiplash Injuries: Current Concepts in Prevention, Diagnosis, and Treatment of the Cervical Whiplash Syndrome, edited by Robert Gunzburg and Marek Szpalski. Lippincott–Raven Publishers, Philadelphia © 1998.

13

Eye Movement Disorders after Whiplash Injury

Christian Van Nechel, Mireille Soeur, Monique Cordonnier, and Andre Zanen.

C. Van Nechel: Neuro-Ophthalmology Unit, Erasme Hospital, Free University of Brussels; and Neurological Rehabilitation Department, Brugmann University Hospital, Brussels, Belgium.
M. Soeur: Department of Neurology, Centre Hospitalier Molière Longchamp, Brussels, Belgium.
M. Cordonnier and A.P. Zanen: Neuro-Ophthalmology Unit, Erasme Hospital, Free University of Brussels, Brussels, Belgium.

Visual disturbances are quite frequent after whiplash injury (23), and most of them result from eye movement disorders. These disorders are usually considered to be caused by brainstem or cerebellar lesions (21), but voluntary eye movements are perceptivo-motor processes and some of the dysfunctions may have their origin in the sensorial and cognitive steps. This pre-motor stage can be easily assessed by evaluating the efficiency of different stimuli that would generate the same eye movement. In this study, we have modulated the presentation time-of-target for visually guided saccades in patients suffering from the consequences of a whiplash injury.

METHODS

Eye movement disorders were assessed by clinical examination and oculography in 50 patients (mean age, 39.3 years) referred to our neuro-ophthalmological unit after a whiplash injury. The selection was made according to a history of sudden head acceleration relative to the trunk, without head trauma or cervical fracture. Most patients were victims of rear-end car collisions. The median delay between the injury and the examination was 12.4 months (range, 3 weeks to 113 months). Adequate questions were asked to specify the visual complaints; for instance, does the disorder affect near or distance vision, or fixed or moving visual targets?

The clinical examination searched for ocular lack of alignment (phoria or tropia), spontaneous eye instability (during fixation or with Frenzel lenses), fusional amplitude, and convergence power. When the neck movements were well tolerated, the eye stability was also assessed after the head-shaking test and in different head positions known to induce positional vertigo.

Ocular pursuit and visually guided saccades were recorded by DC-electro-oculography. The targets (Nicolet light bar controlled by a computer) were randomly presented at

10°, 20°, and 30° to the right or to the left of a central fixation point. A succession of 40 stimulations was carried out in accordance with two paradigms. First, the lateral target was switched on for 1 sec after the extinction of the central fixation point. Second, the target was switched on for 10 msec after the disappearance of the central fixation point and then switched on again 1 sec later for 1 sec in the same position. The subject was warned of the lighting of the target by a nonlateralized sound. Horizontal eye movements were recorded for 2 sec after the central point was switched off. The data were then digitalized at a sampling time of 2 msec. The amplitude and velocity measurements were computed on the basis of the initial calibration and the stable position of the eyes at the end of the 1-sec target presentation. The automatic analysis was visually controlled for each saccade off-line. The computer then calculated the theoretical velocity–amplitude relationship (VAR) that best fit the velocity data, with the function

$$Velocity = a[1 - e^{(b.amplitude)}]$$

using an algorithm that minimizes the residual sum of squares. The amplitudes and velocities considered were those of the first saccade phase that followed the first modality target presentation. This VAR was then used to compute a theoretical velocity for the first phase amplitude of the saccade generated after the 10-msec stimulus. Differences between these theoretical velocities and the measured velocities for the short stimuli were assessed with a nonparametric permutation test for paired observations (19). These data were calculated independently for each eye in each direction.

The accuracy, latencies, and velocities of these visually guided saccades for sustained (1 sec) and short (10 msec) stimuli were quantified and compared with a control group of 36 subjects (mean age, 32.6 years) without neurologic or neuro-ophthalmological history. Latencies and amplitudes must be characterized by an asymmetric distribution, whereas velocity distributions are Gaussian. Using these various distributions, we computed the limits including 95% (l_{95}) and 99% (l_{99}) of the control group data. The normative data were also analyzed according to age. No significant change was observed within the range of patient age. Our normative data were computed separately for each eye in each direction and published previously (24). We have considered that a saccade parameter was impaired for a given subject when it was outside the l_{99} for at least 5 of the 40 saccades. This takes the distribution flattening of these parameters into account, which is not always reflected by means comparisons.

RESULTS

Because of the neuro-ophthalmological recruitment, most of these patients (73%) complained of visual disorders (Table 1). Impaired near-sight, diplopia, oscillopsia, wrong distance evaluation, and intolerance to moving objects in the visual field were the more frequent visual symptoms. Most diplopias were intermittent and, at the time of examination, an ocular misalignment was observed in only 20 patients: 3 with convergence spasms, 4 with hypertropia of one eye, and 13 with horizontal diplopia for near or distance vision. One case of hypertropia resulted from trauma to the fourth cranial nerve, but increased vertical fusional power beyond 5 diopters in the two other cases did not allow us to establish the difference between a decompensated congenital fourth nerve palsy and a posttraumatic but long-lasting fourth nerve palsy (17). The fourth patient presented with a left hypertropia with right extorsion and shift of the subjective visual vertical of both eyes suggesting an ocular tilt reaction.

TABLE 1. *Complaint frequencies*

Complaint	Patients with complaint (out of a total of 50) (N)	Complaints seen after a delay < 12.4 mo (total, 33 examinations) (%)	Complaints seen after a delay > 12.4 mo (total, 34 examinations) (%)
Headaches	36	88	72
Impaired near-sight	21	40	34
Diplopia	20	40	32
Unsteadiness	17	21	35
Positioning vertigo	10	21	20
Nucalgia	10	24	11
Oscillopsia	10	21	29
Wrong distance evaluation	10	21	18
Intolerance to moving objects in the visual field	10	21	29
Rotational vertigo (nonpositioning)	4	12	5
Linear vertigo	3	3	5
Topographical disorientation	2	9	5
Scotoma	2	3	8
Acrophobia	2	6	3
Intolerance to acceleration	2	3	3

Only seven patients were examined on several occasions. Two were free of symptoms between 15 and 20 months but one of them kept saccadic impairments. The five remaining patients continued to have visual complaints and eye movement disorders. Therefore, we tried to document the possible evolution of the complaints and related eye movement disorders by splitting the patient group according to the median of examination delay from the whiplash injury. Except for postural and visual instability, the complaint frequencies remained quite similar. Findings of clinical examination and eye movement recordings (Table 2) showed the same invariability except for paroxystic positional vertigo and convergence spasms, which were more frequent, and fusional vergence disorders, which were less common in the second subgroup. Saccade impairments were the most frequently recorded abnormalities, especially for short targets, and they persisted for a long time after the injury for some patients.

Table 3 shows the incidence of impaired parameters in relation to the side and presentation time of the saccade stimuli, or the direction of the pursuit stimulus. There was a significant asymmetry with a left-side predominance of the latency increase and saccade hypometry but not for saccade hypermetry and pursuit. These latency and amplitude asymmetries were accentuated when the shorter stimuli were used. Although these stimuli also induced a further saccade slowing, this was not significantly asymmetric.

DISCUSSION

The specific recruitment of a neuro-ophthalmological unit clearly explains the higher incidence of visual disturbances seen there compared with a neurology department (23).

TABLE 2. *Eye movement disorders*

Disorder	Patients seen with the disorder after a delay < 12.4 mo (total, 33 examinations) (%)	Patients seen with the disorder after a delay > 12.4 mo (total, 34 examinations) (%)
Decreased fusional vergence	13 (39%)	6 (18%)
Convergence insufficiency	8 (24%)	5 (15%)
Horizontal misalignment	7 (21%)	6 (18%)
Positioning nystagmus	3 (9%)	7 (21%)
Spontaneous nystagmus	3	3 (9%)
Abnormal head shaking test	1	2
Convergence spasm		3 (9%)
Vertical misalignment	2	2
Abnormal accommodation	1	
Voluntary nystagmus		1
Disorders of eye movement recordings:		
Pursuit	20 (61%)	15 (44%)
Saccades (target of 1 sec)		
Latencies	19 (58%)	15 (44%)
Accuracy	14 (42%)	17 (50%)
Velocities	7 (21%)	6 (18%)
Saccades (target of 10 msec)		
Latencies	32 (97%)	26 (76%)
Accuracy	31 (93%)	29 (85%)
Velocities	26 (79%)	24 (76%)

The most striking result of this study is the predominance of saccade impairment for visual targets appearing in the left hemifield. It is unlikely that this results from an asymmetry of lesions along the anatomic pathways that generate visually guided saccades. We suggest that it is related to the different skills governed by the right and left brain hemispheres. Symmetrical dysfunctions of both hemispheres have different consequences on perceptive performances within the left or right hemispace. In fact, the eye movement is the last step of the perceptivo-motor program generating visually guided saccade. The further impairment of saccade parameters when using shorter targets at the same location suggests that this lack of efficiency lies at a pre-motor level. The occurrence of a new target in the visual field periphery during a central point fixation triggers at first an attentional process. The attention must be disengaged from the central fixation and then reengaged to the new peripheral stimulus. This is performed without any eye movement (15). This attentional process would depend of a cortico-limbo-reticular loop (25). A second process must then decide whether this new stimulus is sufficiently interesting to be accurately analyzed by the central portion of the retina. Simultaneously, the target position in space is computed. If the decision process gives an affirmative answer, a saccade is performed. This decision process would be performed in a part of the loop (i.e., the posterior parietal cortex) (12).

Inattention is dependent on the disruption at any level of these cortico-limbo-reticular loops. Lesions of mesencephalic reticular formation, thalamus, or frontal lobes also induce attentional deficits. An attentional deficit would explain why saccade latencies and accuracies are the most asymmetrically impaired. Pursuit of a moving target does not require this attentional engagement and disengagement process, because it remains projected in the center of the visual field.

Although less sensitive to hemispheric dysfunctions, saccade velocities may also be slowed by supracollicular lesions (24). The hypothesis that an attentional deficit is at the

TABLE 3. *Frequency of impaired saccades or pursuits*

Saccades	Left side only (%)	Both sides (left > right) (%)	Right side only (%)	Both sides (right > left) (%)	Both sides (symmetric) (%)	Probability
1-sec stimulus						
Latencies						
Increased	22	6	4	2	22	< .01
Normal					44	
Amplitudes						
Decreased	20	4	4		10	< .01
Increased	6		4		6	n.s.
Normal					50	
Velocities						
Decreased	10		2		8	< .05
Normal					80	
10-msec stimulus						
Latencies						
Increased	16	20		2	46	< .01
Normal					16	
Amplitudes						
Decreased	32	12	4	2	32	< .01
Increased		2	4		6	n.s.
Normal					14	
Velocities						
Decreased	18	10	18	2	26	n.s.
Normal					26	
Pursuit						
Saccadic aspect	22	2	6	4	16	n.s.
Normal					50	

Frequencies of impaired saccade or pursuit parameters in relation to the presentation side (saccades) or direction (pursuit) of the stimulus. Pure and predominantly unilateral impairments were pooled to test the significance of the asymmetry.

N = 50 patients.

root of eye movement disorders after whiplash injuries is also consistent with other neuropsychological studies (5,16). In a prospective study by Di Stefano and Radanov (4), pain and medication were not found to be major factors in explaining the cognitive impairment.

The question is now, why does this attention disorder prevail for visual targets in the left hemispace? Some hypothetical mechanism may be formulated.

Loops of both hemispheres are not equally efficient for the attention in the ipsi- and contralateral visual hemispace. The right hemisphere seems to modulate the attention in both ipsi- and contralateral hemispaces, whereas the left hemisphere is less efficient for attentional processing in the left hemispace (25). This could explain why left attentional deficit is more pronounced in patients with mild bilateral hemispheric dysfunction.

Another proposal is that left hemispheric dysfunction induces a right inattention for verbal task, whereas a left inattention for space-perceptual task would be more the consequence of the right hemispheric dysfunction (11). Kinsbourne (10) conjectured that the verbal communication occurring between the doctor and the patient would result in the activation of the patient's left hemisphere and would foster an increase of his tendency of gaze to the right.

Pre-motor skills for eye movements are also not symmetric between the two hemispheres. The incidence of conjugate head and gaze deviation, with preserved reflex eye movements, after a stroke is significantly higher in the right-brain-damaged group than in the left-brain-damaged group, and the sign recovers slowly in the former (3). Hemi-inattention was still present in many of these patients who had recovered from gaze palsy. This supports a relationship between attentional mechanisms and oculomotor balance. These authors also showed that gaze paresis appears predominantly associated with parietal injury in the right brain or with a widespread involvement of the left hemisphere. In that way, bilateral parietal dysfunctions after whiplash injuries may impair more markedly leftward saccades. Such bilateral parietal dysfunction is supported by brain single-photon emission computed tomography (SPECT) in late whiplash syndrome (13,14).

Finally, depressive disorders may modify the balance between the cerebral hemispheres, but the attentional direction shift remains controversial and very dependent on the stimulus and gender (2,18,20). Moreover, we would expect that this effect would increase with delayed recovery and this was not obvious in our group.

Posttraumatic impaired near-sight has been known for a long time (26). It is generally attributed to convergence insufficiency, poor accommodation, and fusional vergence. These functions depend on volitional effort and subject attention capacity. Lesions at midbrain level but also at hemispherical levels (9,22) may induce convergence and fusional disorders. It is interesting to note that acquired parietal lobe lesions may lead to impaired stereopsis and fusional vergence (6). In that way, hemispheric arousal deficits may also partly explain these disorders.

The spasm of the near reflex characterized by pseudomyopia, convergent strabismus, and miosis is more often related to functional than organic disorders (7). This etiologic aspect and its poor spontaneous remission probably explain their later occurrence in the group we studied.

Vestibular problems are quite frequent after whiplash injuries (8), especially benign positional vertigo (1). Its tendency to recur accounts for the persistence of the 20% positive tests we recorded 1 year after the injury.

From this study, it can be concluded that near-sight, pursuit, and saccade impairments are long-drawn-out deficits after a whiplash injury. Attentional dysfunctions probably explain the asymmetric (prevailingly left-sided) impairment of saccade latencies and accuracies. Similar hemispheric arousal deficits are likely to interfere with nonlateralized tasks such as convergence, accommodation, and visual fusion, which are related to the impaired near-sight, the most frequent visual complaint of our patients after a whiplash injury. Many brain structures, from midbrain to parietal cortex, are involved in these attentional processes and a restricted location could not be stated precisely, whereas diplopia and nystagmus are more related to brainstem, cranial nerve, or vestibular lesions.

REFERENCES

1. Barber HO, Leigh RJ. Benign (and not so beningn) postural vertigo: diagnosis and treatment. In: Barber HO, Sharpe A, eds. *Vestibular disorders.* Boca Raton, FL: CRC Press, 1988:215–232.
2. Crews WD, Harrison DW. Cerbral asymmetry in facial affect perception by women: neuropsychological effects of depressed mood. *Percept Mot Skills* 1994;79(3):1667–1679.
3. De Renzi E. Disorders of space exploration. In: De Renzi E, ed. *Disorders of space exploration and cognition.* New York: John Wiley & Sons, 1982;57–125.
4. Di Stefano D, Radanov BP. Course of attention and memory after common whiplash: a two-year prospective study with age, education and gender pair-matched patients. *Acta Neurol Scand* 1995;91:346–352.
5. Ettlin TM, Kischka U, Reichmann S, et al. Cerebral symptoms after whiplash injury of the neck: a prospective clinical and neuropsychological study of whiplash injury. *J Neurol Neurosurg Psychiatr* 1992;55:943–948.
6. Fowler S, Munro N, Richardson A, Stein J. Vergence control in patients with lesions of the posterior parietal cortex. *J Physiol* 1989;417:92.

7. Goldstein JH, Schneekloth BB. Spasm of the near reflex: a spectrum of anomalies. *Surv Ophthalmol* 1996;40(4):269–278.

8. Hinoki M. Vertigo due to whiplash injury: a neurotological approach. *Acta Otolaryngol* 1985;419(suppl):9–29.

9. Kerkhoff G, Stogerer E. Treatment of fusional disorders in patients with brain damage. *Klin Monatsbl Augenheilkd* 1994;20(2):70–75.

10. Kinsbourne M. In: Kinsbourne M, Smith WL, eds. *Lateral interactions in the brain.* 1972;239–259.

11. Leicester J, Sidman M, Stoddard LT, Mohr JP. Some determinants of neglect. *J Neurol Neurosurg Psychiatr* 1969;32:580–587.

12. Lynch JC, McLaren JW. Deficits of visual attention and sacadic eye movements after lesions of parieto-occipital cortex in monkey. *J Neurophysiol* 1989;61:74–90.

13. Otte A, Mueller-Brand J, Fierz L. Brain SPECT findings in late whiplash syndrome. *Lancet* 1995;345: 1513–1514.

14. Otte A, Ettlin T, Fierz L, Mueller-Brand J. Parieto-occipital hypoperfusion in late whiplash syndrome: first quantitative SPECT study using tecchnetium-99m bicisate. *Eur J Nucl Med* 1996;23(1):72–74.

15. Posner MI, Walker JA, Friedrich FJ, Rafal RD. Effects of parietal injury on covert orienting of attention. *J Neurosci* 1984;4(7):1863–1874.

16. Radanov BP, Di Stefano G, Schnidrig A, Sturzenegger M, Augustiny KF. Cognitive funtioning after common whiplash. A controlled follow-up study. *Arch Neurol* 1993;50:87–91.

17. Rutstein RP, Corliss DA. The relationship between duration of superior oblique palsy and vertical fusional vergence, cyclodeviation and diplopia. *J Am Optom Assoc* 1995;66(7):442–448.

18. Sackeim HA, Decina P, Epstein D, Bruder GE, Malitz S. Possible reversed affective lateralization in a case of bipolar disorder. Presented at the annual meeting of the International Neuropsychological Society, Pittsburg, 1982.

19. Siegel S, Castellean NJ. The case of on sample, two measures or paired replicates. In: Siegel S, Castellan NJ, eds. *New parametric statistics for the behavioral sciences.* New York: McGraw-Hill, 1988;73–101.

20. Silberman EK, Weingartner H, Stillman R, Chen HJ, Post RM. Altered lateralization of cognitive processes in depressed women. *Am J Psychiatr* 1983:140;1340–1344.

21. Spanio M, Rigo S. Voluntary eye movements in whiplash injuries. In: Cesarani A, Alpini D, Boniver R, et al., eds. *Whiplash injuries. Diagnosis and treatment.* New York: Springer, 1996.

22. Spierer A, Huna R, Rechtman C, Lapidot D. Convergence insufficiency secondary to sudural hematoma. *Am J Ophthalmol* 1995;120(2):258–260.

23. Sturzenegger M, DiStefano G, Radanov BP, Schnidrig A. Presenting symptoms and signs after whiplash injury: the influence of accident mechanisms. *Neurology* 1994;44:688–693.

24. Van Nechel C, Cordonnier M. Electro-oculography of saccades to flashed target. *J Neuroophthalmol* 1991; 11(2):77–86.

25. Watson RI, Miller BD, Heilman KM. Nonsensory neglect. *Ann Neurol* 1978;3:505–508.

26. Westcott V. Concerning accomodative asthenopia following head injury. *Am J Ophthalmol* 1936;19:385–391.

Whiplash Injuries: Current Concepts in Prevention, Diagnosis, and Treatment of the Cervical Whiplash Syndrome, edited by Robert Gunzburg and Marek Szpalski. Lippincott–Raven Publishers, Philadelphia © 1998.

14

The Whiplash Syndrome: Neurolinguistic and Attention Disorders

Anne de Heering

A. de Heering: Centre Hospitalier Molière Longchamp, Brussels, Belgium.

Language problems are not uncommon among whiplash patients with cognitive complaints, but they are usually of shorter duration than memory and concentration problems. They include expression as well as comprehension difficulties for oral and written language.

Word-finding difficulties, pseudostuttering, and sequence errors of the dyslexic type may be observed, along with a global inability to express elaborate thoughts. Patients may also complain of auditory filtering inefficiency in social meetings (cocktail-party effect) or of more elementary comprehension troubles in simple conversation.

Some whiplash patients are worried when they have to write a simple letter, either because they cannot remember what exactly has to be written or because they feel unable to organize their thoughts; in some cases, they make unusual spelling mistakes without being able to detect them. Also, reading may become difficult because of a visual attention deficit or because no new information can spontaneously be kept in memory.

Classic neurolinguistic and neuropsychological tests often fail to contribute in such matters; the source of the disorder is located at a general attention level, attention failures being responsible for language as well as for memory difficulties. The attentional function allows us to select and to integrate relevant information among several perceptual or representational fields. Attention is thus a mechanism of control and integration that is bound to interact with every other cognitive function.

CONTEMPORARY MODELS OF ATTENTION

Attention allocation also means brain activation. According to Posner and Rothbart (9) and other contemporary researchers, there are three basic attentional systems responsible for selective attention:

The *posterior attentional network* has been investigated mainly in relation to visual and spatial attention. This system is globally involved in the selection of sensorial stimuli. It includes areas of the parietal cortex associated with certain subcortical structures (thalamic areas, pulvinar, reticular structures, and parts of the superior colliculus). Its functioning is essentially unconscious. Patients with parietal lesions show specific inability to disengage from a stimulus once attention has been committed in that direction.

The *anterior attentional network* involves areas of the medial prefrontal cortex (cingular gyrus and supplementary motor area) that are active in situations associated with event detection and often result in a conscious verbal or manual response. There is an indication that such an attentional command in the left hemisphere would be necessary not only to trigger a spatial orientation but also to draw the subject's attention to a verbal task.

The *vigilance network* is important in situations where an alert state must be maintained (e.g., during a brief delay between trials). Its proper functioning depends on the lateral parts of the right frontal lobe. This network works in conjunction with the cingular gyrus and the subcortical arousal systems. The alert system has direct action on neither the motor reaction nor the information processing, but on a central mechanism allowing the programming of a response.

A dichotomy such as that between the anterior and the posterior systems has also been seen in the cortical control of saccades: the parietal eye field (PEF) could be more involved in the reflexive exploration of the visual environment, and the frontal eye field (FEF) could be more involved in the intentional exploration of this environment (7).

Attention can thus be involved both in early visual processing (posterior network) and in selection of information for output (anterior network); the integrity of the alert system is a prerequisite for normal functioning of both systems.

Various positron-emission tomography (PET) studies implicate a wide spectrum of cortical areas in the attentional effects on language. The processing of semantic associations seems to be related to the anterior system: to inferior regions such as the anterior cingular gyrus and superior regions such as the supplementary motor area, which becomes increasingly active when a real motor action such as speech is required (8). Frontal areas may thus be important in general functions of attention common to both spatial voluntary orienting and language control. On the other hand, there is growing evidence for linking the posterior mechanisms involved in spatial orientation to the processes used for orientation to mental structures. It seems reasonable to suppose that automatic orientation in semantic memory, for instance, will take advantage of these same principles (8). Finally, it should be noted that, according to recent PET scan studies, several right hemisphere areas are activated during linguistic motor tasks (6).

In this framework, spatial attention could be considered a module within a more general system of attention that extends to other cognitive systems such as language or memory. The information provided by visual attention tests should prove especially interesting in the case of whiplash patients, who often complain of various visual problems.

We chose to work with the ocular motility test from the TEA computer attention battery designed by P. Zimmerman and B. Fimm (10). Despite the fact that full statistical data obtained for control subjects are still unpublished, we decided to apply it at once to whiplash patients, hoping to be able to detect general trends that could later be confirmed by a careful statistical analysis. This is thus a preliminary study.

THE OCULAR MOTILITY TEST (TEA)

The ocular motility test was designed to investigate the attentional component of horizontal saccades selectively performed in response to a certain type of visual stimulus.

The subject is seated at a distance of about 60 cm from the computer screen and requested to keep his gaze fixed on a central point unless something new appears left or right of that point. He is asked to press a button with his preferred hand at the occurrence of open squares, but he must not react to the occurrence of similar closed squares.

Squares may appear on the right, on the left, or in the middle of the screen. There are 100 successive trials, 40 involving closed and 60 involving open squares (Fig. 1).

Two types of visually guided saccades are elicited in this test. In the first condition, the Gap condition, the fixation point disappears 200 msec before the appearance of the target. Disengagement from fixation is thus performed before the occurrence of the following eye movement. In the second condition, the Overlap condition, which is supposed to be more demanding, the fixation point remains visible when the lateral target occurs. Active disengagement from this point is then required before the saccade can be triggered.

In spite of its apparent simplicity, this test involves a whole range of operations, each of them more or less lateralized in the brain. Also, when active central fixation is required, laterality effects are enhanced for visual tasks where brain activation is known to repeatedly shift over time, depending on the hemifield where the target occurs. In such a case, activation of one hemisphere normally inhibits potentially analogous functions in the other hemisphere (3).

As far as laterality components are concerned, the theoretical considerations for right-handers using their right hand and presenting a left lateralization for language include the following:

1. *Bihemispherical activation,* resulting from the requirement to fixate a central target, fixation being mediated by the prefrontal cortex (1).

2. *Right hemisphere activation,* resulting from the need to prepare and sustain alertness, which is known to be related to the lateral parts of the right frontal lobe.

3. *Left hemisphere activation,* related to the ability to activate an attentional command, resulting in the understanding of the task, the conscious selection of the proper stimuli, and the execution of a right hand movement.

4. *Shifting activation,* depending on the global ability to focus attention on, or to select a specific type of, visual stimulus, namely the open squares; the posterior attentional network is responsible for the unconscious selecting of specific information in the contralateral hemifield.

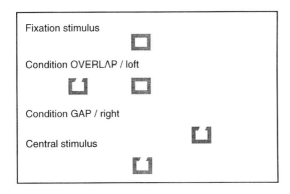

FIG. 1. Fixation stimulus, Overlap condition/left, Gap condition/right, central stimulus.

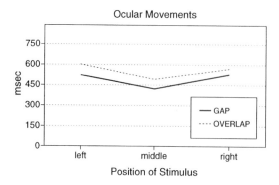

FIG. 2. Ocular motility: typical Gap and Overlap curves for a right-hander using his/her right hand.

Results in Control Subjects

In normal subjects and 29 orthopedic patients, saccades performed under the Gap condition are quicker than those obtained under the Overlap condition, implying refixation of a new target. In the Gap and in the Overlap conditions, there is an advantage of the central targets because adducting and centripetally directed saccades generally tend to be faster (4). In the Gap condition, manual responses to open squares appearing at the central fixation point are the quickest when no eye movement is needed.

On the whole, reactions for right visual hemifield stimuli are faster than responses for left visual hemifield targets. Left hemisphere activation, probably enhanced by the use of the right hand in the majority of subjects, appears to be dominant in this test (Fig. 2).

RESULTS IN WHIPLASH PATIENTS

Fourteen right-handed whiplash patients [4 men and 10 women; median age, 42 (range, 16 to 70)] without known neurologic illness were given the ocular motility test and the simple motor reaction time test (alert test) of the same attentional program, on average 17.2 months after the accident (range, 1 to 66). Four patients were involved in sport accidents and 10 in car accidents, with a rear-end (five cases), lateral (three cases), or frontolateral (two cases) impact direction. Three patients had only visual complaints; 11 suffered only from cognitive or from cognitive and visual disorders, four of them in association with language difficulties.

Five patients found the two tasks hard and two found them very hard to perform because of obvious visual problems. No patient had a completely typical pattern of curves. Only striking deviations from the norm have been taken into account.

No evident anomalies could be discovered for the three patients with visual complaints apart from increased latencies for the central target in one patient.

However, in the 11 patients with only cognitive or with cognitive and visual complaints, the following results were found:

1. An overall pathologic slowing of responses in the reaction time test and in the ocular test was discovered in three subjects; one patient had extremely slow reactions ranging from 464 to 1890 msec in the saccade test in association with a strongly reversed Overlap curve (Fig. 3).

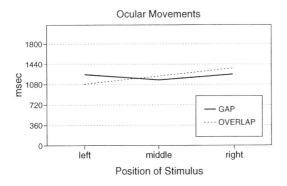

FIG. 3. Strongly reversed pattern of the Overlap curve in 1 patient, along with very slow reaction times in the saccade and in the alert test.

2. A reversed pattern of the Gap curve was found in two patients whose reaction times were increased for the saccades but not for the alert test (Fig. 4).

3. Increased latencies for central targets were elicited for one subject in the Gap condition alone and for another subject in the two conditions.

The five patients with pathologic reaction times or abnormalities of the Gap curve were involved in car accidents with a lateral or frontolateral impact. They included the four subjects with language complaints.

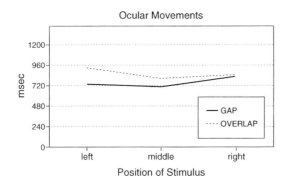

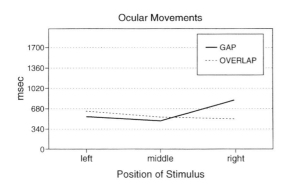

FIG. 4. Reversed pattern of the Gap curve in two patients whose reaction times were increased for the saccade but not for the alert test.

DISCUSSION

1. Except for one case with higher latencies for the central targets, the results obtained by patients with pure visual complaints were not very specific.

2. Three patients with pathologic latencies in the alert test and in the ocular motility test—one of them with only memory, two of them with memory and language complaints—seemed to suffer from a lack of activation in the right hemisphere. Their vigilance network might have been unable to maintain a normal level of visual arousal and motor activation.

3. Two patients with memory and language difficulties showed a dissociation between normal results at the alert test and delayed right hemifield responses in the Gap condition of the ocular motility test. There are reasons to think that they did not suffer from a right hemisphere but from a left hemisphere impairment of the attentional command responsible for the triggering of an active response when a target has to be really selected. The advantage for the left targets in the Gap condition could reflect contralateral hypometria and/or an increased percentage of express saccades directed towards the less activated hemisphere. The normal pattern of the Overlap curve could be explained by the fact that express saccades are largely suppressed in this condition, even in patients with a lesion in the frontal eye field (2).

4. Unlike patients who are helped by fixation, subjects showing a typical Gap but an atypical Overlap curve seem too sensitive to the occurrence of left hemifield targets when another square remains visible on the screen, perhaps because of an inability to actively engage or maintain long-lasting fixation towards central and (especially) right stimuli. Along with abnormal latencies for Overlap central targets, such a response pattern could reflect another, more diffuse type of left hemisphere hypoactivation, which might also be present in several other conditions including depression or simple fatigue.

5. Lack of advantage of the central targets in the Gap condition could result from fixation instabilities or other visual disorders.

Despite the fact that cases of parieto-occipital hypoperfusion in whiplash patients have been recently described (5), typical slowing of attentional disengagement in the Overlap curve could not be discovered, probably because of the importance of the frontal components of the task.

CONCLUSIONS

Anomalies have been found only for subjects involved in car accidents with a side impact. Four such patients had language complaints. A comparison with electro-oculographic recordings would be of great interest.

The TEA ocular motility test does seem useful to test whiplash patients. Further research in this field is needed. It will be prospective and will include a large number of right- but also left-handers with and without visual and cognitive complaints. Along with extensive questioning about the accident mechanisms and the patients' emotional state, attention and memory testing will be part of the study. Matched orthopedic patients will be selected as control subjects.

REFERENCES

1. Anderson TJ, Jenkins IH, Brooks DJ, Hawken MB, Frackowiak RSJ, Kennard C. Cortical control of saccades and fixation in man, a PET study. *Brain* 1994;117:1073–1084.

2. Braun D, Weber H, Mergner TH, Schulte-Mönting J. Saccadic reaction times in patients with frontal and parietal lobe lesions. *Brain* 1992;115:1359–1386.
3. Kinsbourne M. The cerebral basis of lateral asymmetries in attention. *Acta Psychol* 1970;33:193–201.
4. Leigh RJ, Zee DS. *The neurology of eye movement*. Philadelphia: FA Davis, 1983;40.
5. Otte A, Ettlin T, Fierz L, Mueller-Brand J. Parieto-occipital hypoperfusion in late whiplash syndrome: first quantitative SPECT study using technetium-99m bicisate (ECD). *Eur J Nucl Med* 1996;23(1):72–74.
6. Petersen SE, Fox PT, Posner MI, Mintun M, Raichle ME. Positron emission tomographic studies of the cortical anatomy of single word processing. *Nature* 1988;331:1627–1631.
7. Pierrot-Deseilligny C, Rivaud S, Gaymard B, Müri R, Vermersch AI. Cortical control of saccades. *Ann Neurol* 1995;37(5)557–567.
8. Posner MI. Orienting of attention. *Q J Exp Psychol* 1980;32:3–25.
9. Posner MI, Rothbart MK. Les mécanismes de l'attention et l'expérience consciente. (Translated: Attentional mechanisms and conscious experience in the neuropsychology of consciousness.) *Rev Neuropsychol* 1991;2(1): 85–115.
10. Zimmermann P, Fimm B. *Tests d'évaluation de l'attention (TEA), Version 1.02.* Adaptés en français par North P, Leclercq M, Crémel N, Tassi P, Jeronim D. Brussels: Psytest, 1994.

*Whiplash Injuries: Current Concepts in
Prevention, Diagnosis, and Treatment
of the Cervical Whiplash Syndrome,*
edited by Robert Gunzburg and Marek Szpalski.
Lippincott–Raven Publishers, Philadelphia © 1998.

15

Course of Psychological Variables in Whiplash Injury*

Bogdan P. Radanov, Stefan Begré, Matthias Sturzenegger, and Klaus F. Augustiny

*B. P. Radanov and K. F. Augustiny: Department of Psychiatry,
University of Berne, Berne, Switzerland.
S. Begré: Department of Internal Medicine, Psychosomatic Unit, University of Berne,
Berne, Switzerland.
M. Sturzenegger: Department of Neurology, University of Berne, Berne, Switzerland.*

Different psychological symptoms have been documented during the course of whiplash injury (1,8,10,13,14). However, studies on psychological problems in these patients had two serious limitations: unclear definition of whiplash (e.g., patients with head injuries were included) and consideration of preselected patients (e.g., litigation cases). Recently published follow-up studies using nonselected patients (11,18) suggested that psychological symptoms of whiplash patients may reflect difficulties in adjusting to trauma-related symptoms, of which neck pain and headache are the most prominent (19). The fact that long-term follow-up studies focusing on the relationship between somatic and psychological symptoms are lacking has recently been emphasized (2). The principal focus of the present study was to evaluate the course of psychological variables during a 2-year follow-up using a nonselected sample of recently injured patients with common whiplash.

In accord with previous reports (9), common whiplash in this study was considered a medical trauma leading to musculoligamental sprain or strain of the cervical spine as a result of hyperflexion/hyperextension, without fractures or dislocations. To preclude an overlap with head injury, any head impact or traumatic loss of consciousness (including posttraumatic amnesia) was an exclusion criterion.

PATIENTS AND METHODS

As reported previously (16–19), a nonselected sample was obtained by announcing the study in the *Swiss Medical Journal,* and by distribution of letters to primary care physicians in our catchment area (population, about 800,000, about 15% non-Swiss people and

*Reprinted from: *Pain,* 64, Radanov BP, Begré S, Sturzenegger M, Augustiny KF, Course of psychological variables in whiplash injury—a two-year follow-up with age, gender and education pair-matched patients, 429–434, 1996, with kind permission of Elsevier Science—NL, Sara Burgerhartstraat 25, 1055 KV Amsterdam, The Netherlands.

about an additional 20% French-speaking). Physicians were asked to refer patients who had suffered whiplash injury within the shortest possible interval. Inclusion criteria were (a) injury according to the definition; (b) German as native language; (c) age less than 55 years (because of neuropsychological testing) (16); (d) no trauma to other parts of the body; and (e) negative history of neurologic dysfunctions (i.e., neuralgia, multiple sclerosis). The study was designed to investigate patients as soon as possible after trauma and at 3, 6, 12, and 24 months. All patients were examined at referral, and at 3 and 6 months. Patients who at 6 or 12 months were fully recovered from trauma-related symptoms were released from the study, with the possibility of being re-referred by their physicians if any symptom recurred. From a total of 164 referred patients, 27 did not meet the criteria and 20 dropped out at follow-ups. The final initial sample consisted of 117 patients [mean age, 30.8 ± 9.6 (range, 19 to 51 years); average educational attainment, 12.7 ± 2.7 years; women, 58%). From a retrospective study using the register of the Swiss Accident Insurance Company (6) during the sampling period in our catchment area, the total number of whiplash patients (probably including an unknown number of patients with head injury or injury to other parts of the body as well as patients with a native language other than German) could be estimated to be 205 to 210. All patients were injured in automobile accidents and were fully and equally covered by accident insurance according to the country-wide conditions. (According to the Swiss Accident Insurance Company, if the patient loses time from work because of injury, the patient receives a proportional amount of salary regardless of liability. Certification of disability is the task of the treating physician. The system does not provide compensation for noneconomic loss such as pain or suffering.) As reported previously (16–19), all patients underwent assessment of subjective complaints, neurologic and physical investigation, radiologic assessment of the cervical spine, and a detailed assessment of personal and family history with focus on factors possibly influencing illness behavior. As previously described (16,17,19), all patients at all investigations rated the intensity of neck pain and headache on a point scale from 0 (no pain) to 10 (maximal pain).

PSYCHOLOGICAL ASSESSMENT

Psychological assessment included *self-rated well-being,* assessed using the well-being scale (20,21), a valid, reproducible, and sensitive test for assessing changes in patients' well-being on repeated measures (18,20). This has been used previously in numerous studies including those on patients with somatic illness or chronic pain (18,20,24). The test–retest reliability has been established at 0.96 to 0.99 (20). The well-being scale consists of a list of 28 pairs of adjectives polarizing the positive and negative aspects of a particular affective state (e.g., fresh versus dull, pleased versus melancholy, jolly versus whiny) (18,20). Subjects are asked to choose one of the extremes from each pair. The higher the score on the well-being scale, the greater the impairment of the subjects' well-being. Scores greater than 17 (normal range, 4 to 17 points) (i.e., *t*-values greater than 56) reflect a significantly impaired well-being. Pathologic scores may be observed during the course of a somatic illness or a depressive episode (20).

Personality traits were examined using the Freiburg Personality Inventory (7), which is a well-validated and widely used assessment scale in clinical routine in German-speaking areas. The answer analysis of the Freiburg Personality Inventory reveals scores of different personality traits, which are transformed into standardized values (STANINE) (7). A STANINE value of between 4 and 6 occurs in 54% of a random sample, whereas scores above 6 are pathologic. This inventory is composed of the following scales: (a) nervousness, which identifies subjects prone to develop psychosomatic conditions (elevated scores on this scale, however, may also be observed during the course of a serious somatic illness); (b) spontaneous aggressiveness, a scale on which high scores may reflect emotional imbalance thought to be a facet of neurotic behavior; (c) depression, on which elevated scores are indicative of depressed mood (i.e., negative affectivity thought to influence the course of recovery) (22); (d) excitability, on which high scores indicate a low frustration level and thus may reflect a compound of neurotic behavior; (e) social withdrawal, on which high scores may be found in individuals with problems in establishing social relationships; (f) irritability, a scale on which high scores indicate irritation, anxiety, or despair; (g) reactive aggressiveness, high scores on which are indicative of the ability to be assertive; (h) inhibition, on which high scores indicate a timidity and reserve in establishing interpersonal relationships; (i) closed-mindedness, on which high scores may indicate a tendency towards deception; (j) extraversion, assessing this particular personality trait; (k) neuroticism, a personality trait thought to be a sensitive indicator of the manner and seriousness with which symptoms are reported (4); and (l) passivity, a scale on which high scores indicate a tendency towards passive or resignative behavior. Extraversion and neuroticism have been found to be stable personality traits (3).

The social withdrawal scale was originally entitled sociability scale, the irritability scale was the calmness scale, the closed mindedness scale was the openness scale and, the passivity scale was originally entitled the masculinity scale (7). For consistency of data presentation, scores on these scales have been reversed so that a STANINE value over 6 on all scales are pathologic.

To avoid response bias at subsequent follow-ups, parallel versions of personality inventory and well-being scale were used, which have been shown to have a high test–retest reliability (7,20).

EVALUATION STRATEGY

For each patient who still suffered from trauma-related symptoms at the end of the 2-year follow-up (symptomatic group), an age-, gender-, and education-pair-matched counterpart was chosen from those individuals who were symptom free at the investigation 6 or 12 months after injury and in whom symptoms did not recur during the follow-up period of 2 years (i.e., the asymptomatic group). Thus, all patients considered for the present analysis were investigated at referral (T1), and at 3 (T2), 6 (T3), and 24 months (T4).

The statistical analysis employed used BMDP Statistical Software (5).

RESULTS

Two years after the initial trauma, 21 patients still suffered from trauma-related symptoms (symptomatic group). Out of 96 individuals who had recovered, 21 patients were pair-matched with regard to age, gender, and education to establish the asymptomatic group for comparison.

Initially (T1), the symptomatic group scored on average 5.3 ± 2.2 with regard to neck pain intensity, and at the final investigation (T4), 4.8 ± 2.1. The same patients on headache rating initially scored an average of 4.8 ± 3.4, and, at T4, 5.6 ± 2.5. The Wilcoxon matched-pair signed-ranks test revealed neither with regard to neck pain rating ($z = 0.8928$, two-tailed $p = .372$) nor headache rating ($z = 0.6097$, two-tailed $p = 0.542$), a significant difference between the initial and final investigations. The presentation of respective results of the asymptomatic group appears obsolete, because these patients at T4 were completely recovered.

Scores for the two groups obtained at T1, T2, T3, and T4 regarding the well-being scale and the Freiburg Personality Inventory were analyzed (Table 1). Furthermore, a one-factor analysis of variance with repeated measures was employed to evaluate differences between the groups and the deviation of scores over time (Table 2). This analysis included the following: (a) for each patient, the deviation from the average score over time has been calculated for every scale [i.e., well-being scale and the Freiburg Personality Inventory (Time)]. The level of significance on this analysis (Time) indicates a significant deviation of scores within the groups between the initial (T1) and the final (T4) investigations. Whether this deviation is based on an increase or a decrease in scores must be analyzed according to the respective scores; (b) for scores on the well-being scale and Freiburg Personality Inventory, symptomatic and asymptomatic groups were compared. The level of significance on this analysis (Sympt) indicates that over the follow-up period, groups significantly differed from each other. A level of significance for both analyses (Sympt and Time) suggests that groups differ significantly over time and one of the groups shows significant deviation regarding the initial (T1) and final score (T4); (c) furthermore, the interaction between the factors (Time × Sympt) was analyzed. This analysis assesses whether scores of both groups over time are parallel or overlap. The level of significance regarding this analysis indicates the inability to designate patients to one of the two groups (i.e., symptomatic or asymptomatic) according to test scores. In

TABLE 1. *Scores (mean ± SD) on psychological testing at the initial and follow-up investigations (T1-T4)*

Scale	Group	T1	T2	T3	T4
Well-being scale	Symptomatic	59.50 ± 9.76	58.02 ± 11.30	54.17 ± 8.91	55.41 ± 9.26
(*t* values)	Asymptomatic	53.17 ± 10.42	48.19 ± 11.11	45.66 ± 8.96	44.81 ± 6.97
Nervousness scale	Symptomatic	5.38 ± 1.69	5.95 ± 1.72	5.52 ± 1.78	6.19 ± 1.99
	Asymptomatic	4.05 ± 1.40	2.95 ± 1.53	3.33 ± 1.88	3.33 ± 1.88
Spontaneous	Symptomatic	4.14 ± 1.85	3.62 ± 1.88	3.90 ± 1.79	4.10 ± 1.58
aggressiveness scale	Asymptomatic	4.24 ± 1.64	3.57 ± 1.57	4.43 ± 2.01	4.71 ± 1.98
Depression scale	Symptomatic	4.48 ± 1.78	4.24 ± 2.36	4.57 ± 2.18	4.52 ± 2.25
	Asymptomatic	3.86 ± 1.56	2.95 ± 2.11	3.71 ± 1.82	3.76 ± 1.84
Excitability scale	Symptomatic	4.29 ± 1.90	4.76 ± 2.19	4.57 ± 2.23	4.67 ± 2.33
	Asymptomatic	4.43 ± 1.36	3.24 ± 1.34	3.90 ± 1.55	3.95 ± 1.77
Social withdrawal	Symptomatic	5.24 ± 1.55	4.76 ± 1.67	5.38 ± 1.94	5.14 ± 1.74
scale	Asymptomatic	5.00 ± 1.48	4.19 ± 2.18	4.95 ± 1.47	4.43 ± 1.43
Irritablility scale	Symptomatic	4.43 ± 1.72	5.38 ± 1.69	4.81 ± 1.83	5.67 ± 2.29
	Asymptomatic	4.90 ± 2.0	4.05 ± 1.60	5.48 ± 1.91	4.19 ± 2.16
Reactive	Symptomatic	4.52 ± 1.60	4.43 ± 2.29	4.00 ± 1.97	3.62 ± 1.83
aggressiveness scale	Asymptomatic	3.67 ± 1.79	2.76 ± 1.97	3.33 ± 1.53	4.00 ± 1.26
Inhibition scale	Symptomatic	4.67 ± 2.03	4.90 ± 1.79	5.14 ± 1.49	5.90 ± 1.97
	Asymptomatic	5.19 ± 1.63	4.38 ± 1.90	4.71 ± 1.95	4.62 ± 2.06
Closed-mindedness	Symptomatic	6.43 ± 1.78	6.00 ± 2.02	5.90 ± 2.34	6.19 ± 2.04
scale	Asymptomatic	5.81 ± 1.89	5.90 ± 2.21	5.86 ± 2.35	5.71 ± 2.17
Extraversion scale	Symptomatic	4.62 ± 1.80	4.71 ± 1.93	4.71 ± 1.95	4.38 ± 1.99
	Asymptomatic	4.76 ± 1.58	4.71 ± 1.90	4.57 ± 1.78	5.05 ± 1.63
Neuroticism scale	Symptomatic	4.14 ± 1.71	4.39 ± 2.08	4.43 ± 1.91	4.52 ± 2.11
	Asymptomatic	4.14 ± 1.68	3.19 + 2.11	3.00 ± 2.25	3.67 ± 1.84
Passivity scale	Symptomatic	5.05 ± 1.63	5.38 ± 1.72	576 ± 1.57	6.24 ± 2.02
	Asymptomatic	4.81 ± 1.44	4.76 ± 1.76	4.57 ± 1.94	3.86 ± 1.88

TABLE 2. *Deviation over time (Time), group differences according to test scores (Sympt), and statistical interaction (Time × Sympt)*

Scale	Time		Sympt		Time × Sympt	
Well-being scale	$x2 = 16.96$	$p < .001$	$x2 = 20.46$	$p < .0001$	$x2 = 1.90$	ns
Nervousness scale	$x2 = 1515.92$	$p < .0001$	$x2 = 13.11$	$p < .0001$	$x2 = 10.48$	$p < .015$
Spontaneoous aggressiveness scale	$x2 = 2.59$	ns	$x2 = 32.19$	$p < .0001$	$x2 = 12.49$	$p < .006$
Depression scale	$x2 = 12.75$	$p < .005$	$x2 = 0.43$	ns	$x2 = 2.79$	ns
Excitability scale	$x2 = 6.05$	ns	$x2 = 3.11$	ns	$x2 = 1.61$	ns
Social withdrawal scale	$x2 = 3.12$	ns	$x2 = 1.95$	ns	$x2 = 14.0$	$p < .002$
Irritability scale	$x2 = 10.30$	$p < .016$	$x2 = 1.39$	ns	$x2 = 1.03$	ns
Reactive aggressiveness scale	$x2 = 3.02$	ns	$x2 = 0.92$	ns	$x2 = 20.74$	$p < .0001$
Inhibition scale	$x2 = 5.18$	ns	$x2 = 2.39$	ns	$x2 = 15.38$	$p < .002$
Closed-mindedness scale	$x2 = 6.54$	ns	$x2 = 0.77$	ns	14.04	$p < .003$
Extraversion scale	$x2 = 1.09$	ns	$x2 = 0.30$	ns	$x2 = 1.09$	ns
Neuroticism scale	$x2 = 0.10$	ns	$x2 = 0.14$	ns	$x2 = 2.78$	ns
Passivity scale	3.10	ns	$x2 = 1.94$	ns	$x2 = 4.88$	ns

case a significant interaction between factors is found, a *post hoc* analysis for determining the source of the interaction (i.e., T1, T2, T3, or T4) is calculated.

Well-Being Scale

Scores for the symptomatic group on this scale at the initial investigation (T1) were generally pathologic (T > 56), and they remained in the upper normal range over follow-up (see Table 1). In contrast, the average scores of the asymptomatic group on this scale at T1 were in the upper normal range but decreased considerably within the first 6 months after trauma (T1-T3) (see Table 1). A significant deviation over time and a significant difference between the groups was found on this scale. However, a significant interaction between factors could not be established.

Personality Inventory

With regard to the nervousness scale from the personality inventory, the symptomatic group on average showed increased scores during follow-up (see Table 1). During this period, there was a significant deviation and a significant difference between groups. Furthermore, a significant interaction between factors was found for, which T1 contributed ($z = 3.055$, $p < .003$).

Regarding the spontaneous aggressiveness scale, a significant deviation over time was not found, but there was a significant difference between groups. In addition, there was a significant interaction between factors, which was due to T1 ($z = 3.131$, $p < .002$) and T2 ($z = 2.026$, $p < .05$).

Scores on the depression scale showed a significant deviation over the follow-up period. However, the groups did not differ significantly from each other, and a significant interaction between factors could not be established.

With the excitability scale, there was neither significant difference between groups, nor significant deviation over time or between factors.

On the social withdrawal scale, there were no significant differences between groups or with regard to deviation over time. However, a significant interaction between factors was found, the sources of which were T1 ($z = 3.097$, $p < .002$) and T2 ($z = 3.097$, $p < .002$).

On the irritability scale, there was a significant deviation over time but neither a significant difference between groups nor a significant interaction between factors could be established.

There were neither significant group difference nor significant deviation during the follow-up period on the reactive aggressiveness scale. However, a significant interaction between factors was found with contributions from all investigations [i.e., T1 ($z = 2.367$, $p < .02$), T2 ($z = 2.430$, $p < .02$), T3 ($z = 2.872$, $p < .005$), and T4 ($z = 2.809$, $p < .005$)].

On the inhibition scale, groups did not significantly differ from each other and there was no significant deviation during follow-up period. For this scale, a significant interaction between factors was established, the sources for which were T2 ($z = 3.083$, $p < .002$) and T4 ($z = 3.306$, $p < .001$).

With regard to the closed-mindedness scale, neither a significant difference between groups nor a significant deviation over time was found. There was, however, a significant interaction between factors resulting from T1 ($z = 3.207$, $p < .002$) and T4 ($z = 2.886$, $p < .004$).

For the extraversion, neuroticism, and passivity scales, there was neither significant difference between groups, significant deviation over time, nor significant interaction between factors.

DISCUSSION

The present study assessed the course of psychological variables during a 2-year follow-up period after whiplash injury. In contrast to previous reports (17), the present study represents the first long-term prospective analysis of the relationship between somatic and psychological symptoms of whiplash patients. Defined injury criteria were chosen for screening and sampling procedures to provide a nonselected sample. Patients with cervical spine fracture or dislocation, head injuries, and injuries to other parts of the body were excluded to ensure homogeneity of the sample. Based on a previous retrospective report of cervical spine injuries in Switzerland (6), and taking into account the chosen exclusion criteria in our study, the initial number of patients enrolled here likely reflects a representative sample of total whiplash injuries occurring in our catchment area. All patients were injured in automobile accidents, had similar socioeconomic background and educational attainment, and were fully covered by accident insurance. Since the insurance scheme provides only for economic loss, bias due to compensation-seeking behavior is improbable.

Two aspects appear to be of particular interest: (a) whether there were deviations of scores in the symptomatic and asymptomatic groups over time (Time), and (b) whether groups differed significantly from each other regarding test scores (Sympt). In consideration of the evaluation strategy, which was based upon age, gender, and education pair-matched individuals, both analyses (i.e., Time and Sympt) should not reach significance. As the only difference between the groups over time was that one of these complained of trauma-related symptoms at 2 years, the level of significance regarding both analyses could be interpreted as being dependent on differences in somatic outcome. Accordingly, in cases of significant interaction between factors (Time × Sympt) the crucial factor is the source of the interaction. Of particular relevance for interpreting the relationship between test scores and course of recovery is the possibility of multiple sources of interaction (i.e., groups could not be distinguished according to test scores) or interaction resulting from later investigations (i.e., T3 or T4). In the latter case, this may suggest that the inability to distinguish between the groups is based on other causes (e.g., life circumstances) rather than somatic outcome.

Significant differences with regard to Time were found for the well-being, nervousness, depression, and irritability scales. Elevated scores on the well-being scale may indicate impaired general well-being resulting from somatic or psychological causes (such as depression) (20). We believe that the significant deviation over time (Time) and particularly the significant difference between groups (Sympt) on the well-being scale are a result of somatic complaints in the symptomatic group. In support of this view is the evidence that there were neither significant differences between the groups nor significant interactions between the factors regarding the depression scale. The average scores on the well-being scale decreased during follow-up, albeit to different levels in symptomatic and asymptomatic groups. This result indicates a time-related adaptation in both groups, which in the symptomatic group occurred at a delayed rate.

Interactions were found on the social withdrawal, reactive aggressiveness, inhibition, and closed-mindedness scales. In a case of the three last-mentioned scales, interactions may indicate a dependence on factors other than somatic outcome. For the social withdrawal scale, sources of interaction were identified at T1 and T2. Later in the follow-up period, groups on this scale could be distinguished according to test scores, suggesting that potentially symptomatic patients may show disruption of normal behavior that may manifest itself by an increasing tendency to express resignation concerning social interactions.

A significant deviation over time and significant differences between groups were found regarding the nervousness scale. High scores on this may be observed during the course of somatic illness (7). In addition, a significant interaction between factors on this scale was found at T1. However, at T1, groups could not be distinguished from each other based on scores, which may indicate that in the early posttraumatic phase the asymptomatic group also scored high because of trauma-related symptoms. Furthermore, findings on this scale in the symptomatic group are in accordance with results on the well-being scale, because ratings of both well-being and nervousness assess similar correlates. Thus, results on these scales suggest an imbalance resulting from somatic complaints in the symptomatic group.

An important finding is the lack of significant difference between groups on the depression scale. Many items assessing depression may overlap with those frequently found in painful conditions, notably sleep disturbances, lack of energy, increased fatigability, and poor concentration. It is thus reasonable not to overemphasize depression in posttraumatic conditions such as whiplash, because the diagnosis of depression in these patients may be based on the consideration of somatic symptoms. This is also important from the therapeutic point of view for the following reason: some patients, because of some trauma-related symptoms, may show the tendency to develop a somatization reaction. Such a reaction may be exacerbated as a side effect of antidepressants, which, if not prescribed according to a reliable diagnosis of depression, may contribute to an iatrogenic worsening of a primarily benign condition.

Regarding extraversion and neuroticism scales, neither significant difference between the groups nor significant deviation over time was calculated. Because these personality traits have been found to be stable (3), a lack of significant deviation over time is indicative of good construct validity of the inventory used in this investigation. Based on this, the following points emerging from the results deserve particular attention: (a) in accordance with previous reports (4,15,23), personality traits such as neuroticism do not appear of primary relevance for the course of recovery; (b) psychological symptoms observed during the course of posttraumatic conditions are likely dependent on somatic symptoms; and (c) impaired psychological functioning observed in retrospective studies (1,10,13,14), which was interpreted as the cause of poor recovery, may have reflected the consequence of traumatic injury. Thus, evidence of psychological problems in the course of posttraumatic conditions does not necessarily imply that these factors have predictive relevance.

In accordance with previous reports (11,12,18), present results indicate that psychological symptoms in posttraumatic conditions are not the cause but rather the consequence of somatic symptoms.

ACKNOWLEDGMENTS

This study was supported by the Swiss National Science Foundation (project number 3. 883-0.88) and the Swiss Accident Insurance Company (Schweizerische Unfallversicherungsanstalt) regional agency, Berne.

REFERENCES

1. Balla JI. The late whiplash syndrome. *Aust N Z J Surg* 1980;50:610–614.
2. Barnsley L, Lord S, Bogduk N. Whiplash injury. *Pain* 1994;58:283–307.
3. Costa PT, McCrae RR, Zonderman AB, Barbano HE, Lebowitz B, Larson DM. Cross-sectional studies of personality in a national sample: 2. Stability in neuroticism, extraversion, and openness. *Psychol Aging* 1986;1: 144–149.
4. Costa PT, McCrae RR. Neuroticism, somatic complaints, and disease: is the bark worse than the bite? *J Pers* 1988;55:299–316.
5. Dixon WJ. *BMDP statistical software, P5V repeated measures analysis of variance, Wald tests of significance of fixed effects.* University of California, Berkeley, 1988.
6. Dvořák J, Valach L, Schmid S. Injuries of the cervical spine in Switzerland. *Orthopade* 1987;16:2–12.
7. Fahrenberg J, Hampel R, Selg H. In: Hogrefe CJ, ed. *Das Freiburger Persönlichkietsinventar (FPI)*, 4th ed. Göttingen, 1984.
8. Farbman AA. Neck sprain. Associated factors. *JAMA* 1973;223:1010–1015.
9. Hirsch SA, Hirsch PJ, Hiramoto H, Weiss A. Whiplash syndrome, fact or fiction? *Orthop Clin North Am* 1988; 19:791–795.
10. Hodge JF. The whiplash neurosis. *Psychosomatics* 1971;12:245–249.
11. Mayou R, Bryant B, Duthie R. Psychiatric consequences of road traffic accidents. *Br Med J* 1993;307:647–651.
12. Merskey H. Psychological consequences of whiplash. *Spine State of the Art Rev* 1993;7:471–480.
13. Miller H. Accident neurosis. *Br Med J* 1961;1:919–925, 992–998.
14. Pearce JM. Whiplsh injury: a reappraisal. *J Neurol Neurosurg Psychiatry* 1989;52:1329–1331.
15. Radanov BP, Di Stefano G, Schnidrig A, Ballinari P. Role of psychosocial stress in recovery from common whiplash. *Lancet* 1991;338:712–715.
16. Radanov BP, Di Stefano G, Schnidrig A, Sturzenegger M, Augustiny KF. Cognitive functioning after common whiplash: a controlled follow-up study. *Arch Neurol* 1993;50:87–91.
17. Radanov BP, Sturzenegger M, Di Stefano G, Schnidrig A, Aljinovic M. Factors influencing recovery from headache after common whiplash. *Br Med J* 1993;307:652–655.
18. Radanov BP, Di Stefano G, Schnidrig A, Sturzenegger M. Common whiplash—psychosomatic or somatopsychic? *J Neurol Neurosurg Psychiatry* 1994;57:442–448.
19. Radanov BP, Sturzenegger M, Di Stefano G, Schnidrig A. Relationship between early somatic, radiological, cognitive and psychosocial findings and outcome during a one-year follow-up in 117 common whiplash patients. *Br J Rheumatol* 1994;33:484–488.
20. von Zerssen D. *Befindlichkeitsskala.* Beltz: Weinheim, 1976.

21. von Zerssen D. Self-rating scales in the evaluation of psychiatric treatment. In: Helgason T, ed. *Methodology in evaluation of psychiatric treatment.* Cambridge: University Press, 1983; 183–204.
22. Watson D, Pennebaker JW. Health complaints, stress, and distress: exploring the central role of negative affectivity. *Psychol Rev* 1989;96:234–254.
23. Weighill VE. "Compensation neurosis." A review of the literature. *J Psychosom Res* 1983;27:97–104.
24. Westhoff G. *Handbuch psychosozialer Messinstrumente: ein Kompendium für epidemiologische und klinische Forschung zu chronischer Krankheit.* CJ Hogrefe, Göttingen, 1993.

Whiplash Injuries: Current Concepts in
Prevention, Diagnosis, and Treatment
of the Cervical Whiplash Syndrome,
edited by Robert Gunzburg and Marek Szpalski.
Lippincott–Raven Publishers, Philadelphia © 1998.

16

The Controversy over Late Whiplash: Are Chronic Symptoms after Whiplash Real?

Michael D. Freeman and Arthur C. Croft

M. D. Freeman: Department of Public Health, Oregon State University,
Salem, Oregon 97303.
A. C. Croft: Department of Orthopaedics, Los Angeles College of Chiropractics,
Whittier, California 90609.

The prevalence of chronic symptoms after whiplash, or "late whiplash" (3), is a topic that has been examined numerous times over the past 40 years. Different groups have vested economic interest in diametrically opposing outcomes of these studies: insurers and defense attorneys and their medical experts appear to believe that there is no relationship between acute whiplash injuries and chronic neck pain and other chronic symptoms. The familiar adage that whiplash injuries resolve in 6 to 8 weeks is rarely heard outside of medicolegal defense circles.

Conversely, plaintiff attorneys, health care providers, and, most significantly, the injured individuals themselves, are more likely to believe that acute whiplash injuries can produce chronic symptoms. To date, no broad consensus on the subject exists.

This controversy has been fueled by two recent publications regarding the subject of late whiplash. The first publication, a text entitled *Whiplash-Associated Disorders (WAD)—Redefining "Whiplash" and Its Management,* was authored by the Québec Task Force (QTF) on Whiplash-Associated Disorders. The QTF was chaired by Walter O. Spitzer M.D., M.P.H., F.R.C.P.C., and consisted of a panel of eminent experts in medicine, epidemiology and biostatistics, chiropractic, and other disciplines. The text was published in January 1995 and was accompanied by a condensed version that was published as a supplement to the journal *Spine* in its April 15, 1995 issue (17). The text consisted of a retrospective cohort study, a literature search, and a set of guidelines and recommendations. Among other things, the QTF concluded that whiplash injuries were "short-lived," involving "temporary discomfort," that the pain resulting from whiplash was "not harmful," and that whiplash injuries have a "favorable prognosis."

The second publication was a paper by Schrader et al. (16) that appeared in *Lancet* (May 4, 1996) and was entitled "Natural Evolution of Late Whiplash Syndrome Outside the Medicolegal Context." The authors conducted a retrospective cohort study in which they surveyed 202 individuals in Kaunas, Lithuania, who had been involved in car accidents. The subjects were surveyed an average of 21.7 months after the accident to determine if they had any residual symptoms associated with the accident. Because the rate of chronic neck symptoms matched that of the control group, the authors concluded that chronic symptoms were not caused by the accident. The authors attributed the difference between their findings and those of prior authors, who had found a relationship between automobile accident injuries and chronic neck pain, to the lack of financial incentive present in Lithuania. The implication was obvious: in industrialized countries, avarice is the cause of chronic neck pain after whiplash.

The conclusions of these studies were widely reported in the popular press under headlines such as "Whiplash is all in the head" (19) and "Whiplash treatments found to be ineffective" (1).

In this chapter, we report the results of an examination of both studies for methodologic flaws and potential sources of bias.

RESULTS

Police Reports as a Selection Criterion

One flawed methodology employed by both studies was the use of police records to identify whiplash-injured individuals. This method of study selection is dependent on the criteria by which police reports are generated, after an appearance by the police at the accident scene. In Quebec and in Kaunas, the police come to an accident scene if there is substantial visible damage to the vehicle or if immediate medical attention is required for any of the accident victims (6,16). This criterion eliminates all potentially whiplash-injured individuals who do not require immediate medical attention and who were in vehicles that did not sustain significant structural damage.

To understand the way many potential cohort enrollees are eliminated from consideration by this selection criterion, we examined the literature on the subject of delayed symptoms, the collision velocity at which vehicle damage occurs, and the percentage of whiplash injuries that occur at speeds below the threshold of vehicle damage.

Several authors have reported delay of symptoms in whiplash-injured individuals (3,6,8,9). For example, Hildingsson and Toolanen (8) reported the delay of symptom onset in their cohort of 93 whiplash-injured patients: 65 patients were symptomatic within 1 hour, 77 patients were symptomatic within 5 hours, and 85 patients were symptomatic within 15 hours. Of their cohort, 32% were not symptomatic within the first hour and would not have needed immediate medical attention. Therefore, approximately one out of three whiplash-injured individuals in this study would potentially not have a police report associated with their injury.

Several studies have reported damage thresholds for various vehicles (for front- or rear-end impacts). For example, Szabo and Welcher (18) found that 1981 to 1983 Ford Escorts could withstand multiple impacts at 16.1 kph without sustaining damage. Bailey et al. (2) reported the damage thresholds for a 1980 Toyota Tercel, a 1977 Honda Civic, a 1980 Chevrolet Citation, and a 1981 Ford Escort as 13.0 kph, 13.2 kph, 13.5 kph, and 16.4 kph, respectively.

Wooley et al. (20) tested a 1979 Pontiac Grand Prix, a 1979 Ford E-150 van, a 1978 Honda Accord, a 1979 Ford F-250 pick-up, a 1983 Ford Thunderbird, and a 1989 Chevrolet Citation and reported damage thresholds at 15.9 kph, 15.9 kph, 17.7 kph, 18.8 kph, 19.5 kph, and 20.4 kph, respectively.

The rate of injury for accidents occurring at velocity changes of less than 15.0 kph was reported to be 36% by Foret-Bruno et al. (5). Olsson et al. (12) found that 18% of injuries occurred at velocity changes of less than 10.0 kph, and that 60% of injuries occurred between 10.0 and 20.0 kph. It is reasonable to conclude from these data that a substantial proportion of whiplash injuries occur in accidents in which there is little or no structural damage.

It is not readily apparent from the literature whether the approximately one third of whiplash-injured individuals who have delayed symptom onset are a subpopulation of the more than one third of whiplash-injured individuals who were injured at subvehicular-damage speeds. However, it is reasonable to assume that the police record criterion for cohort inclusion eliminates a significant minority of whiplash-injured individuals. This unstudied subpopulation may have a different history of chronicity than the cohort that was studied, resulting in study results that are difficult to interpret and that lack external validity.

Selection Bias

The retrospective cohort study design utilized in the Schrader et al. (16) study calls for the assembly of a cohort that has been exposed to a biologically credible causative agent, followed by examination of the subjects of the cohort for the presence of the disease thought to be linked to the exposure. To track the natural progression of a disease from acute to chronic, the selection criteria must primarily include the existence of the disease in its acute form. Yet the authors of this study used exposure to an automobile accident for their inclusion criterion, not the presence of acute whiplash. To use involvement in an automobile accident for a selection criterion, Schrader et al. (16) needed to first establish the nature of the relationship between automobile accidents and acute neck injuries. If the relationship was very weak, then a history of an automobile accident would not be a reliable predictor of an acute neck injury, and it would be an even poorer predictor of a possible chronic sequela of the acute injury.

When the accident-exposed cohort was examined for subjects who had been exposed to acute whiplash, we found that only 15% (31 of 202) of this cohort gave any indication of neck pain after their accident. We rejected 22 of the 31 who had neck pain for less than a week, because, by any definition, this is an atypically brief recovery time for a whiplash injury, and these individuals could not be considered at risk for chronic symptoms. Further, using a typical definition of what constitutes a primary risk factor for the development of late whiplash [i.e., persistent symptoms arising from an acute whiplash injury that has not resolved after 6 months or more (14)], we would then have to reject seven of the remaining nine subjects who became asymptomatic within 1 month. This leaves two subjects (1%) who were probably appropriate for selection for the exposed cohort.

From this analysis, it is evident that in Kaunas, Lithuania, an automobile accident is a very poor predictor of acute neck injury, and, thus, chronic neck pain. As a result, the authors' conclusions about this cohort relating to the natural progression of late whiplash are invalid as a result of severe and fatal selection bias.

Methodologic Flaws in the Quebec Task Force Study on Whiplash-Associated Disorders

Selection Bias

Aside from potential bias from the use of police records to identify whiplash-injured individuals for the QTF cohort study, substantial selection bias was introduced into the study by including only whiplash-injured individuals who drew compensation for time lost from work. Additionally, individuals who had any diagnosis in addition to neck strain (e.g., neck strain and lumbar strain), were eliminated from the analysis of injury recurrence. The resulting subpopulation that was ultimately studied comprised only 35% of an already biased subpopulation of whiplash-injured individuals. The results of such a study are virtually meaningless because the study population is so highly selected.

The QTF further erred when they compared the results of their cohort study to those of other authors. Because the study population is so selected, lack of generalizability (external validity) in the QTF cohort study prohibits meaningful comparison with other studies.

Improper Use of Terminology

The Results and Discussion section of the cohort study (section 6, pages 5 to 15) contains numerous references to the percentage of the study population "recovered" at the time of cessation of compensation. However, the QTF did not gather any data regarding the symptoms, level of treatment, or functional impairment of their cohort, all factors necessary to determine the level of recovery after an injury. The QTF chose to define *recovery* unconventionally as cessation of compensation. Not surprisingly, the QTF found that 87% and 97% of their cohort were "recovered" at 6 and 12 months after the accident, respectively. To refer to these individuals as "recovered" is misrepresentative of the data collected.

Unsupported Conclusions and Recommendations

The QTF set out to use what they termed the "preeminence of evidence" to develop their guidelines and recommendations. Yet they made the following unsupported statements in their Recommendations and Conclusions section: "Whiplash-associated disorders are usually self-limited," "Patients should be reassured that most WAD are benign and self-limiting," "All interventions . . . should be accompanied by reassurance about the favorable prognosis," "The key message to the WAD patient is that the pain is not harmful, is usually short-lived," and "most incidents of WAD are self-limited, involving temporary discomfort and rarely resulting in permanent harm."

These conclusions are misrepresentative of the literature that the QTF reviewed.

In the text in table 5.3.4.4 labeled "Prevalence of symptoms at follow-up," the four studies on prognosis that were accepted for review are listed along with their findings. These included Norris and Watt (11), who found that 66% of their cohort had neck pain at an average of 2 years after injury; Radanov et al. (13), who found that 27% of their cohort were symptomatic 6 months after the accident, and who, in another study 2 years later (15), reported that 27% of their cohort had headaches 6 months after the accident; and Hildingsson and Toolanen (8), who found 44% of their cohort symptomatic at an average of 2 years after the accident.

The terms *self-limited, short-lived,* and *temporary discomfort* are not applicable to the cohorts that were studied in the literature the QTF deemed acceptable for review. Nor do they apply to the injuries studied in the QTF cohort study, as the QTF did not gather evidence regarding actual recovery rates. As a result, it is reasonable to state that some of the most crucial and oft-repeated conclusions and recommendations of the QTF are not supported by their research, making this section of the publication speculative, at best.

CONCLUSION

The issue of greatest concern surrounding these two publications is not that they are methodologically flawed, but that this fact has gone unrecognized by the popular press and in the medical literature, and that they continue to be viewed as landmark studies in the field of whiplash. In reality, these two studies have only acted to obscure the true nature of chronic whiplash.

Chronic symptoms resulting from whiplash, or late whiplash, is a complex subject requiring extensive study. The epidemiology of the condition defies phraseology such as short-lived or all in the head. Such characterizations do little to comfort the patient with chronic pain after a whiplash injury. Only carefully designed, powerful, population-based studies will allow a more complete understanding of the condition, and, in doing so, limit speculation on the subject.

REFERENCES

1. Altman LK. Whiplash treatments found to be ineffective. *New York Times* 1995;May 2, section C:1,6.
2. Bailey MN, Wong BC, Lawrence JM. Data and methods for estimating the severity of minor impacts. Society of Automotive Engineers Technical Paper Series 1995;950352:139–174.
3. Balla JI. The late whiplash syndrome. *Aust NZJ Surg* 1980;50:610–614.
4. Deans GT, Magalliard JN, Kerr M, Rutherford WH. Neck sprain—a major cause of disability following car accidents. *Injury* 1987;18:10–12.
5. Foret-Bruno JY, Dauvilliers F, Tarriere C. Influence of the seat and head rest stiffness on the risk of cervical injuries. *Proceedings of the 13th international technical conference on experimental safety vehicles.* 1991;S-8-W-19:968–974.
6. Gagne S. Conversation with Officer Sylvain Gagne of the Quebec Police Department, July 15, 1996.
7. Gotten N. Survey of one hundred cases of whiplash after settlement of litigation. *JAMA* 1956;162(9):865–867.
8. Hildingsson C, Toolanen G. Outcome after soft-tissue injury of the cervical spine. A prospective study of 93 car-accident victims. q*Acta Orthopod Scand* 1990;61:357–359.
9. Kischka U, Ettlin T, Heim S, Schmid G. Cerebral symptoms following whiplash. *Eur Neurol* 1991;31(3): 136–140.
10. Larder DR, Twiss MK, Mackay GM. Neck injury to car occupants using seat belts. *Proceedings of the 29th annual meeting of the American Association for Automobile Medicine* 1985:153–165.
11. Norris SH, Watt I. The prognosis of neck injuries resulting from rear-end vehicle collisions. *J Bone Joint Surg Br* 1983;65:608–611.
12. Olsson I, Bunketorp O, Carlsson G, et al. An in-depth study of neck injuries in rear end collisions. 1990 International IRCOBI Conference, Bron, Lyon, France. 1990;Sept 12–14:1–15.
13. Radanov BP, Di Stefano G, Schnidrig A, Sturzenegger M, Augistiny KF. Cognitive functioning after common whiplash. *Lancet* 1991;338:712–715.
14. Radanov BP, Sturzenegger M, Stefano GD. Long-term outcome after whiplash injury: a two-year follow-up considering features of injury mechanism and somatic, radiologic, and psychosocial factors. *Medicine* 1995;74(5): 281–297.
15. Radanov BP, Sturzenegger M, Di Stefano G, Schnidrig A, Aljinovic M. Factors influencing recovery from headache after common whiplash. *Br Med J* 1993;307:652–655.
16. Schrader H, Obelieniene D, Bovim G, et al. Natural evolution of late whiplash syndrome outside the medicolegal context. *Lancet* 1996;347:1201–1211.
17. Spitzer WO, Skovron ML, Salmi LR, Cassidy JD, Duranceau J, Suissa S, Zeiss E. Scientific monograph of the Quebec Task Force on Whiplash-Associated Disorders: redefining whiplash and its management. *Spine* 1995; 20(8S):1S–73S.
18. Szabo TJ, Welcher J. Dynamics of low speed crash tests with energy absorbing bumpers. Society of Automotive Engineers Technical Paper Series 1992;921573:1–9.
19. Schoene M, ed. Traffic accidents are rarely the cause of persistant whiplash symptoms, says groundbreaking new study. *The backletter.* 1996;11(6):61–69.
20. Wooley RL, Strother CE, James MB. Rear stiffness coefficients derived from barrier test data. Society of Automotive Engineers Inernational Congress, Detroit, MI 1991:910120.

SECTION 4

Treatment Modalities

Whiplash Injuries: Current Concepts in Prevention, Diagnosis, and Treatment of the Cervical Whiplash Syndrome, edited by Robert Gunzburg and Marek Szpalski. Lippincott–Raven Publishers, Philadelphia © 1998.

17

Emergency Care and Surgery for Whiplash Injuries to the Cervical Spine

H. Michael Mayer

H. M. Mayer: Department of Orthopaedic Surgery, Free University of Berlin, Berlin, Germany.

There is general agreement that the outcome of treatment in patients with whiplash injuries to the cervical spine strongly depends on the initial medical care. Especially in patients with severe trauma to the cervical spine associated with neurologic deficit, the prevention of further lesions to the damaged neural tissue is paramount. Although emergency care for the patient suffering from spinal cord injury has been optimized in the industrial countries, about 30% of patients suffering from spinal cord injury expire before they reach the hospital (4,5,12,14).

Thus, the critical period of patient management does not start at the emergency room but at the accident scene, and it includes the transport period as well as postemergency care in the hospital.

In traumatic instabilities of the cervical spine, the indications for surgical intervention have been well defined for the different types of bony and/or ligamentous lesions. However, the timing of surgery as well as the surgical approaches and techniques are still a matter of debate.

This chapter describes the general principles of emergency care in patients with severe whiplash injuries as well as the surgical strategies which are applied at the Department of Orthopaedic Surgery of the Free University of Berlin.

INITIAL MANAGEMENT IN CERVICAL SPRAIN SYNDROME

The majority of whiplash injuries to the cervical spine result from car accidents (7). About 66% of the accidents are rear collisions and rear–head-on collisions resulting in the typical hyperflexion–hyperextension movement of the cervical spine that may also be associated with a rotational component. This chain of nonphysiologic motions can lead to different types of injury in different regions of the cervical spine affecting different anatomic structures (1,8,9). More than 80% of these accidents result in more or less severe soft-tissue injuries without involvement of the bony structures. In only 13% do they lead to fractures with or without neurologic deficit (8,9). The mildest clinical forms are known as cervical sprain syndrome (10) (Table 1). The clinical symptoms consist mainly of neck pain, stiffness, and muscle spasms (62% to 100%), headaches (up to 82%), back pain (35% to 42%), paraesthesias of the upper extremities (up to

TABLE 1. *Symptoms in cervical sprain syndrome*

Symptom	Frequency (%)
Neck pain, stiffness, muscle spasms	62–100
Headaches	Up to 82
Back pain	35–42
Paraesthesias upper extremities	Up to 45
Dysphagia	7–18
Neurologic deficits	12–20

From Cabbell K, Papadopoulos SM. Whiplash syndrome. In: Menezes AH, Sonntag VKH, eds. *Principles of spinal surgery.* New York: McGraw-Hill, 1996;801–806; LaRocca H. Cervical sprain syndrome. In: Frymoyer JW, ed. *The adult spine: principles and practice.* New York: Raven Press, 1991;1051–1061; and McAfee PC. Cervical spine trauma. In: Frymoyer JW, ed. *The adult spine: principles and practice.* New York: Raven Press, 1991;1063–1106.

45%), dysphagia (7% to 18%), and neurologic disturbances (12% to 20%) (3,10). The aims of initial management are pain reduction, prevention of deterioration, and the exclusion of severe pathology such as fractures or ligamentous instabilities. After a thorough clinical–neurologic examination, anteroposterior (AP) and lateral x-rays should be performed, as well as odontoid views when trauma to the upper cervical spine is suspected. The cervicothoracic junction (C7) must be seen on the radiograph. In case of technical difficulties, a computed tomography (CT) scan of C7-T1 may be necessary to exclude any lesion in this anatomic region. If there are no obvious signs of severe ligamentous or bony pathology, symptomatic therapy can be started. Pain reduction is achieved with the application of a soft collar and the administration of analgesics as well as nonsteroidal anti-inflammatory drugs. Moreover, physical therapy such as hot-packs or ultrasound may be helpful. Chiropractic manipulations should be strictly avoided.

INITIAL MANAGEMENT OF SEVERE WHIPLASH-TYPE CERVICAL SPINE INJURIES

Accident Scene

Initial management (Table 2) is determined by the type and the severity of the lesion to the cervical spine and spinal cord, as well as by associated injuries. This information is usually not available on arrival at the accident scene. However, if a cervical spine injury with or without associated injuries is suspected, initial management concentrates on (a) the preservation of life, (b) the prevention of further insult to the spine and spinal cord, (c) the preservation of vital and spinal functions, and (d) the definition of pathology. The accident scene management consists of steps 1 to 3. After initial evaluation, the vital functions must be preserved. This may include the application of oxygen, the prevention of aspiration, and intubation. Because the latter often requires manipulation of the cervical spine, all accident victims must be assumed to have an unstable spine and/or a spinal cord lesion until proven otherwise (use caution with unconscious patients with associated head injuries). Aspiration is prevented with only slight manual traction and chin lift. For intubation, either the nasotracheal route or the awake translaryngeal route may be prefer-

TABLE 2. *Initial management of whiplash injury*

Accident scene

Initial evaluation
Preservation of life
Oxygen
Prevention of aspiration (slight manual traction, chin lift)
Intubation routes
  Nasotracheal
  Orotracheal (use caution with hyperextension–hyperflexion)
  Awake translaryngeal
Avoid cricothyroidotomy
Therapy for shock symptoms
Methylprednisolone [according to NASCIS II (2)]
Secure patient (sandbags, tape, backboard)
Head-to-toe secondary evaluation

Attention: The cervical spine is assumed to be unstable until proven otherwise! All patients with head injuries are assumed to have spinal cord injury until proven otherwise!

Transport

Secure immobilization of the spine/patient
Prevent or treat regurgitation/aspiration
Preserve vital parameters

Emergency room

Preservation of vital and specific functions
  Cardiovascular system
  Urinary system
  Pulmonary system
  Gastrointestinal system (nasogastric tube)
  Prophylaxis of venous thromboembolism
  Emotional support
Definition of spine pathology

From Chesnut RM, Marshal LF. Early assessment, transport, and management of patients with post-traumatic spinal instability. In: Cooper PR, ed. *Management of posttraumatic spinal instability.* Park Ridge, IL: American Association of Neulogical Surgeons, 1990;1–17.

able. Cricothyroidotomy should be avoided so as not to interfere with possible anterior surgical approaches to the cervical spine. Therapy for shock syndrome and the administration of steroids to prevent secondary damage to the spinal cord follow the rules according to the results of the U.S. National Acute Spinal Cord Injury Study (NASCIS II) (2,15,16).

The patient then should be secured "as he lies" with sandbags placed alongside the head and neck (fixed with tape) and should be prepared for transport. Fixation of the patient on a backboard is advisable.

TRANSPORT

The preparation of the patient for transport should be so as to avoid the possibility of the immobilization device breaking free during car or helicopter transport. Besides immobilization, the avoidance of regurgitation and aspiration is paramount on the way to the hospital. Facilities needed to treat regurgitation and to prevent aspiration should be available in the transport medium.

EMERGENCY ROOM

The general management after arrival in the hospital aims to maintain the vital functions, to rule out other injuries, and to initiate specific diagnosis and therapy for the cervical trauma. The exclusion of other injuries includes a trauma skeletal x-ray series, abdominal ultrasound or CT scan, and a diagnostic peritoneal lavage. Head injury is ruled out by CT scan of the skull and brain. General care also includes immobilization in a special bed (e.g., Stryker Frame or Rotobed), pulmonary care, a nasogastric tube, a Foley catheter, and deep venous thrombosis prophylaxis. In the conscious patient with an obvious severe neurologic deficit, emotional support should begin immediately, as it influences all subsequent diagnostic and therapeutic measures. Under specific management, the exact diagnosis as well as the underlying pathology must then be established.

In conscious patients without neurologic deficit, radiographs of the cervical spine (AP, lateral, and odontoid views) are obtained. If they are normal despite considerable clinical neck pain, pillar and oblique views are performed. If there is no fracture, the patient receives a hard collar. After 24 to 48 hours under analgesic and anti-inflammatory medication, flexion–extension views are obtained and magnetic resonance imaging (MRI) is performed to rule out ligamentous injury and instability. If the radiographic series ascertains a fracture, a CT scan or MRI is performed to define the fracture type.

In patients with neurologic deficits, the diagnosis, the definition, and the level of the underlying pathology must be enforced by the various imaging techniques mentioned. Special interest should be concentrated on the cervicothoracic junction and the thoracic spine.

EMERGENCY SURGERY

A considerable number of severe whiplash injuries result in fractures or ligamentous lesions that are associated with segmental instability or deformity. A variety of lesions at different anatomic regions of the cervical spine can result from whiplash mechanisms (12). The goals of any surgical intervention are always the restoration of normal anatomy and stability, the prevention of neurologic deficits, or the promotion of neurologic recovery. This is achieved by surgical realignment, decompression, and fixation and fusion techniques.

The general principles of emergency treatment are early reduction (before the CT scan) in cases of fracture–dislocations proven by radiograph. In the majority of dislocated fractures or subluxations, these goals can be achieved by early manual reduction with or without the help of traction devices (e.g., Halo-rings, Gardner-Wells tongs, Crutchfield tongs) of which the principles, indications, contraindications, and hazards are well described (5). They should result in neutral anatomic positioning in which the patient should be immobilized by sandbags, collars, or a halo until the decision for definitive treatment has been made. In all cases of unstable spine or neurologic deficits, the patient should be referred to the intensive care unit (ICU).

The indication for emergency surgery is driven by anatomic and functional parameters (Table 3). If associated injuries and the general condition of the patient allow surgical intervention, this should be performed as early as possible in all cases of spinal cord or root compression caused by bone fragments, hematoma, or ruptured intervertebral disc material. Emergency surgery is also indicated in all cases of irreducible fracture–dislocations such as uni- or bilateral interlocked facet fracture–dislocations. It is also indicated

TABLE 3. *Indications for emergency surgery in severe whiplash injury*

Based on underlying pathology
Spinal cord compression caused by
Bone fragments
Hematoma
Ruptured disc material
Unreducible fracture–dislocation
Uni- or bilateral facet block
Open or penetrating injuries

Based on clinical function
Impaired but residual neurologic function below level of injury
Deterioration of neurologic symptoms
Complete or incomplete neurologic deficits at C5-C6

in all types of open or penetrating injuries to the cervical spine. The surgical technique depends on the fracture type as well as on the individual treatment philosophy of the spine center involved (see Chapters 24 through 26 on surgical techniques).

Impaired but residual neurologic function below the level of a subluxation, and deterioration of neurologic symptoms, are absolute indications for early surgical intervention. This is also true for complete or incomplete neurologic deficit close to the "key segment" C4 (note: ventilation).

Even if it has not been proven scientifically that improvement of neurologic deficits or cervical function is significantly influenced by emergency, or at least early, surgical intervention, it has been shown recently that general complications such as deep venous thrombosis as well as pulmonary complications can be decreased significantly if early surgical intervention (i.e., less than 72 hours after the accident) is performed in cervical trauma associated with neurologic deficits (13). Moreover, hospital stay, ICU stay, days of required mechanical ventilation, and overall costs can be significantly reduced (2,6,11,13,15).

Except for the situations previously mentioned, it is rarely necessary to operate for cervical trauma on an emergency basis, and we are very reluctant to perform surgery within 72 hours, except to avoid secondary complications.

REFERENCES

1. Braakman R. Mechanisms of injury. In: Findlay G, Owen R, eds. *Surgery of the spine.* Oxford: Blackwell Scientific, 1992;989–998.
2. Bracken MD, Shepard MJ, Collins WF, et al. Methylprednisolone or naloxone treatment after acute spinal cord injury: one year follow-up data. Results of the second National Acute Spinal Cord Injury Study. *J Neurosurg* 1992;76:23–31.
3. Cabbell K, Papadopoulos SM. Whiplash syndrome. In: Menezes AH, Sonntag VKH, eds. *Principles of spinal surgery.* New York: McGraw-Hill, 1996;801–806.
4. Chesnut RM, Marshal LF. Early assessment, transport, and management of patients with posttraumatic spinal instability. In: Cooper PR, ed. *Management of posttraumatic spinal instability.* Park Ridge, IL: American Association of Neulogical Surgeons, 1990;1–17.
5. Cooper PR. Stabilization of fractures and subluxations of the lower cervical spine. In: Cooper PR, ed. *Management of posttraumatic spinal instability.* Park Ridge, IL: American Association of Neulogical Surgeons, 1990; 111–133.
6. Duh MS, Bracken MD, Shepard MJ, Wilberger JE. Surgical treatment of spinal cord injury—The National Acute Spinal Cord Injury Study II experience. Presented at the annual meeting of the American Association of Neurological Surgeons. Boston, April 1993 (abst).

7. Dvořák J, Panjabi MN, Gerber M, Wichmann W. CT-functional diagnostics of the rotatory instability of upper cervical spine. *Spine* 1987;12:197–205.
8. Dvořák J, Valach L. Cervical spine injuries in Switzerland. *J Manual Med* 1989;4:7–16.
9. Dvořák J. Soft tissue injuries of the cervical spine. In: Findlay G, Owen R, eds. *Surgery of the spine.* Oxford: Blackwell Scientific, 1992;1037–1042.
10. LaRocca H. Cervical sprain syndrome. In: Frymoyer JW, ed. *The adult spine: principles and practice.* New York: Raven Press, 1991;1051–1061.
11. Levi L, Wolf A, Rigamonti D, et al. Anterior decompression and cervical spine trauma: does the timing of surgery affect the outcome? *Neurosurgery* 1991;29:216–222.
12. McAfee PC. Cervical spine trauma. In: Frymoyer JW, ed. *The adult spine: principles and practice.* New York: Raven Press, 1991;1063–1106.
13. Schlegel J, Bayley J, Yuan H, Fredricksen B. Timing of surgical decompression and fixation of acute spinal fractures. *J Orthop Trauma* 1996;10:323–330.
14. Sonntag VKH, Hadley MN. Management of nonodontoid upper cervical spine injuries. In: Cooper PR, ed. *Management of posttraumatic spinal instability.* Park Ridge, IL: American Association of Neulogical Surgeons, 1990; 99–110.
15. Wilberger JE. Diagnosis and management of spinal cord trauma. *J Neurotrauma* 1991;8:S521–S530.
16. Wilberger JE. Acute spinal cord injury. In: Menezes AH, Sonntag VKH, eds. *Principles of spinal surgery.* New York: McGraw-Hill, 1996;753–767.

Whiplash Injuries: Current Concepts in
Prevention, Diagnosis, and Treatment
of the Cervical Whiplash Syndrome,
edited by Robert Gunzburg and Marek Szpalski.
Lippincott–Raven Publishers, Philadelphia © 1998.

18

Pharmacologic Interventions in Whiplash-Associated Disorders

Marek Szpalski, Robert Gunzburg, Mireille Soeur, Georges Bauherz,
Jean-Pierre Hayez, and Françoise Michel

*M. Szpalski, J.-P. Hayez and F. Michel: Department of Orthopaedic Surgery,
Centre Hospitalier Molière Longchamp, Brussels, Belgium.
R. Gunzburg: Department of Orthopaedics, Centenary Clinic,
Antwerp, Belgium.
M. Soeur and G. Bauherz: Department of Neurology, Centre Hospitalier
Molière Longchamp, Brussels, Belgium.*

Surprisingly, very little has been published about pharmacologic interventions, whether locally or generally administered, in acute or chronic whiplash disorders. Furthermore, true controlled studies are even rarer. This chapter will review the current literature on the subject and present the first placebo-controlled study of the effect of a nonsteroidal anti-inflammatory drug (NSAID). In this study, assessment was performed with a pain scale and with an objective measure of neck function.

LOCALLY ADMINISTERED PHARMACOLOGIC INTERVENTIONS

There are few if any studies published dealing with epidural or intrathecal injections of corticosteroids or any other drug, or with topical treatments.

Intraarticular Steroids

A controlled double-blind study was reported by Barnsley et al. (1) on 41 patients presenting chronic zygapophyseal pain after automobile accidents. The mean duration of symptoms was 39 months. Patients were randomly assigned to receive intraarticular injections of bupivacaine or betamethasone. The median time for a return to a pain level equal to 50% of the pretreatment pain level was 3.5 days in the anesthetic group and 3 days in the corticosteroid group. This difference was minimal and statistically not significant. The authors concluded that betamethasone injection certainly did not appear to be an effective treatment. They also hypothesized that the beneficial effect in some patients might be caused by the stretching of the capsule, irrespective of the nature of the injected product. Interestingly, similar results have been reported for lumbar facet joint injections (8).

Intracutaneous and Subcutaneous Sterile Water Injections

While not strictly speaking a pharmacologic intervention, we feel that sterile water injection therapy may, nevertheless, be discussed in this chapter. The use of intracutaneous sterile water injections over the sacrum has been described as effective for relieving low back pain during labor and urolithiasis attack (12).

Byrn et al. studied (2,3) the intracutaneous injection and subcutaneous injection (the latter being more bearable by patients) in trigger points, tender to pressure, in patients with chronic pain after whiplash from car accidents. Pressure on trigger points provokes tenderness and a radiating effect. The trigger points appear to correlate with pain and dysfunction in whiplash patients (17).

In their preliminary uncontrolled study (2) on a small number of subjects, the authors found that intracutaneous injections were dramatically effective. They then conducted a controlled study (3) comparing subcutaneous sterile water with saline solution in 40 patients. Although controlled, this study was not a true double-blind assessment, because of the patients' painful reaction to the injection of sterile water. The authors found improved benefit of sterile water at 3 months for pain score, mobility, and self-assessment of improvement. At 8 months, there was a more limited effect on minimum pain score and mobility, but not on maximum pain score and self-assessment of improvement.

It appears that sterile water injections at trigger points may have a certain efficacy in whiplash-associated pain. However, it is associated with severe immediate pain.

GENERALLY ADMINISTERED PHARMACOLOGIC INTERVENTIONS

Intravenous Corticosteroids in the Acute Phase

Corticosteroids have a neuroprotective effect (13). Petterssen (14) conducted a randomized double-blind study of the effect of high dose methylprednisolone administered intravenously in the very early phase of whiplash injuries. Forty patients seen within 8 hours of injury were included in the study and randomized to receive either methylprednisolone (30 mg/kg bolus followed by 5.4 mg/kg/hr) or placebo during a 24-hour infusion. The presence of disabling symptoms and duration of sick-leave periods were used as assessment criteria.

At the 6-month follow-up, there was a significant difference in favor of the corticosteroids group for all the measured parameters.

This study shows that this very early intervention may be beneficial in the long term for reducing disabling symptoms and work incapacity. However, patients must be seen very early after the accident, and often the complaints do not appear for 24 to 48 hours.

Orally Administered Drugs

We did not find (and neither did the Quebec Task Force) any studies on the use of myorelaxant or antidepressant drugs for whiplash. No study has been conducted on the effect of analgesics or NSAIDs in either the acute or the chronic phase of whiplash-associated disorders. The use of these drugs associated with other treatment modalities has shown a limited efficacy in the acute phase of whiplash (5,6,9,10). However, because of the associated treatment it is not possible to determine the real effect of the pharmacologic intervention by itself. There is a need for controlled studies of pharmacologic intervention in acute whiplash.

THE TENOXICAM CONTROLLED STUDY

It has been shown that early mobilization and return to activity are highly beneficial in whiplash-associated disorders (9,11). Furthermore, studies have shown that in terms of the psychological and psychosocial components of whiplash injuries (16), the early suffering and impairment of function may perhaps affect the later feeling of sickness behavior. Therefore, it is of interest whether an early and easy pharmacologic intervention may have an effect on pain and function in the acute phase, helping earlier and faster return to activity. Furthermore, the pain score seems to be a useful indicator of prognosis (9).

We have conducted a controlled double-blind study to assess the effect of tenoxicam, an NSAID with a long duration of action on pain and motion in the early phase of whiplash injuries. NSAIDs have been chosen as they allow an easy single daily intake, which improves patient compliance (7).

Materials and Methods

Patients

Fifty-one patients presenting with whiplash injuries less than 72 hours after the accident were included in the study. All were classified as groups I and II on the Quebec Task Force scale. All underwent cervical spine and skull x-ray to exclude fracture or dislocation, which were exclusion criteria. Other exclusion criteria were pregnancy or lactation, history of hypersensitivity to NSAIDs, history of gastrointestinal ulceration, and current treatment with NSAIDs or anticoagulant drugs.

Methods

The study followed randomized, double-blind, parallel groups, using a comparative study design. There were 25 patients allocated to the tenoxicam group (group T), and 26 to the placebo group (group P). The groups were similar in terms of demographic characteristics (Table 1).

Patients were given 20 mg a day of tenoxicam or placebo administered as a single dose taken in the morning for 14 days. Pain was assessed with a horizontal, 10-cm visual analog scale (VAS) which was simple and effective to administer (15). The VAS score was assessed on day 1 and on day 15.

The assessment of function was realized with a three-dimensional motion-measuring device, the CA 6000 Spine Motion Analyzer (Orthopaedics Systems Inc., Hayward, CA) (Fig. 1). The device consists of a linkage system with six high-precision potentiometers connected by a series of seven bars. The system allows unrestricted three-dimensional motion. The device is linked to an IBM-compatible computer through a 12-bit

TABLE 1. *Demographics of the patients in the tenoxicam group (T) and the placebo group (P)*

	Group P	Group T
Men	7	9
Women	18	17
Mean age ± SD	35.1 ± 9.6	37.8 ± 10.2

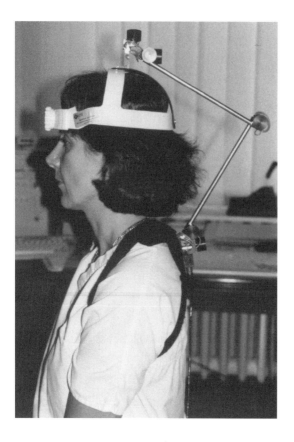

FIG. 1. CA 6000 device attached to a patient.

analog/digital converter board. It enables the measurement of ranges of motion, and velocities and accelerations at a sampling rate of 100 Hz. The reliability and validity of the system has been established previously (4).

Patients were assessed on day 1 and day 15. Maximum range of motion (degrees) in the three planes (sagittal, frontal, and transverse) as well as velocity (degrees/sec) and acceleration (degrees/sec^2) were recorded (Fig. 2).

Results

Two patients, both in the tenoxicam group, were lost to follow-up. No patient presented with any side effect leading to exclusion from the study. Thus, 49 patients (25 in the placebo group, 24 in the tenoxicam group) were included in the final analysis.

VAS Pain Assessment

The results of the VAS readings are shown in Table 2. The Student's *t* test was used to analyze improvement in the two groups. Both groups showed a highly significant improvement during the study period. However, there appears to be a significant differ-ence (p = .034) between the two treatments in favor of the NSAID.

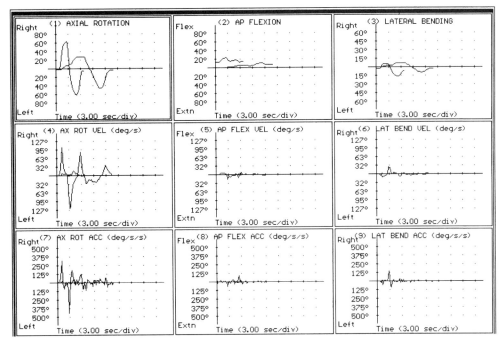

FIG. 2. Graphs of position, velocity, and acceleration for one patient, before and after treatment. The left column shows values for the principal axis of motion (in this case, rotation) and the other graphs represent the secondary axis of motion (flexion–extension and lateral flexion).

Function Assessment

The results are expressed as percentage improvements between day 1 and day 15 (Table 3). A Student's *t* test was used to analyze those results, because those percentages showed a normal distribution pattern.

Here, also, both groups show a very significant improvement of function between day 1 and day 15. However, the results showed a significant difference in favor of the tenoxicam group for all variables except extension velocity and rotation acceleration. Those differences were most marked for the measures of acceleration.

DISCUSSION

Both groups showed a favorable evolution during the study period for the measure of pain (VAS) as well as for the measure of function. This confirms that the natural history of whiplash injuries has a relatively favorable evolution.

TABLE 2. *Visual analog scale (VAS) measurements of pain in the tenoxicam group (T) and the placebo group (P) over time*

	Group P (mean ± SD)	Group T (mean ± SD)
Day 1	4.95 ± 1.22	5.58 ± 1.09
Day 15	2.95 ± 1.23	2.06 ± 1.15

TABLE 3. *Percentage improvement (mean ± SD) in functions after 15 days of tenoxicam (T) or placebo (P)*

Function		Group T	Group P	Significance
Range of motion	Flexion	136 ± 18.4	116.5 ± 15.1	$p < .05$
	Extension	127 ± 28.1	111.8 ± 24.9	$p < .05$
	Rotation	127.2 ± 17.5	105.8 ± 14.6	$p < .01$
	Lateral flexion	136.6 ± 27	120.4 ± 25.9	$p < .05$
Velocity	Flexion	109.7 ± 13.4	103.5 ± 15.2	ns
	Extension	154.8 ± 31.5	124.4 ± 27.8	$p < .01$
	Rotation	125.8 ± 27.1	114.5 ± 24.4	$p < .05$
	Lateral flexion	136.9 ± 25.4	116.5 ± 23.4	$p < .05$
Acceleration	Flexion	150.8 ± 33.2	124.5 ± 30.1	$p < .01$
	Extension	183.4 ± 36.2	136.2 ± 29.1	$p < .01$
	Rotation	119.4 ± 18.5	111.4 ± 13.9	ns
	Lateral flexion	145.2 ± 34.1	121.9 ± 26.5	$p < .01$

Nevertheless, it appears from our results that the use of tenoxicam, an NSAID, has a beneficial effect on pain and neck function in the acute phase of whiplash injuries. This has implications in the ability of patients to begin an early activation program, which has been shown to improve long-term outcome.

The marked effect on movement acceleration implies that the anti-inflammatory and analgesic effect is mostly effective on the movement starter, thus mostly helping the initial phase of the movement during position changes. This may have a favorable effect on the patients' feeling of their own pathology, reducing the impression of severity associated with restricted movement, which induces a poor functional status.

Whereas the influence of this treatment on long-term outcome has still to be investigated, it appears that an early anti-inflammatory treatment helps the patient move with less pain, enabling earlier and easier mobilization.

REFERENCES

1. Barnsley L, Lord SM, Wallis BJ, Bogduk N. Lack of effect of intraarticular corticosteroïds for chronic pain in the cervical zygoapophyseal joints. *N Engl J Med* 1994;330:1047–1050.
2. Byrn C, Borenstein P, Linder LE. Treatment of neck and shoulder pain in whip-lash syndrome patients with intracutaneous sterile water injections. *Acta Anaesthesiol Scand* 1991;35:52–53.
3. Byrn C, Olsson I, Falkheden L, et al. Subcutaneous sterile water injections for chronic neck and shoulder pain following whiplash injuries. *Lancet* 1993;341:449–452.
4. Dvořák J, Antinnes JA, Panjabi M, Loustalot D, Bonomo M. Age and gender related normal motion of the cervical spine. *Spine* 1992;17:S393–398.
5. Foley-Nolan D, Moore K, Codd M, et al. Low energy high frequency pulsed electromagnetic therapy for acute whiplash injuries. *Scand J Rehabil Med* 1992;24:51–59.
6. Foley-Nolan D, Barry C, Coughlan RJ, O'Connor P, Roden D. Pulsed high frequency electromagnetic therapy for persistent neck pain. A double blind placebo controlled study of 20 patients. *Orthopedics* 1990;13:445–451.
7. Gately MS. To be taken as directed. *J R Coll Gen Pract* 1968;16:39–42.
8. Lillius G, Laasonen EM, Myllynen P, Harilainen A, Gronlund G. Lumbar facet syndrome. A randomized clinical trial. *J Bone Joint Surg* 1989;71B:681–684.
9. McKinney LA. Early mobilisation and outcome in acute sprains of the neck. *Br Med J* 1989;299:1006–1008.
10. McKinney LA, Dornan JO, Ryan M. The role of physiotherapy in the management of acute neck sprains following road-traffic accidents. *Arch Emerg Med* 1989;6:27–33.
11. Mealy K, Brennan H, Fenelon GCC. Early mobilisation of acute whiplash injuries. *Br Med J* 1986;292:656–657.
12. Odent M. La réflexothérapie lombaire. Efficacité dans le traitement de la colique néphrétique et en analgésie obstétricale. *Nouv Presse Med* 1975;4:188.
13. Olmarker K, Byröd G, Cornefjord M, Nordborg C, Rydevik B. Effects of methyl-prednisolone on nucleus pulposus induced nerve root injury. *Spine* 1994;19:1803–1808.

14. Pettersson K. High dose methyl-prednisolone prevents extensive sick-leave after whiplash injury. Doctoral dissertation, University of Umea, 1996.
15. Scott J, Huskisson E. Graphic representation of pain. *Pain* 1976;2:175–185.
16. Schrader H, Obelienene D, Bovim G, et al. Natural evolution of late whiplash syndrome outside the medico-legal context. *Lancet* 1996;347:1207–1211.
17. Travell JG, Simons DG. Myofascial pain and dysfunction. In: *Myofascial pain and dysfunction. The triggerpoint manual.* Baltimore: Williams & Wilkins, 1983;44.

*Whiplash Injuries: Current Concepts in
Prevention, Diagnosis, and Treatment
of the Cervical Whiplash Syndrome,*
edited by Robert Gunzburg and Marek Szpalski.
Lippincott–Raven Publishers, Philadelphia © 1998.

19

Chronic Symptoms after Whiplash: A Cognitive Behavioral Approach

Pieter F. van Akkerveeken and Alexander A. Vendrig

*P. F. van Akkerveeken and A. A. Vendrig: Rug AdviesCentra Nederland B.V.,
Zeist, The Netherlands.*

The term whiplash is often used in the sense of a diagnosis. As has been discussed in previous chapters, however, it indicates merely a trauma mechanism. According to the Quebec Task Force on Whiplash-Associated Disorders (18), patients without neurologic signs, fractures, or dislocations have a simple neck sprain with muscle spasm secondary to soft-tissue injuries (grades 1 and 2). Therefore, one may expect healing within a couple of weeks. And indeed hospital-based prospective studies demonstrated that about two-thirds of all patients became free of symptoms within 2 years after the accident (5,7,10). Of these patients, 88% were free of symptoms within 2 months, but on the other hand, 86% of the patients who had still symptoms at 2 months after the trauma, still had symptoms at 2 years (10). Furthermore, 93% of patients who are symptom free at 3 months after the accident will still be free of symptoms 2 years later. These figures support the statement that the trauma in the majority of patients results in a simple physical lesion: a sprain of the neck (18).

The question arises, why do a number of patients become chronic sufferers? And, which mechanisms are involved in the process towards chronicity? It seems unlikely that physical pathology is causing this persistence of symptoms. Only in grade 3 and grade 4 lesions is this probably the case. In analogy with other types of chronic benign pain of the musculoskeletal system, the authors postulate that conditioning processes, in particular operant conditioning, play a role in the process towards chronicity. In these processes, the patient's health beliefs may also be significant. On the basis of these theories, a multidisciplinary team of the Rug AdviesCentra in Zeist, the Netherlands, consisting of an orthopedic surgeon, a psychologist, a physiotherapist, and an occupational therapist, developed a diagnostic protocol to assess a number of parameters. Following inclusion and exclusion criteria, patients were chosen and subsequently offered a cognitive behavioral program. This program was aimed at a functional restoration of the patient. The program was considered a success when the patient had regained his normal daily activities, including work.

To evaluate the efficacy of this program, a prospective study was set up. The outcome data of the program will be compared with Dutch and other statistics on whiplash-associated disorders.

In this chapter, we present the preliminary results of this study. First, however, the literature with respect to psychological factors and whiplash is reviewed, and the relationship of whiplash to psychophysiologic reactions (or somatizing), operant conditioning, and health beliefs is discussed.

FROM ACUTE TO CHRONIC SYMPTOMS

The question of whether or not psychological factors are involved in patients with chronic symptoms after whiplash trauma is loaded with speculations and contradictions. For most patients, however, the answer to this question is rather simple: "the symptoms started after the accident, and besides, before the accident I didn't have neck pain or problems with my memory. So the cause of my symptoms cannot be psychological." Also, for many patients the term *psychological* has the connotation of *not real* or *malingering,* implying that the patient may be blamed for the symptoms. Therefore, it is not surprising that many patients dislike an explanation of their chronic symptoms that takes into account psychological factors.

The question of whether or not psychological factors are involved in whiplash is not new. As early as 1953, Gay and Abbott (4) mentioned "neurotic reactions" in "common whiplash injuries." Hodge (6) went a step further: patients with chronic symptoms after whiplash trauma should have psychopathologic problems even before the accident. The accident offers some kind of solution for their preexisting neurosis. Others speak of "litigation neurosis" (11). In this concept, symptoms are exaggerated to receive secondary gain, particularly financial gain. Unfortunately, in early publications, psychopathologic issues have been poorly defined and most statements are based on speculations or retrospective descriptive data.

Recently, some attempts have been made to study prospectively the influence of psychological factors on the course of symptoms after whiplash trauma. Radanov and co-workers examined patients early after the accident. The assessment included psychological tests for personality, psychopathologic symptoms, and cognitive (neuropsychological) functioning. Those patients who improved (e.g., returned to work, reported fewer symptoms) were compared with respect to baseline data with those who did not improve. Their main finding was that neither personality traits nor psychopathologic symptoms measured at baseline predicted patients' functioning in any respect (pain symptoms, psychopathologic symptoms, cognitive functioning) at follow-up varying from 6 months to 2 years (14–17). Do these findings imply that psychological factors are not important for the development of chronic symptoms after whiplash trauma? The answer is no. Radanov and co-workers demonstrated only that neither psychopathology nor personality traits predicted the course of symptoms after the accident. But, theoretically, it is conceivable that other psychological factors or mechanisms, such as conditioning processes and the role of the patient's health beliefs, are significant in this respect.

To understand these other psychological factors, it is worthwhile to look at chronic back pain. A substantial body of research has been conducted over the past three decades on the relationship between psychological factors and chronic back pain, mainly inspired by the classic work of Fordyce (3), who developed the concept of operant pain behavior. Furthermore, based on this wealth of empirical research, so-called cognitive behavioral treatment programs have been developed and have turned out to be well studied and successful (2).

From several perspectives, three response systems have been described that may contribute to the experiencing of pain and other chronic symptoms. These are respondent reactions (also called psychophysiologic reactions, or somatizing), overt (operant) behavior, and cognitions (here meaning catastrophizing thoughts and health beliefs). With regard to whiplash, it is important to recognize these factors because they can exist without psychological symptoms. First, processes of somatizing, operant conditioning, and health beliefs will be discussed in general. Next, some suggestions will be made for how these processes can be recognized in patients with chronic symptoms after whiplash trauma. These suggestions are based on our clinical experience, because until now no empirical research on these factors in relation to whiplash-associated disorders has been published.

Somatizing

Patients may suffer an illness without a known disease as proven by careful medical examination according to the current state of knowledge. This discrepancy may be explained psychologically by the concept of somatizing. An example of extreme somatizing is the somatization disorder as described in the Diagnostic and Statistical Manual of Mental Disorders (DSM-IV). To consider this diagnosis, patients should have or should have had several somatic symptoms such as headache, gastrointestinal symptoms, and dizziness since early adulthood.

Tension headache is a well known example of "common" somatizing. Pathophysiologically, tension headache and neck pain seem to be the consequence of muscle spasm and abnormal vascular activity.

Similar mechanisms have been demonstrated in back pain patients who showed a higher paravertebral muscle activity when under emotional stress, for example speaking in public, but not under neutral stress situations, for example while performing arithmetic tasks (1).

Regarding acute whiplash, it may be speculated that the trapezius muscle reacts in a physiologic manner (with hypertonicity) to immobilize and protect the neck. This is indeed a normal protective reaction, as was demonstrated experimentally in the 1930s (15).

However, persisting hypertonicity is not functional and may result in pain. Pain may sensitize this system, which results in increasing muscle hyperactivity. Because of the interactions between pain and muscle activity, the patient finds him- or herself in a vicious circle. It may be speculated that patients with difficulties in coping with, for example, the whiplash-associated symptoms are more prone to be trapped in this vicious circle. However, this does not necessarily means that they have or develop psychological symptoms!

Operant Conditioning

The concept of pain behavior has been studied quite extensively in patients with chronic back pain. Pain behavior has been defined as the communication of pain (3) and also, in a broad sense, as all those actions that characterize chronic pain patients, also called illness behavior (12). Fordyce (3) stated that pain behavior, like all other behavior, increases if it is followed by some kind of reward (positive reinforcement) or by the avoidance of a negative agent (negative reinforcement). An example of negative reinforcement is the avoidance of physical activities that have resulted previously in an increase of pain. The patient has learned that these activities result in pain and will persist in avoiding them. Some authors speak in this context even of kinesiophobia (8).

Regarding whiplash-associated disorders, no attempts have been made yet to apply the concept of pain behavior. In our clinical experience with patients with chronic back pain and those with whiplash-associated symptoms, we observed pain behavior in both groups. There is one type of pain behavior in particular: many patients are afraid to use their neck, and by keeping their trapezius muscle tight, they rigidly fix their neck. They are not aware of doing this: it is an automatic reaction to their anxiety about the status of their neck. This behavior may reduce blood flow in the trapezius muscle, leading to a decrease of the muscle strength endurance and increase in pain (9).

Health Beliefs

Many types of behavior, including pain behavior, are the result of the ideas (or cognitions) people have. For example, a patient with chronic back pain who thinks that the pain is the result of some kind of disc pathology that may lead to paralysis, will act completely differently from a patient who thinks that the pain is merely the result of a simple muscle sprain. The former patient commonly believes that activity is harmful (21) and thus has to be avoided. This so-called fear-avoidance belief appears to be associated with a reduced behavioral performance in chronic back pain patients (20).

Regarding whiplash-associated disorders, it is, in our experience, very important to assess the cognition of patients about the nature of their symptoms. Do they think in terms of lesions or in terms of dysfunctions? And what have other health-care providers told them regarding the cause of their persisting symptoms? In our view, the "lesion view" does more harm than good because it induces several kinds of illness behavior, which creates new problems such as inactivity and loss of perspective, which may trigger depressive states, and so on.

PATIENT MANAGEMENT

Diagnostic Assessment

Patients are assessed in our institution multifactorially by a multidisciplinary team. The aim of this intake examination is to define mechanisms involved in the process towards chronicity and to compare patient characteristics with inclusion and exclusion criteria.

The assessment is set up as follows:

1. Orthopedic/neurologic medical specialist examination, to rule out a neurologic deficit or fracture–dislocation indicating a Quebec Task Force grade 3 or 4 lesion.

2. Radiologic examination consisting of plain radiographs including extension–flexion films, and, when in doubt, magnetic resonance imaging (MRI) to rule out physical pathology. Degenerative changes are considered coincidental findings.

3. Bicycle ergometry as a baseline measure for the operant physical training program. A submaximal protocol was used (13).

4. Psychological assessment, including an interview, the Minnesota Multiphasic Personality Inventory (MMPI), and pain drawing, to provide answers to the question of whether psychophysiologic reactions (somatizing) and operant conditioning are present, and to gain insight into the reinforcing factors in the latter, and, furthermore, to exclude psychopathology.

5. Neuropsychological screening (about 1.5 to 2 hours) is used to rule out neuropsychological disturbances. When findings indicate a possibility of a focal lesion, a complete assessment is performed later.

6. When patients have a job, reintegration in their work is a goal. Therefore, the work situation was evaluated by an occupational therapist, using a standard protocol to assess the physical and mental work load.

The inclusion criterion is persisting symptoms 3 months or longer after whiplash trauma.

The exclusion criteria are symptomatic pathology in the neck, psychopathology related to the problem, and gross neuropsychological deficits. Mild attention or memory problems were not regarded as an exclusion criteria.

The involvement of a lawyer is a relative exclusion criterion in the sense that an attempt was made to involve the lawyer in the problem-solving process. If the lawyer definitely refused and advised the patient accordingly, participation of that patient in a program is bound to be unsuccessful.

Patients generally had suffered a Quebec Task Force grade 1 or 2 lesion. Patients fulfilling the inclusion and exclusion criteria were subsequently offered a cognitive behavioral training program that included reintegration into their own work. Patients either agreed to participate or chose not to. Those who could not believe that anything could help them did not participate.

Cognitive Behavioral Training

The intervention program is based on cognitive and operant conditioning theories. It aims at a change of the cognition of the patient, in particular in the perception of the persisting nature of the symptoms in relation to the accident. Furthermore, the daily activity pattern of the patient is changed by operant conditioning techniques based on the graded activity principle of Fordyce (3): activities are set up in a weekly schedule on a time-contingent basis and not the pain-contingent basis that the patient has used since the accident. The program is given to a group of about six patients by a multidisciplinary team, which preferably also did the diagnostic assessment.

The program consists of three phases: a preparatory phase, an intensive phase, and a follow-up phase.

During the preparatory phase, two or three members of the team discuss with the patient and his or her partner the aims of the program, the set-up of the program, and practical points related to the program.

The intensive phase lasts 3 to 4 weeks, with four sessions a day from 9:30 AM till 5:30 PM, and the first aim is to change the belief system of the patient related to the symptoms. Patients are taught that pain should not be the guide for activities, and that chronic pain is not a warning sign indicating a need for rest. By using a graded activity build up on a time-contingent basis, patients experience that pain is not harmful and presents no danger or risk, although it is annoying and irritating. The patient is gradually weaned from pain killers and when they use a soft collar, it is worn on a time-contingent basis.

The partner must take part in the program for half a day per week: the partner must gain insight into the mechanisms involved in the chronicity of the symptoms. Besides, he or she can act as a reinforcer for healthy behavior!

The follow-up phase is aimed at checking functional progress of the patient, and it is also meant to provide guidance in the process of work reintegration. This includes at least one visit of the occupational therapist to the work site to discuss together with the patient matters with the company doctor and the supervisor or manager. When successful, the patient will be back to normal daily activities including full-time work in about 3 months after the start of the program. After that, a number of follow-up visits are made, the last 1 year after the intensive phase.

PRELIMINARY RESULTS OF AN ONGOING PROSPECTIVE STUDY

Method

Population

Patients with chronic symptoms after an extension-acceleration injury (whiplash) lasting 6 months or more were included in this study. Retrospectively, they should have a Quebec Task Force grade 1 or 2 lesion and should not display any symptoms or signs indicating a neurologic deficit, either in the physical examination or with imaging, including MRI.

Outcome Measures and Evaluation

Participants to the program were assessed before treatment, after treatment, and at follow-up 4 months after treatment. The most important criteria were those related to the daily functioning of the participants. Four objective, rather strict criteria were used to assess whether or not the participant met each of these criteria during these 4 months.

These criteria were (a) complete return to work, (b) no sick leave resulting from whiplash-related complaints, (c) no use of analgesics for whiplash-related complaints, and (d) no medical or paramedical treatment because of whiplash-related complaints.

Furthermore, the MMPI-2 and the Quebec Back Pain Disability Scale (Quebec BPDS) were administered. On the MMPI, the scales Hs, D, Hy, and HEA were used. These four scales can be regarded as a general measure of distress and health concern. Scores above 65T are regarded as clinically significant. The Quebec BPDS was used because specific neck pain disability scales are not available. Patients were asked to answer the questions about functional limitation regarding their neck pain instead of back pain. The Quebec BPDS measures self-reported functional limitation. Scores varies between 0 and 100.

Results

So far, 26 participants (13 male, 13 female) have been included in this study. The mean age of participants is 35.8 (SD = 8.7). The mean duration of symptoms since the accident is 20.8 months (SD = 10.2). Of the participants, 36% had high education (high school and university) and 64% had low education (lower than high school).

In Table 1, participants' scores on the MMPI-2 and Quebec BPDS measured before and after treatment and at follow-up are presented. It can be seen that participants' level of distress and health concern decreased dramatically during treatment. The *t*-tests for

TABLE 1. *Mean scores (± SD) on the MMPI-2 and Quebec BPDS before and after the intensive phase and at follow-up*

Assessment scale	Before intensive phase	After intensive phase	At follow-up
Quebec BPDS	34.4 ± 14.2	16.6 ± 8.3	15.9 ± 15.1
MMPI-2 Hs	73.2 ± 8.7	58.3 ± 9.9	57.5 ± 11.3
MMPI-2 D	64.1 ± 9.7	50.0 ± 10.4	47.9 ± 8.2
MMPI-2 Hy	78.6 ± 12.6	59.8 ± 11.6	58.4 ± 12.3
MMPI-2 Health Concern	66.5 ± 7.1	55.5 ± 9.1	52.3 ± 8.1

paired differences showed all changes to be highly significant ($p < .001$). Comparison of the scores after treatment and at follow-up shows that the changes of test scores are rather stable.

In Table 2, the number and percentages of participants are presented who met the criteria of "normal" functioning at follow-up 4 months after the intensive phase. Because not all participants had finished this 4-month period, the number of participants is below the total number of participants of the entire sample (21 versus 25). With some reservations in mind, it may be concluded that for each criterion, about two thirds of participants were at a normal level of functioning. Further analysis revealed that most participants met all four criteria. So, the distribution of the participants regarding normal functioning is rather one-sided (i.e., most participants have function normally in nearly all respects, while some participants fail to do so in most respects).

DISCUSSION

The preliminary results of this ongoing study evaluate the efficacy of a cognitive behavioral intervention program in patients with chronic symptoms after a whiplash trauma. The aim of the program was a normal pattern of daily activities, including reintegration at work. The preliminary results are promising: about two thirds of patients achieved a complete functional restoration including a normal pain-free daily activity pattern, and more than two out of three patients demonstrated no sick leave caused by whiplash-related symptoms. These results are in accordance with the efficacy of multidisciplinary treatment programs for chronic pain problems (2). In this project's favor, it should be said that the outcome criteria used were rather strict. All subjects returned to work, but the ones who were not working completely normally were regarded as failures. When those patients who returned to work for 50% or more of their normal employment were considered a 50% success, the return-to-work rate was slightly over 80%.

An interesting finding was that most patients reported a variety of somatic symptoms at treatment admission as measured with the MMPI-2 scales Hs, Hy, and Health Concern (HEA). However, after treatment, a substantial decrease in these complaints was ob-

TABLE 2. *Functioning of participants at follow-up 4 months after the intensive phase of a cognitive behavioral program*

Criteria met?	Yes (%)	No (%)
Complete return to work	15 (68)	7 (32)
No sick leave because of whiplash-related disorders	15 (68)	7 (32)
No use of analgesics because of whiplash-related disorders	16 (73)	6 (27)
No medical treatment because of whiplash-related disorders	19 (86)	3 (14)

served while the mode of treatment was behavioral and not directed at somatic pathology. Therefore, it can be concluded that the concept of a physical lesion explaining the chronic symptoms after whiplash trauma is unlikely. In other words, it is unlikely that symptoms disappear by behavioral interventions if these symptoms are the only and direct consequence of an anatomic lesion.

The cognition of the patient in relation to the symptoms is indeed significant. It appears that all of the failures could not believe that they would ever get rid of their symptoms. They tried everything in the first half year after the accident, but nothing worked. This shaped their cognition in such a way that, from then on, they considered themselves helpless. Furthermore, in their understanding, their symptoms are related to an up-to-now undefined anatomic lesion. Because the intervention team was apparently unable to change that belief, they became failures.

No empirical research has been conducted in this realm. In only one case study has the cognitive behavioral treatment of a patient with chronic symptoms after whiplash trauma been described, in which special attention was paid to neuropsychological dysfunction (19). The number of subjects in this preliminary study is much too small to lead to firm conclusions. So, no generalizations can be made. More empirical research in this realm is absolutely needed!

However, these early results are very promising. One has to take into consideration that they are the results of a professional team applying a cognitive behavioral approach to chronicity after whiplash injury. Therefore, it can be speculated that the results will improve with time, and also when the intervention is carried out earlier instead of nearly 2 years after the injury.

CONCLUSIONS

Chronic symptoms after whiplash injury may be persistent as a result of psychophysiologic processes such as conditioning. The majority of patients do not seem to have preexisting psychological problems. Patients with chronic symptoms after a Quebec Task Force grade 1 or 2 lesion of the neck seem to benefit from cognitive behavioral intervention. Early results are very encouraging and suggest a success rate of about 75% or higher when an experienced team applies this approach about 6 months after the injury.

REFERENCES

1. Flor HC, Turk DC, Birbaumer N. Assessment of stress-related psychophysiological reactions in chronic back pain patients. *J Consult Clin Psychol* 1985;53:3654–3664.
2. Flor HC, Fydrich TH, Turk DC. Efficacy of multidisciplinary pain treatment centers: a meta-analytic review. *Pain* 1992;49:221–230.
3. Fordyce WE. *Behavioral methods of chronic pain and illness.* St. Louis: CV Mosby, 1976.
4. Gay JR, Abbott KH. Common whiplash injuries of the neck. *JAMA* 1953;152:1698–1704.
5. Gargan F, Bannister GC. The rate of recovery following whiplash injury. *Eur Spine J* 1994;3:162–164.
6. Hodge JR. The whiplash neurosis. *Psychosomatics* 1971;12:245–249.
7. Hohl M. Soft-tissue injuries of the neck in automobile accidents. Factors influencing prognosis. *J Bone Joint Surg* 1974;56A:1675–1681.
8. Kori SH, Miller RP, Todd DD. Kinesiophobia: a new view of chronic pain behavior. *Pain Management* 1990;35–43.
9. Larsson SE, Ålund M, Cai H, Åke Öberg P. Chronic pain after soft-tissue injury of the cervical spine: trapezius muscle blood flow and electromyography at static loads and fatique. *Pain* 1994;57:173–180.
10. Maimaris C, Barnes MR, Allen MJ. "Whiplash injuries" of the neck: a retrospective study. *Injury* 1988;19: 393–396.

11. Miller H. Accident neurosis. *Br Med J* 1961;1:919–925, 992–998.
12. Pilowsky I. Abnormal illness behavior. *Br J Med Psychol* 1969;42:347–351.
13. Pollock ML, Schmidt DH. Measurement of cardiorespiratory fitness and body composition in the clinical settings. *Comp Ther* 1980;6:12–27.
14. Radanov BP, Di Stefano G, Schnidrig A, Sturzenegger M. Psychosocial stress, cognitive performance and disability after common whiplash. *J Psychosom Res* 1992;57:1–10.
15. Radanov BP, Di Stefano G, Schnidrig A, Sturzegger M. Cognitive functioning after common whiplash: a controlled follow-up study. *Arch Neurol* 1992;50:87–91.
16. Radanov BP, DiStefano G, Schnidrig A, Aljinovic M. Factors influencing recovery from headache after common whiplash. *Br Med J* 1993;307:652–655.
17. Radanov BP, Di Stefano G, Schnidrig A, Sturzenegger M. Common whiplash—psychosomatic or somatopsychic? *J Neurol Neurosurg Psychiatry* 1994;57:486–490.
18. Scientific Monograph of the Quebec Task Force on Whiplash Associated Disorders. *Spine* 1995;20(8S):21–24.
19. Vendrig AA. Cognitieve gedragstherapie bij chronische klachten na een whiplashtrauma. *Gedragstherapie* 1997;30:19–33.
20. Vlaeyen J, Kole-Snijders A, Boeren R, Eek H. Fear of movement/(re)injury in chronic low back pain and its relation to behavioral performance. *Pain* 1995;62:363–372.
21. Waddell G, Newton M, Henderson I, Somerville D, Main C. A fear-avoidance beliefs questionnaire (FABQ) and the role of fear-avoidance beliefs in chronic pain and disability. *Pain* 1993;52:157–168.

Whiplash Injuries: Current Concepts in Prevention, Diagnosis, and Treatment of the Cervical Whiplash Syndrome, edited by Robert Gunzburg and Marek Szpalski. Lippincott–Raven Publishers, Philadelphia © 1998.

20

Whiplash and Spinal Manipulation

Jean-Yves Maigne

J.-Y. Maigne: Department of Rehabilitation and Physical Medicine, Hôtel-Dieu Hospital, Paris, France.

Cervical spine trauma as a result of whiplash is a frequently encountered injury. Hyperextension–hyperflexion may result in a variety of spinal lesions, injuring the vertebrae themselves (fractures) or damaging the motion segment. The severity of the trauma varies considerably between different patients. The most serious injuries (fractures, severe sprains with cervical spine instability, large intervertebral disk herniations with neurologic signs) are managed with orthopedic surgery. The other, more frequently encountered and more diverse, lesions are treated non-operatively. Among the many modalities suggested, manipulation plays a considerable role. This chapter looks at the utility of the technique in whiplash patients.

WHAT IS MANIPULATION, AND HOW DOES IT WORK?

Vertebral manipulation consists in the direct or indirect application to the spine of a forced movement directed to one or more motion segments. The joints involved are taken past their usual range of motion, but not beyond their anatomic range (5). After the joint has been taken through its normal passive range, a single short, sharp thrust is delivered. Manipulation is associated with an audible cracking noise from the joint. The mechanism of action of manipulation is as yet but incompletely understood. According to Shekelle (6), it may involve the release of entrapped synovial folds, the relaxation of hypertonic muscle by sudden stretching, the disruption of articular or periarticular adhesions, and the unbuckling of motion segments that have undergone disproportionate displacements.

This author has performed (unpublished) cadaver studies. In a first study, an intradiscal pressure sensor was inserted at the centers of the lumbar disks from L1-2 to L4-5, and an accelerometer was placed between the bodies of L3 and L4. This set-up was linked to a computer that allowed the two parameters to be monitored continuously. Two fresh cadavers were instrumented with this system and subjected to two kinds of lumbar manipulation. The recordings showed a sudden drop in intradiscal pressure during the manipulative thrusts, with the pressure falling to or below zero. Within a few seconds, the pressure returned to its baseline value.

In another four cadavers, erector spinae stretching was measured. On one side, the muscle was stretched to about 20% beyond its baseline length; on the opposite side, the muscle relaxed by the same amount. In cadavers, the joints do not crack. However, it is likely that the physiologic process described in other joints, a sudden opening of the joint surfaces (7), occurs also in the facets when they are submitted to a cavitation phenomenon. What appears to happen is that the high-velocity movement imparted to the spine by the manipulator (the manipulative thrust) is not transmitted in its entirety to the target motion segment. Energy is stored in the facet joint. At the end of the movement, when the tensile forces become overwhelmingly strong, the joint surfaces suddenly snap apart. This separation happens at great speed and gives additional impetus to the manipulative thrust. It follows that the cracking of the joint should not be interpreted as a sign of therapeutic benefit being conferred to the facet joint, but as audible evidence of a movement that makes the facet joints the driving unit of manipulation. These findings made in the lumbar spine probably apply to the cervical spine as well. Thus, the sudden sharp stretching of the paraspinal muscles, which are often found to be tense in back pain patients (4), may make these muscles relax. The equally sudden lowering of the intradiscal pressure may lead to a redistribution of the pressures acting on the anulus, leveling off the stress peaks that are notoriously adverse (1).

INDICATIONS FOR VERTEBRAL MANIPULATION IN RECENT CERVICAL SPINE TRAUMA PATIENTS

Indications and Precautions

Acute stage. Great care must be taken to ensure that patients with lesions that may be made worse by manipulation are not treated with this modality. Neurologic abnormalities, neck stiffness, or severe pain constitute clinical contraindications to manipulation.

Stress (flexion–extension) radiographs should routinely be obtained to screen for instability. As a general rule, manipulation should be performed early after high-energy whiplash trauma. In such cases, the patients should wear a collar for 1 to 3 weeks. This time may be used to perform magnetic resonance imaging (MRI), if required, to obtain a full picture of the lesions sustained. A slightly bulging disc is not a contraindication to manipulative treatment, but a herniated nucleus pulposus, with or without nerve root involvement, would definitely rule out manipulation.

Subacute stage. At a later stage, manipulation may be offered. Vertebral manipulation appears to be beneficial in moderately severe muscle contractions (spasm, tension, trigger points, taut bands) regardless of origin (frequently, after vertebral trauma) and in painful minor intervertebral dysfunction (PMID). The clinical patterns associated with these lesions are very varied. Patients may complain of simple neck pain or pain radiating into the shoulder blade, headaches, or pain between the shoulder blades associated with the back muscles.

Chronic pain. Chronic symptoms may also be managed with spinal manipulation. However, it should be borne in mind that in chronic cases there may be an underlying legal problem (unsettled compensation or insurance claims) or a psychogenic element, which tends to make the treatment less effective.

How to Manipulate

The mobility of the cervical spine is studied to establish the painful as well as the completely free directions. The findings are plotted in a star diagram with six branches

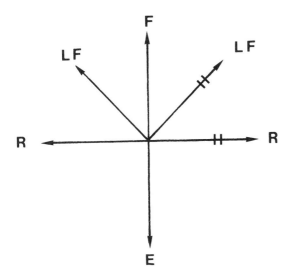

FIG. 1. Diagram of motion for the cervical spine. Each branch may be crossed out by one, two, or three bars, according to the intensity of the pain. Here, right rotation and lateral flexion are painful. (*F*, flexion; *E*, extension; *R*, rotation; *LF*, lateral flexion.)

(Fig. 1) that signify the six degrees of freedom of the spine (flexion, extension, lateral flexion to left and to right, rotation to left and to right). Each branch may be crossed out once, twice, or three times, depending on the severity of the pain encountered. If three or more of these directions are found to be painful or blocked, manipulation should not be performed. Otherwise, the joint is manipulated in the direction opposite to the most painful movement. Thus, if rotation to the right is painful, manipulation should be in rotation to the left (Fig. 2). The rule—established by R. Maigne and followed by the French school—is that of no pain and of opposite movement (5). Manipulation must be preceded by stretching maneuvers, in order to condition the tissues and to prevent damage. The patient must trust the manipulator, be relaxed, and know how and why the procedure is going to be performed. Main maneuvers consist in a rotational or a lateral thrust (Fig. 3). Flexion is possible on the upper thoracic spine, where the major cervical dorsal muscles attach.

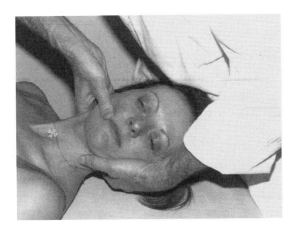

FIG. 2. A cervical manipulation in a left rotation.

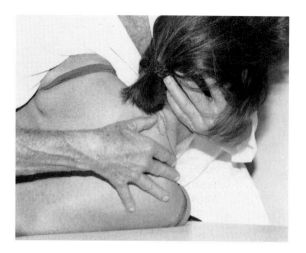

FIG. 3. A manipulation of the cervicothoracic junction in a left lateral flexion.

Each session should consist of one to four manipulations. The result may be seen immediately, or it may not manifest itself for up to 3 days. A good course of treatment should, on average, comprise between two and four sessions. If, after two sessions, no result has been seen, the patient should be changed over to a different treatment modality.

Other Contraindications to Cervical Spine Manipulation

Contraindications may be related to trauma (instability, fractures, herniated nucleus pulposus), or they may be of a technical kind (very severe neck pain in fewer than three free directions). The patient may refuse manipulation (from apprehension, or because of adverse past experience). Also, there are certain general contraindications to be borne in mind: high-grade osteoporosis, old age (although very gentle maneuvers are possible even in the very old), and vascular problems (atherosclerosis, history of stroke).

RESULTS

In a systematic review of the literature, Hurwitz et al. did not find any studies comparing the efficacy of manipulation with that of other treatments in the management of pain after whiplash syndrome (3). In nonspecific neck pain, the authors concluded that manipulation was probably more effective than conventional treatments at least in the short term.

Cassidy et al. found an immediate benefit in terms of pain reduction and range of motion after manipulation in patients with whiplash-related disorders (2).

This author's experience shows that, in minor motion segment disorders without any underlying psychologic or compensation-related problems, manipulation is a treatment modality that can benefit the patients.

REFERENCES

1. Adams MA, McMillan DW, Green TP, Dolan P. Sustained loading generates stress concentration in lumbar discs. *Spine* 1996;21:434–438.

2. Cassidy JD, Lopes AA, Young-Hing K. The immediate effect of manipulation versus mobilization on pain and range of motion in the cervical spine: a randomized controlled trial. *J Manipulative Physiol Ther* 1992;15: 570–575.
3. Hurwitz EL, Aker PO, Adams AH, Meeker WC, Shekelle PG. Manipulation and mobilization of the cervical spine. A systematic review of the literature. *Spine* 1996;21:1746–1760.
4. Indahl A, Kaigle A, Keikeras O, Holm S. Electromyographic response of the porcine multifidus musculature after nerve stimulation. *Spine* 1995;20:2652–2658.
5. Maigne R. *Diagnosis and treatment of pain of vertebral origin. A manual medicine approach.* Baltimore: Williams & Wilkins, 1995;191–197.
6. Shekelle PG. Spinal manipulation. *Spine* 1994;19:858–861.
7. Unsworth A, Dowson D, Wright V. Cracking joints. *Ann Rheum Dis* 1971;30:348.

Whiplash Injuries: Current Concepts in
Prevention, Diagnosis, and Treatment
of the Cervical Whiplash Syndrome,
edited by Robert Gunzburg and Marek Szpalski.
Lippincott–Raven Publishers, Philadelphia © 1998.

21

Education and Return to Work

Margareta Nordin

M. Nordin: Occupational and Industrial Orthopaedic Center, Hospital for Joint Diseases;
and Department of Environmental Medicine, New York University School of Medicine,
New York, New York 10012.

The neck structure is intricate and is composed of 37 joints and 20 pairs of muscles. A complex system of muscles, ligaments, discs, neural network, and vascular structures make the neck susceptible to injury. Impact on the head and the whiplash exposure are examples. The role of the cervical spine is to give strong support to the skull, to protect the neural components and vascular structures, and to provide muscle attachments. Yet the neck must have the flexibility afforded by the extensive range of motion to integrate the head with the body and the environment (6,22). The neck must also act as a shock absorber to protect the brain. It must provide portals of entry, exit, and passage for neurovascular structures. The cervical spine is structured to allow mutual functioning under normal physiologic circumstances. A car accident that involves the rear or side impact of a vehicle is not a normal circumstance. A whiplash exposure of the neck with or without head impact can occur. This mechanism is described in Chapters 8 and 9. Injuries to the neck are commonly perceived to have a dismal prognosis leading eventually to death. The reason for this perception is not completely understood. Through the efforts of the Québec Task Force, a better understanding was gained of the impact of auto accident–induced whiplash-associated disorders (24,25). This chapter will focus on early mobilization and return to usual activity of the patient with a whiplash exposure without head impact, and the need for education of the health care provider and the patient.

DEFINITION OF WHIPLASH-ASSOCIATED DISORDERS

Whiplash is an acceleration–deceleration mechanism of energy transfer to the neck. It may result from rear-end or side-impact motor vehicle collisions, but it can also occur during diving or other mishaps. The impact may result in bony or soft-tissue injuries (whiplash injury), which may in turn lead to a variety of clinical manifestations [whiplash-associated disorders (WAD)] (24,25). This definition does not include patients with whiplash injuries and head impact. Individuals who during the accident suffered a head impact may need a different clinical approach, depending on the symptomatology.

CLASSIFICATION OF WHIPLASH-ASSOCIATED DISORDERS

The Québec Task Force has suggested a clinical classification of WAD (24,25). The suggested classification is perhaps the most important contribution of the Task Force.

TABLE 1. *The Québec Task Force—suggested clinical classification of whiplash-associated disorders*

Grade	Clinical presentation[a]
0	No complaint about the neck No physical sign(s)
I	Neck complaint of pain, stiffness, or tenderness only No physical sign(s)
II	Neck complaint AND musculoskeletal sign(s)[b]
III	Neck complaint AND neurologic sign(s)[c]
IV	Neck complaint AND fracture or dislocation

[a] Symptoms and disorders that can be manifest in all grades include deafness, dizziness, tinnitus, headache, memory loss, dysphagia, and temporomandibular joint pain.

[b] Musculoskeletal signs include decreased range of motion and point tenderness.

[c] Neurologic signs include decreased or absent deep tendon reflexes, weakness and sensory deficits.

Reprinted with permission from Spitzer WO, Skovron ML, Salmi LR, et al. Scientific monograph of the Québec Task Force on whiplash-associated disorders: redefining whiplash and its management. *Spine* 1995;20(8S): 10S–73S.

Clinicians and researchers in the future will decide if the proposed classification needs refinement. For now, it is the only classification available based on an extensive literature investigation and synthesis of the best evidence. The clinical classification is meant to provide categories that are mutually exclusive, that are clinically meaningful, that stand the test of common sense, and that are user-friendly. The clinical classification has two axes: (a) a clinical anatomic axis, and (b) a time axis. The clinical–anatomic axis has five grades that correspond roughly to the degree of clinical severity (Table 1).

This chapter will consider only WAD grades I, II, and III. These are the most common clinical complaints. Grade 0 is important for insurance purposes and for research, but it may be less frequently seen by a clinician. However, a patient with a grade 0 WAD may show up in the emergency room for various reasons.

The time axis suggested by the Québec Task Force is classified within each clinical grade (I to III) as follows: Patients exposed to whiplash presenting within less than 4 days of date of injury, in 4 to 21 days, in 22 to 45 days, and in 46 to 180 days, and finally those patients with exposure duration of more than 180 days. The Task Force by consensus designated patients with symptomatology or residual disability more than 6 months to be chronic. Continued complaint and residual disability from a patient in more than 45 days in grades I, II, and III injuries are important warnings of chronicity and permanent disability. Patients still experiencing problems after 45 days should receive expanded clinical interventions and mandatory interdisciplinary clinical consultation to prevent chronicity and permanent disability.

CLINICAL SPECTRUM OF WAD GRADES I, II, AND III

The clinical spectrum of the WAD-related diagnosis is large. Table 2 is not meant to be exhaustive but to give examples of commonly used clinical terms. It is adapted from Spitzer et al. (24,25).

TABLE 2. *Nonexhaustive clinical spectrums of whiplash-associated disorders without head impact*

WAD grade I: Neck complaint of pain, stiffness, or tenderness only; no physical sign(s)
  Common synonyms
    Whiplash injury
    Minor whiplash
    Minor cervical sprains or strains
    Neck tension
  Presumed pathology
    Microscopic or multimicroscopic lesions
    Lesion is not serious enough to cause muscle spasms
  Clinical presentation
    Usually presents to a physician more than 24 hours after an accident
WAD grade II: Neck complaint and musculoskeletal sign(s)
  Common synonyms
    Whiplash
    Cervical sprain
    Cervicalgia with headaches
    Headache of cervical origin
    Traumatic cervicalgia
    Cervicoscapulalgia
    Minor intervertebral dysfunction
    Sprained cervical facet joints
  Presumed pathology
    Neck sprain and bleeding around soft-tissue (articular capsules, ligaments, tendons, and muscles)
  Clinical presentation
    Usually presents to a physician in the first 24 hours after an accident
    Nonspecific radiation to the head, face, occipital region, shoulder, and arm from soft-tissues injuries
    Neck pain with limited range of motion due to muscle spasms
WAD grade III: Neck complaint and neurologic sign(s)
  Common synonyms
    Whiplash
    Cervicobracialgia
    Cervical herniated disc
    Cervicalgia with headaches
    Headaches of cervical origin
    Cervicoscapulalgia
  Presumed pathology
    Injuries to the system by mechanical injury or by irritation secondary to bleeding or inflammation
  Clinical presentation
    Presents to a physician usually within hours after an accident
    Limited range of motion combined with neurologic symptoms and signs

Adapted from Spitzer WO, Skovron ML, Salmi LR, et al. Scientific monograph of the Québec Task Force on whiplash-associated disorders: redefining whiplash and its management. *Spine* 1995;20(8S):10S–73S.

Epidemiologic Support for Early Activity or Mobilization of WAD Grades I, II, and III

The natural history of WAD is of interest when recommending activity or prescribing mobilization for the patient with WAD complaints. Suissa et al. studied a large cohort of patients (N = 2810) exposed to collision in the province of Québec (28). They showed that 22% of the patients recovered within 1 week of collision. Fifty percent recovered within 1 month and 64% recovered within 60 days. At 6 months, 87% had returned to activity and approximately 3% of the population were still absent from work or normal activity after 1 year (Fig. 1). Prospective studies have showed that delayed recovery is associated with initial neck pain intensity, injury-related cognitive impairment, female

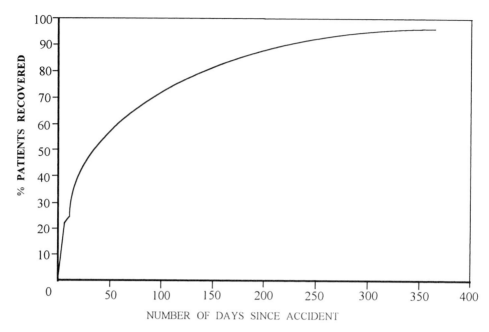

FIG. 1. Overall 1-year cumulative return to activity of cohort of patients with whiplash. Adapted from Spitzer WO, Skovron ML, Salmi LR, et al. Scientific monograph of the Québec Task Force on whiplash-associated disorders: redefining whiplash and its management. *Spine* 1995; 20(8S):10S–73S.

sex, older age, increased numbers of dependents, marital status, multiple injuries, greater collision severity, collisions other than rear-ended, vehicle other than car or taxi, and nonuse of seat belt (20,27,28). The recurrence rate of individuals analyzed in one cohort was close to 7% (28). Other studies (8,10,20) found that up to 27% of their patient series were still symptomatic after 1 year. The difference in recovery results can be attributed to the difference in the capture area of patients and representativeness of the population at large. Long-term (6 months) chronic WAD and/or permanent disability may or may not be related to the whiplash injury itself (21).

Clinical Biomechanical Support for Early Mobilization of WAD Grades I, II, III

Exposure to whiplash may or may not lead to injury. The amplitude of the impact is not directly related to the severity of the injury (18). A host of factors may modify the severity of the injury, such as the car design, bumper design, type of head rest, head rest adjustment, seat design, vehicle speed, passenger position and posture during collision, and passenger age (18,28). Nevertheless, the patient seeking care has been exposed to an energy transfer and the aim is to determine the extent of tissue damage, if possible. Patients presenting with WAD grades I, II, and III most likely have a soft-tissue injury. The exact structure damaged may be clinically difficult to locate.

The Québec Task Force therefore synthesized knowledge from the sprain and strain models from animal experiments, and from *in vitro* and *in vivo* models (14,31). In WAD grades I and II, the classifications indicate no neurologic symptoms and/or signs. Then the derived animal sprain–strain model on soft tissues can be used. Soft-tissue healing (tendon, ligament/capsule, and muscles) indicates a brief (less than 72 hours) period of acute inflammation and reaction, followed by a period of repair and regeneration (approximately 72 hours to 6 weeks). Finally, a period of remodeling and maturation can last up to 1 year depending on the tissue damage. Using this model, it is reasonable to estimate a healing period and progressive increased well-being of 4 to 6 weeks for most patients (grade I and II) with partial tears of soft tissues. Patients experiencing WAD grade III (including neurologic signs and/or symptoms) may not apply to this model, as a potential nerve injury could prolong recovery.

Long-term immobilization of soft-tissue injuries in any part of the body is a treatment of the past. The consequences of long-term immobilization for a joint complex are devastating, including loss of range of motion, muscle atrophy, and increased perception (by the patient) of illness. Likewise, in WAD grades I, II, and III, prolonged immobilization may increase scar tissue and reduce cervical mobility. The impact of immobilization in WAD grades I to III on the neural and vascular system of the cervical spine is little known and deserves more attention. No randomized controlled prospective trial has been used to examine activity or exercises versus immobilization in patients with WAD grades I through III.

Types of Early Activity and Mobilization for WAD Grades I, II, III

A careful evaluation of the patient with WAD (Chapter 24) must precede all recommendations for resuming normal activity and exercise regimens. Once the patient has been examined and a WAD classification of grade I, II, or III determined, the appropriate activity can be recommended. The overall message is not to immobilize but to promote normal activity. The first encounter with the physician is crucial and time must be allocated to reduce patient fear (19). Return to normal activity, including work, is recommended for patients with WAD grade I. No treatment is necessary. Revisit only if the patient and physician deem it necessary. In patients who display a high fear avoidance behavior, a revisit or a follow-up call may be necessary. In patients with WAD grades II and III, reassurance, prescribed activity, and pain management are appropriate. Again, the message is not to immobilize. The soft collars so commonly used in the management of WAD are not recommended and should be discouraged. The use of soft collars may reinforce the perception of illness and prolong disability.

Patients with WAD grades II and III needing therapy have a choice of physical therapy (physiotherapists) or manipulative therapy (osteopaths, chiropractors, specially trained physical therapists). Physiotherapy should emphasize early return to usual activity and work and promote mobility. The literature is sparse in the field of physiotherapy treatment for WAD injuries. The recommendation was based on cumulative evidence on the beneficial effect of exercises (9,15,16,33) and the harmful effect of disuse (4,32). Reassurance about the good prognosis should accompany all interventions by physiotherapists in pain management and mobility in patients with WAD grades II and III. The goal of the treatment is to resume normal activity. Long-term immobilization and passive modalities are not justified. Stretching, flexibility, and strengthening exercises for the neck, shoulder and back are provided in Appendix 1 (29). These exercises are simple and can be modified according to the patient's tolerance. If no or slow recovery, reevaluation of patient status is recommended at 3 weeks by a specialist and at 6 weeks by a multidisciplinary team. At this time, the patient is at risk for chronicity and permanent disability.

Manipulative therapy can be provided in the early stage of treatment as an alternative. Manipulative treatment should be short term, and the sparse literature indicates a weak association between the reduction of pain and the ease of early mobility (5,17). These findings are currently disputed by Coulter et al. (7), who reviewed over 500 studies related to acute neck pain not necessarily related to WAD. If manipulation is the choice, trained health professionals should provide the treatment. It should always be accompanied by reassurance of the good prognosis and promotion of reassumption of usual activity and work. Long-term, repeated manipulation is not justified without multidisciplinary evaluation. Table 3 shows the operational definitions to be used for the patient-care guidelines recommended by the Québec Task Force.

Patients with non-WAD-related neck pain (i.e., mechanical, occupational, or nonspecific neck pain) perceive decreased pain with strengthening exercises of the neck musculature (3,12,23). Harms-Ringdahl and Ekholm (11) reported neck pain in healthy subjects when maintaining extreme flexion position of the cervical and upper thoracic spine, these postures should therefore be avoided.

Education about Treatment of WAD Grades I, II, and III

The education of patients can be done formally (i.e., in neck school) or in a less formal way including discussion, pamphlets, or advice from the health professional. One of

TABLE 3. *Operational definitions*

Form	Recording information from the history and physical examination, management decisions, and grading of the WAD should be completed for all initial visits for all reassessment visits for grade I to III, and preferably on a standardized form (Appendix 1).
History	Includes characteristics of patient, previous history of medical and other pertinent factors, including neck problems, circumstances, and mechanism of injury, nature and time of onset of all symptoms, and self-assessment of health status.
Isolated	Not associated with other injuries.
Obtunded	Dulled consciousness.
Physical	Includes inspection, palpation, range of motion, neurologic examination, assessment of associated injuries, and examination for general health and mental status: required details can be found on data form for all recommended visits.
Plain radiographs	Include anteroposterior, lateral, and open-mouth views; all seven cervical vertebrae and the C7-T1 level should be included.
Prescribe activity	Interventions should focus on promoting activity. Range of motion exercises should be implemented. Techniques that promote mobility of the cervical spine should be applied by qualified personnel. Interventions that impede active mobilization of the neck are not indicated.
Reassessment	Includes history taking and physical examination as during initial visit, and specialized advice as required from multidisciplinary health professionals with in-depth formal training in musculoskeletal disorders, psychosocial assessment, and other specialties.
Reassurance	Patients should be reassured that most WAD are benign and self-limiting, and they should be encouraged to resume usual activities of life as soon as possible.
Return to usual	Patients should be advised to resume their activities of daily living (work, studying, leisure, social, etc.), as soon as possible (usually immediately for grade I). It should be explained to patients that usual activities may be temporarily painful but not harmful in WAD.
Specialized advice	Consultation with a health professional with in-depth formal training in managing WAD.
Unresolved	Unable to resume usual activities. A patient who still has residual pain or limitation of range of motion but who is able to resume work and other usual activities is considered to have resolved WAD.

the most important recommendations of the Québec Task Force is the reassurance of patients with grades I, II, and III WAD. Patients should be reassured that most WAD is benign and self-limiting. Patients should be encouraged to resume their usual activities of daily life as soon as possible. This recommendation infers that the health professional will initiate a discussion with the patient at the first visit. The discussion should focus on the promotion of regular activity and when and how the patient can resume these activities. It should be explained to the patient that resuming usual activities may be temporarily painful (usually immediately) but not harmful in WAD grade I. These activities in WAD grades II and III can be resumed after discussion and mutual goal setting between the health professional and the patient. This discussion also implies that the care provider may have to change his or her beliefs and accept the underlying theory for promoting activity and well-being. Educational institutions and the directors of clinics and emergency rooms must make an effort to reeducate health professionals.

Health Care Professional Education

Changing the beliefs, practices, and referral system of health care professionals is challenging. The traditional treatment method for WAD grades I, II, and III has been immobilization, pain killers, and refraining from work. The Québec Task Force suggests a radical change from the traditional algorithm for WAD grades I to III, including a careful evaluation, classification, and immediate graded activation or return to work if no treatment is necessary. For the patient, this different approach necessitates some explanation and the health care provider must feel confident in providing the information. Several institutions, insurance companies, and professional organizations have made an effort to provide in-house and external workshops to meet the demands of the new knowledge. These initiatives are commendable. For example, the Societe d'assurance automobile de Québec (SAAQ) has dedicated a group of professionals for education, implementation, data collection, and clinical management of the WAD patient in the province of Québec. In Vancouver, British Columbia (BC), the Physical Medicine Research Foundation has started the BC Whiplash Initiative. This initiative provides workshops and courses in the management of WAD injuries, including course outlines, instructional handbooks, videotapes, and knowledge tests. These initiatives focus on the education of health care providers in the management of patients with WAD. The goals are to prevent chronicity and disability and to save costs. Both goals are equally important.

Patient Education

The first contact between the patient and the health care provider is crucial. The encounter must establish trust and set the tone for eventual need of care. Knowledge can be transferred and patient fears about the presence of a serious condition decreased or even abolished. Studies suggest that for ill-defined symptomatic conditions, communication between the clinician and the patient may have more impact on patient outcomes than the specific treatment choice has. In particular, agreement about the nature of the problem, and the provider's confidence in his or her diagnosis, and optimism about recovery can affect patient outcomes (1,2,26).

Providing information that addresses several basic patient expectations and concerns is important. This information can increase the chances that the consultation will be both satisfying and effective. Information should be given regarding the lack of knowledge about the specific eventual structure damage, a sense of the prognosis (generally most positive in WAD I and II, positive but with a longer recovery time in WAD III), recommendations for controlling symptoms, and early activity guidelines that take into account patient's work and leisure activities. The information can be enhanced by a pamphlet or activity guidance sheet.

Reassuring the patient that a serious condition is not present may be a critical component. If treatment is indicated for patients with WAD grades I to III, set realistic goals and positive expectations for recovery. Discuss follow-up visits and inform the patient about the positive effects of gradually increased activity and return to normal life activities including work. Discuss the length of treatment and expected efficacy. In a randomized controlled study, Thomas (30) demonstrated that patients with nonspecific pain symptoms associated with minor illness were more satisfied with their care and were more likely to recover from their illness within 2 weeks if they received a positive, confident consultation rather than one that highlighted uncertainty. Although this study was not related to patients exposed to whiplash injury, it is valuable in revealing the importance of the educational messages conveyed to the patient.

Neck School

Neck school is a more formal type of educational setting for patients with a delayed recovery or recurrent problem of neck pain. The aim is to educate patients in a group setting of three up to ten individuals. The group meet three to seven times for approximately 1 hour per session over a period of 2 to 3 weeks. The group format, like that used in back schools, provides an economical way of transferring information and fostering a supportive environment in which patients can exchange ideas freely. The term *school* implies that patients are encouraged to ask questions to participate in the class, to learn, and to retain information (29). The content includes anatomy, epidemiology, exercises for the neck and upper extremities, ergonomics, posture, pain medication, and pain management. Some neck schools for patients with chronic neck pain include behavioral techniques such as relaxation techniques, coping mechanisms, and biofeedback. Educational videotapes, brochures, and relaxation tapes may be complements to the teaching format. Neck schools are commonly given by physical therapist or occupational therapist.

The efficacy of neck school for patients with WAD is unknown. There has been only one randomized controlled prospective study (13), and it looked at the effect of neck school on neck and shoulder disorders in 79 medical secretaries in Sweden. The authors concluded that there was a limited effect of neck school in primary prevention. Organizing a neck school for patients with WAD problems is a logistic problem. Most clinics do not encounter enough patients with WAD I to III, and therefore group education may not be feasible. It remains an option for specialized clinics where the patient population is sufficiently large.

CONCLUSIONS

The Québec Task Force studied the optimal treatment for whiplash-associated disorders (24,25). The extensive literature review and best evidence synthesis have changed the recommendations for treatment for patients with soft-tissue whiplash injury. A careful initial evaluation is recommended at the first encounter with a health professional. A new classification of patients' symptom and signs is introduced. If the patient is diagnosed with only soft-tissue injury in the neck (no cervical fracture or dislocation or head trauma present), immediate or early mobilization and return to normal activities is recommended to promote healing and well-being.

APPENDIX 1

Shoulder Shrugs (A). Sitting, standing, or lying, bring both shoulders up to the ears. Hold for 5 seconds and relax. The objective is to relax tense neck muscles.

Shoulder Rolling (B). Sitting or standing, pull both shoulders up, back, and down in a circular motion. The purpose is to relieve muscle tension in the neck, shoulders, and upper back.

Middle Back Stretching (C). Sitting or standing, gently pull one elbow toward the opposite shoulder. Hold 5 seconds and relax. Repeat with the other arm. The purpose is to stretch the muscle in the mid-upper back.

Elbow Press (D). Standing or sitting, bring both elbows up to the chest level. Gently press the elbows backwards. Hold for 5 seconds and relax. The purpose is to decrease tightness in the mid-back and stretch chest muscles.

Pectoral Stretch (E). Standing with the face toward a corner, place the palms against the wall. Keep the hands and elbows at shoulder level. Lean toward the wall, keeping the heels firmly on the floor. Hold for 5 seconds and relax. The purpose is to stretch the chest muscles.

Diaphragmatic Breathing I (F). Standing or sitting, place the hands on the abdomen. Inhale slowly and deeply through the nose, letting the abdomen expand. Exhale slowly through the mouth, deflating the abdomen. The objective is to relieve tension and to maximize oxygen intake for optimal energy.

Diaphragmatic Breathing II (G). Standing or sitting, repeat the directions in diaphragmatic breathing I, but when inhaling, raise both arms over the head, and when exhaling, lower the arms slowly. The objective is to relieve tension and to maximize oxygen intake for optimal energy.

Chin Tucks (H). Standing, sitting, or lying, move the chin straight back without moving the head forward. Keep the eyes focused straight ahead. Hold for 5 seconds and relax. The objective is to improve back and neck posture.

Neck Flexion (I). Standing, sitting, or lying, slowly roll the chin to the chest. Hold for 5 seconds and relax, and move the head back to neutral. The objective is to stretch the muscles in the back of the neck.

Neck Extension (J). Standing or sitting, slowly roll the head back so that the eyes are looking up. Hold for 5 seconds, relax, and move the head back to neutral. The objective is to stretch the muscles in the neck.

Neck Side Bending I (K). Standing or sitting, move the head so that the ear drops toward the shoulder without lifting the shoulder. Hold 5 seconds, relax, and move the head back to neutral. Repeat on the other side. The objective is to stretch the muscle in the side of the neck and the upper shoulder.

Neck Side Bending II (L). Standing or sitting, move the head so that the ear drops toward the shoulder without lifting the shoulder, and at the same time, depress the opposite shoulder. Hold 5 seconds, relax, and move the head back to neutral. The objective is to stretch the muscle in the side of the neck and the upper shoulder.

Neck Rotation (M). Standing, sitting, or lying, turn the head to one side, keeping the eyes level. Hold for 5 seconds, relax, and move the head back to neutral. Repeat on the other side. The objective is to stretch the neck muscles and to improve flexibility.

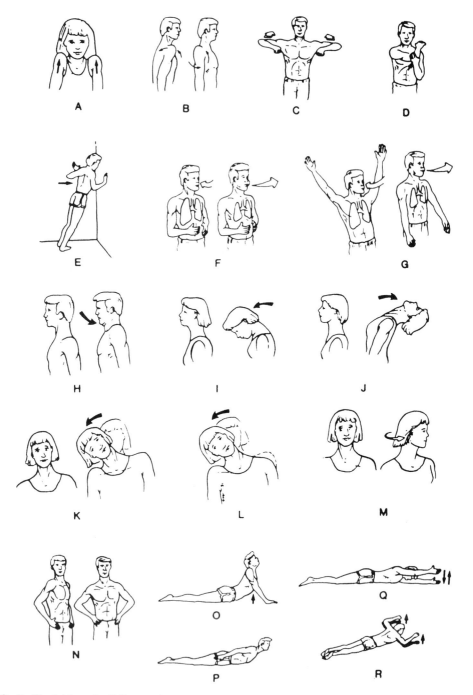

FIG. 2. Stretching, flexibility, and strengthening exercises for the neck, shoulder, and back. From Tan JC, Nordin M. Activation exercises in patients with WAD Grade I, II, III. *Clin Orth North Am* 1992;23(3):437.

Upper Body Rotation (N). Standing or sitting, place the hands on the waist. Turn the upper body gently to one side, keeping the lower body still. Hold for 5 seconds, relax, and move the trunk back to center. Repeat on the other side. The objective is to stretch the neck muscles and to improve flexibility.

Press Up (O). Lying on the stomach, place the hands at shoulder level. Push the upper trunk off the floor, keeping the pelvis on the floor. Hold for 5 seconds, relax, and let the back sag to the floor. The objective is to strengthen the back muscles.

Active Back Extension (P). Lying on the stomach, place the arms at the sides. Tighten the buttocks and raise the head and shoulders off the floor as far as is comfortably possible. Hold for 5 seconds, relax, and let the back sag to the floor. The objective is to strengthen the back muscles.

Upper Back Strengthening (Q). Lying on the stomach, stretch the arms overhead and raise them off the floor one at a time. Position the hands so that the thumbs are pointed up. Hold for 5 seconds, relax, and lower the arm. Repeat the exercise on alternate arms. The objective is to strengthen the upper back muscles.

Mid-Back Strengthening (R). Lying on the stomach, place the hands over the head so that the elbows are at shoulder level. Lift both arms off the floor, hold for 5 seconds, and relax. The objective is to strengthen the muscles in the middle of the back.

ACKNOWLEDGMENTS

I am grateful to Dawn Leger, Ph.D., for editing the manuscript and to Judy Trucios for word processing.

REFERENCES

1. Bass MJ, Buck C, Turner L, et al. The physicians actions and the outcome of illness in family practice. *J Fam Pract* 1986;23:43–47.
2. Battie MC, Nordin M. Education and training. In: Wiesel SW, Wienstein JN, Herkowitz H, Dvořák J, Bell G, eds. *The lumbar spine.* Philadelphia: WB Saunders, 1996;989–998.
3. Berg HE, Berggren G, Tesch PA. Dynamic neck strength training effect on pain and function. *Arch Phys Med Rehabil* 1994;75:661–665.
4. Bortz WM. The disuse syndrome. *West J Med* 1984;141(5):691–694.
5. Cassidy JD, Lopes AA, Yong-Hing K. The immediate effect of manipulation versus mobilization on pain and range of motion in the cervical spine: a randomized controlled trial. *J Manipulative Physiol Ther* 1993;15: 570–575.
6. Conley MS, Meyer RA, Bloomberg JJ, Feeback DL, Dudley GA. Noninvasive analysis of human neck muscle function. *Spine* 1995;20(23):2505–2512.
7. Coulter ID. *The appropriateness of manipulation and mobilization in the cervical spine.* Santa Ana, CA: Rand publication MR-781-CCRM, 1996.
8. Dvořák J, Valach L, Schmid H. Cervical spine injuries in Switzerland. *J Manual Med* 1989;4:7–16.
9. Foley-Nolan D, Barry C, Coughlan RJ, O'Connor P, Roden D. Pulsed magnetic high frequency (27 MHz) electromagnetic therapy for acute whiplash injuries. A double blind randomized controlled study. *Scand J Rehabil Med* 1992,24.51–59.
10. Galasko CSB, Murray PM, Ritcher M, et al. Neck sprains after road traffic events: a modern epidemic. *Injury* 1993;24:155–157.
11. Harms-Ringdahl K, Ekholm J. Intensity and character of pain and muscular activity levels elicited by maintained extreme flexion position of the lower-cervical-upper-thoracic spine. *Scand J Rehabil Med* 1986;18:117–126.
12. Highland TR, Dreisinger TE, Vie LL, Russell GS. Changes in isometric strength and range of motion of the isolated cervical spine after eight weeks of clinical rehabilitation. *Spine* 1992;17(6S):S77–S82.
13. Kamwendo K, Linton SJ. A controlled study of the effect of neck school in medical secretaries. *Scand J Rehab Med* 1992.
14. Woo SL, Buckwalter JA. *Injury and repair of the musculoskeletal soft tissues.* Park Ridge, IL: American Academy of Orthopaedic Surgeons, 1987.

15. McKinney LA, Dornan JO, Ryan M. The role of physiotherapy in the management of acute neck sprains following road-traffic events. *Arch Emerg Med* 1989;6:27–33.
16. Mealy K, Brennan H, Fenelon GC. Early mobilization of acute whiplash injuries. *Br Med J* 1989;292: 1006–1008.
17. Nansel D, Peneff A, Cremata E, Carlson J. Time course considerations for the effects of unilateral lower cervical adjustments with respect to the amelioration of cervical lateral passive end-range asymmetry. *J Manipulative Physio Ther* 1990;13:297–304.
18. Nygren A. Injuries to car occupants—Some aspects of the interior safety of cars. A study of a five-year material from an insurance company. *Acta Otolaryngol* 1984;395(Suppl):1–164.
19. Radanov PR, Di Sefano G, Schnidrig A, Ballinari P. Role of psychosocial stress in recovery from common whiplash. *Lancet* 1991;331:712–715.
20. Radanov BP, Sturzenegger M, Di Stefano G. Long term outcome after whiplash injury. A 2-year follow-up considering features of accident mechanism, somatic, radiological and psychosocial findings. *Medicine* 1995;74: 281–297.
21. Schrader H, Obelieniene D, Bovin G. Natural evolution of late whiplash syndrome outside the medicolegal context. *Lancet* 1996;347:1207–1211.
22. Shapiro I, Frankel VH. Biomechanics of the cervical spine. In: Nordin M, Frankel VH, eds. *Basic biomechanics of the musculoskeletal system,* 2nd ed. Philadelphia: Lea & Febiger, 1989;209–224.
23. Silverman JL, Rodriquez AA, Agre JC. Quantitative cervical flexor strengths in healthy subjects and in subjects with mechanical neck pain. *Arch Phys Med Rehabil* 1991;72:679–681.
24. Spitzer WO, Skovron ML, Salmi LR, et al. Scientific monograph of the Québec Task Force on whiplash-associated disorders: redefining whiplash and its management. *Spine* 1995;20(8S):10S–73S.
25. Spitzer WO, Salmi LR, Skovron ML, et al. Monographie scientifique du groupe de travail Québécois sur les troubles associés à l'entorse cervicale (TAEC). Redéfinir le whiplash et sa prise en charge. *Le Médecin du Québec* 1995;(Suppl):9–76.
26. Starfield B, Wray C, Hess K, et al. The influence of patient-practitioner agreement on outcome of care. *Am J Public Health* 1981;23:127–131.
27. Sturzenegger M, Di Stefano G, Radanov BP, Schnidrig A. Presenting symptoms and signs after whiplash injury: the influence of accident mechanisms. *Neurology* 1994;44(4):688–693.
28. Suissa S, Harder S, Veilleux M. The Québec whiplash-associated-disorders cohort study. *Spine* 1995;20(8S): 12S–20S.
29. Tan JC, Nordin M. Role of physical therapy in the treatment of cervical disk disease. *Orthop Clin North Am* 1992;23(3):435–449.
30. Thomas KB. General practice consultations: Is there any point in being positive? *Br Med J* 1987;294:1200–1202.
31. Woo, SL-Y. The cellular and matrix response of ligaments and tendons to mechanical injury. In: Leadbetter WB, Buckwalter JA, Gordon SL, eds. *Sports Induced Inflammation*. American Orthopaedic Society for Sports Medicine Symposium, 1990;189–224.
32. Zetterberg C, Nordin M, Skovron ML, Zuckerman J. Skeletal effects of physical activity. *Geritopics* 1990;14: 17–24.
33. Zybergold RS, Piper MC. Cervical spine disorders. A comparison of three types of traction. *Spine* 1985;10: 867–871.

Whiplash Injuries: Current Concepts in Prevention, Diagnosis, and Treatment of the Cervical Whiplash Syndrome, edited by Robert Gunzburg and Marek Szpalski. Lippincott–Raven Publishers, Philadelphia © 1998.

22

Cervical Zygapophysial Joint Pain and Percutaneous Neurotomy

An Update to the Québec Task Force Report on Whiplash-Associated Disorders

Nikolai Bogduk

N. Bogduk: Newcastle Bone and Joint Institute, Royal Newcastle Hospital; Faculty of Medicine and Health Sciences, University of Newcastle, Newcastle NSW, Australia.

In its report on whiplash-associated disorders (WAD), the Québec Task Force lamented the paucity of good literature on the diagnosis and treatment of neck pain after whiplash (29). Out of some 10,000 titles, it could find fewer than 300 worthy of review. It had every intention of conducting a meta-analysis of the literature on each topic concerning whiplash but was unable to do so, for there was simply insufficient literature suitable for such analysis. By default, the Task Force had to resort to consensus rather than an evidence-base in its recommendations on how to investigate and treat neck pain after whiplash.

The Québec Task Force completed its literature review in 1993. As a result, it was unaware of developments that had been occurring in Australia, and of literature that appeared in 1994 and that has continued to appear since then. The results of this work fills certain of the voids identified by the Québec Task Force in its report.

HISTORY

At a time when the causes, or even the sources, of neck pain were not known, Bogduk and Marsland raised the proposition that perhaps the cervical zygapophysial joints might be one such source. In 1988, they published the first systematic diagnostic study of cervical zygapophysial joint pain (12). They found 17 out of 24 consecutive patients with chronic, posttraumatic neck pain could have their pain relieved by local anesthetic blocks of one or other of their zygapophysial joints.

This observation ran contrary to traditional wisdom at the time, which was either that chronic neck pain was entirely psychogenic or, at best, was discogenic and due to spondylosis. Detractors at the time would not accept the notion of cervical zygapophysial joint pain, arguing either that these joints could not possibly be a source of pain, or that it was rare, or that investigators could not trust the reports of relief of pain by patients who had diagnostic blocks.

In response, Dwyer et al. (17) demonstrated that the cervical zygapophysial joints could, indeed, be a source of pain in normal volunteers; and Aprill and Bogduk (3) showed that far from being rare, cervical zygapophysial joint pain seemed to affect at least 25% and perhaps as many as 65% of some 300 consecutive patients with chronic, posttraumatic neck pain.

ANATOMY

The cervical zygapophysial joints are paired synovial joints, each about the size of a knuckle, located along the back of the cervical vertebral column, and formed by the infe-

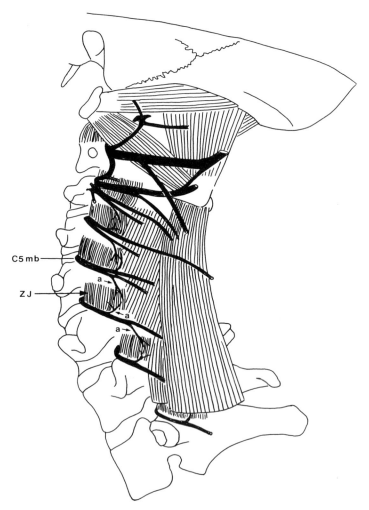

FIG. 1. A sketch of the medial branches of the cervical dorsal rami and the innervation of the cervical zygapophysial joints. Articular branches (*a*) to each joint (*zj*) arise from the medial branch (*mb*) of the dorsal ramus above and below the joint.

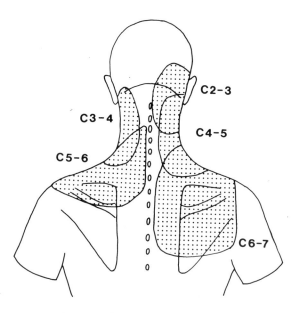

FIG. 2. Referred pain patterns from the cervical zygapophysial joints.

rior and superior articular processes of consecutive cervical vertebrae from level C2-3 to C6-7. Each joint is enclosed by a fibrous capsule and contains fibroadipose meniscoids that protect the articular cartilages that become exposed during movements of the joints (25). At typical cervical levels, the joints are orientated at about 45° to the transverse axis of their vertebrae, but at C2-3 the joint is somewhat more horizontal, and at C6-7 it is somewhat steeper (27). Because of this orientation, the joints are able to sustain axial compression loads and to resist anterior shear.

Each joint is typically supplied by the medial branches of the dorsal rami that bear the same segmental numbers as the joint (11). Each medial branch runs around the waist of the ipsi-segmental articular pillar and sends ascending articular branches to the joint above and descending branches to the joint below (Fig. 1). The exception is the C2-3 joint, which obtains its innervation from the deep surface of the third occipital nerve which crosses the lateral and posterior aspect of the joint (11).

PAIN PATTERNS

In normal volunteers, stressing a cervical zygapophysial joint with intra-articular injections of contrast medium induces pain that is perceived in locations characteristic of the joint stimulated (17) (Fig. 2). These patterns have been corroborated by more recent studies that involved not only physical stimulation of the joints but also electrical stimulation of the nerves that supply them (18). Strikingly, they are patterns that resemble those frequently exhibited by patients with chronic neck pain (12). However, the pain patterns are not diagnostic of zygapophysial joint pain, but they serve as a guide as to which joint should first be suspected and where confirmatory investigations should commence (17).

SYSTEMATIC STUDIES

In 1991, the Motor Accidents Authority of the state of New South Wales in Australia, provided a generous grant that enabled the Cervical Spine Research Unit (CSRU) to be established at the University of Newcastle, which is located in an industrial city some 100 miles north of Sydney. The grant provided scholarships for postgraduate medical research students and part-time support for office staff and medical records expertise. The Unit systematically explored the validity of diagnostic blocks for cervical zygapophysial joint pain, the prevalence of this condition in patients with chronic neck pain after whiplash, and its treatment. For the studies, the Unit drew patients from Sydney, Newcastle, and nearby towns. To be seen by the Unit, patients had to have been suffering neck pain for at least 3 months after a motor vehicle accident, for which no diagnosis had been established despite conventional investigations by their family doctor and at least one specialist.

Diagnostic Blocks

Zygapophysial joint pain cannot be diagnosed clinically. There is no evidence that any particular clinical feature, or any pattern of movement, is characteristic, let alone diagnostic, of pain stemming from one of these joints. Nor can zygapophysial joint pain be diagnosed using medical imaging. There is no feature that might be seen on radiographs, or on computed tomography (CT) or magnetic resonance imaging (MRI) scans that is a valid indication that the particular joint is painful or not.

The only means of establishing if a joint is painful is to anesthetize it. In this regard, local anesthetic blocks are not a test of the patient; they are simply a test of the physician's diagnostic hypothesis. If a joint suspected of being the source of pain is, indeed, the source of pain, anesthetizing it should relieve the pain; but if the physician's guess is wrong, diagnostic blocks will not relieve the pain.

One way of anesthetizing a cervical zygapophysial joint is to block the nerves that supply the target joint, using tiny amounts of local anesthetic delivered onto the course of the nerve, under fluoroscopic guidance (13) (Fig. 3). Such medial branch blocks are easier, faster, and safer to perform that intra-articular blocks of the joint (13).

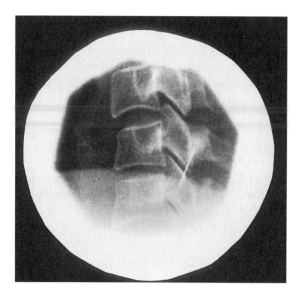

FIG. 3. A lateral radiograph of the lower neck showing a needle in position for a C6 medial branch block, obtained in the course of a C5-6 zygapophysial joint block.

Validity

The first studies of the CSRU established the face-validity of medial branch blocks (4). They showed that the blocks reliably did anesthetize the target nerves, and that they did not consistently anesthetize any other structure that might be relevant to the patient's pain. In particular, the local anesthetic did not spread to affect the spinal nerves, nor did it nonspecifically anesthetize the neck muscles.

The next studies examined construct validity, to test whether a positive response to a diagnostic block really meant that the patient genuinely had zygapophysial joint pain. It was shown that a single diagnostic block was unreliable; single blocks were associated with an unacceptably high false positive rate (5). To ensure validity, some form of control had to be exercised in each and every patient.

The most rigorous form of control would be to administer a placebo block under double-blind conditions, but this is not practical outside a research situation, for it necessitates three diagnostic procedures. The first must be a block using an active agent to determine first if the target joint is at all painful. (There is no point wasting time and resources to perform controlled blocks if the joint is not painful.) Subsequently, the second block cannot routinely be the inactive control, for a mischievous patient could come to know that the second block is always the dummy. To maintain blinding and the element of chance, the second block must randomly be either an active or an inactive agent, and there must be a third block using the reciprocal agent. Although rigorous, such a protocol is unlikely to gain acceptance in conventional clinical practice. Some other more practical, but nonetheless rigorous, form of control was required.

A paradigm of comparative local anesthetic blocks was developed to serve as a control. This paradigm was based on antecedent literature that showed that in the same, normal individuals, the effects of lignocaine did not outlast the effects of bupivacaine (26,28,32). True positive responses to local anesthetic blocks could, therefore, be defined as long-lasting relief when a long-acting agent was administered, and short-lasting relief when a short-acting agent was used (10,14,15). A double-blind study showed that true positive responses were common to cervical zygapophysial joint blocks, and statistical analysis revealed that it was extremely unlikely that these patients could possibly have guessed which agents were used (6).

In that study (6), a substantial proportion of patients were identified who exhibited what seemed to be paradoxical responses to blocks: they had inordinately prolonged responses to lignocaine. This type of response was noted, but it was not classified as positive.

A later study tested the validity of comparative local anesthetic blocks against placebo (21). It found that correct responses to comparative local anesthetic blocks were 83% reliable, but it also found that 65% of patients who had prolonged responses to lignocaine were not placebo responders. Thus, comparative local anesthetic blocks are very specific but lack sensitivity. Patients classified as positive are reliably positive, but comparative blocks may fail to diagnose all patients who genuinely have zygapophysial joint pain.

Prevalence

The first of two prevalence studies used double-blind, comparative local anesthetic blocks in a sample of 50 consecutive patients with chronic neck pain after whiplash (9). It found that zygapophysial joint pain accounted for 54% of these patients. A parallel study (20) determined that in patients in whom headache was the dominant complaint of pain, the pain could be traced to the C2-3 zygapophysial joint in 53%.

A second prevalence study (22), using double-blind, placebo-controlled blocks, confirmed the results of the first study, by showing a prevalence of cervical zygapophysial joint pain of 46%. Collectively, these studies showed, under double-blind conditions in just over 100 patients, the prevalence of zygapophysial joint pain to be 49% with confidence intervals of 40% to 58%.

These studies established that zygapophysial joint pain was the single most common basis of chronic neck pain after whiplash. Moreover, no other diagnostic entity has ever been subjected to such rigorous scientific scrutiny, and no other entity in the field of whiplash has survived such scrutiny. Whatever the beliefs might be that discogenic pain or myofascial pain is the basis of chronic neck pain after whiplash, there is no epidemiologic evidence to substantiate these beliefs, and no evidence that competes with that in support of cervical zygapophysial joint pain (7). The diagnosis of cervical zygapophysial joint pain does not rely on any special manual skills; it is made simply, under double-blind, controlled conditions, using diagnostic blocks. The local anesthetic does the work, and the double-blind conditions prevent either the doctor or the patient from cheating.

TREATMENT

It had been proposed that cervical zygapophysial joint pain could be treated with intra-articular injections of corticosteroids. Accordingly, the CSRU undertook a randomized, double-blind, controlled study of this putative therapy. The results were negative (8). Steroids conferred no therapeutic benefit over injections of local anesthetic alone, and both treatments had no worthwhile clinical effect. Although some patients obtained long-lasting relief, the vast majority had recurrence of their pain within a week. This result left patients with diagnosable zygapophysial joint pain without a proven treatment.

Another treatment that had been postulated for cervical zygapophysial joint pain was percutaneous radiofrequency neurotomy. In this procedure, an electrode is introduced through the skin and neck muscles onto the nerves that mediate the patient's pain, to coagulate those nerves (Fig. 4). The procedure is analogous to the use of radiofrequency lesions in the treatment of trigeminal neuralgia, but there are two differences. First, the target is a medial branch of a dorsal ramus instead of the trigeminal nerve; second, and more important, the target is a peripheral nerve, not the trigeminal ganglion. Consequently, the effect of the operation is not permanent because the cell bodies of the target nerve are not destroyed.

A review of previous reports of this procedure identified many problems (23). There were major problems with patient selection, reliable diagnosis, and accuracy of technique. However, for a pilot study, these were corrected. The pilot showed that technical problems still plagued the effective execution of radiofrequency neurotomy for C2-3 joint pain, but the results at lower cervical levels were sufficiently robust to justify a controlled trial (23).

Twenty-four patients with cervical zygapophysial joint pain proven by double-blind, placebo-controlled diagnostic blocks, volunteered for the study. Twenty-four was the minimum number required to achieve appropriate statistical power in view of the ethical considerations involved for a trial of a neurosurgical therapy. Each patient was randomized to receive either the active therapy or a sham control. The patients and the surgeon remained blind to the randomization until the conclusion of the study. All patients underwent the same 3-hour surgical procedure. Under regional anesthesia, in every

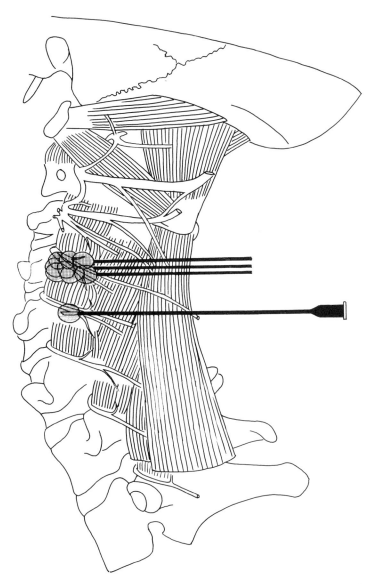

FIG. 4. A sketch of the surgical anatomy of cervical medial branch neurotomy. An electrode is introduced to lie parallel to the target nerve. A small lesion made by the tip of the electrode coagulates the nerve. Several lesions need to be made about the nerve to accommodate variations in its course and to maximize the length of nerve coagulated.

patient, the surgeon correctly placed the electrodes into position and ostensibly coagulated the target nerves. At least six lesions were made around each of the two target nerves in every patient. The only difference between the active and sham procedures was that for the active treatment, lesions were made at 80°C, whereas for the sham procedure, the electrode tip was maintained at 37°C. Because of the local anesthesia, the patients could not feel what temperature was generated, and the surgeon could not see the thermocouple read-out.

Several demanding outcome measures were used. For the procedure to be deemed a success, the patients had to report complete relief of their pain, corroborated by a score of less than 5/100 on a visual analog scale and a total word count of less than 3 on the McGill Pain questionnaire. Moreover, they had to regain the four activities of daily living that previously they had specified as being restricted by their pain and which most dearly they would want restored.

The study showed that the pain relief produced by percutaneous neurotomy was not a placebo effect (24). The median duration of relief obtained by patients undergoing the control treatment was 8 days, whereas in the patients treated with active lesions it was 263 days.

Percutaneous radiofrequency neurotomy is the only treatment for chronic neck pain that has been shown to provide complete relief of pain, even years after its onset. Percutaneous radiofrequency neurotomy is the only treatment for neck pain that has been proved against the strictest form of placebo-control.

Follow-up studies are in progress to establish the durability of the relief. Preliminary experience is very encouraging. Patients maintain their relief for up to a year or more, during which time they can resume a normal, pain-free life (23). If and once the pain recurs, the procedure can be repeated to re-instate relief. No other treatment for neck pain has been shown to have this power.

PATHOLOGY

This series of studies has deliberately been clinical. The cause of cervical zygapophysial joint pain was not explored until it could be shown that cervical zygapophysial joint pain did exist, could be diagnosed, and could be treated.

Studies by others have provided clues as to what might be the cause of cervical zygapophysial joint pain. Biomechanics studies have shown that the cervical zygapophysial joints can be injured in whiplash incidents (1,2,16,33). Postmortem studies have revealed that the joints can be affected by pillar fractures, subchondral fractures, tears of their meniscoids, and intra-articular hemorrhages (19,30,31). Any of these lesions would seem to be a valid explanation of why the joints become painful. Furthermore, such is the nature of the lesions that they are not likely to heal and leave a pristine joint; they are all conditions that in joints of the appendicular skeleton are associated with long-term, destructive changes and chronic pain.

To complete the picture of cervical zygapophysial joint pain, a next step would be to turn high-resolution imaging to joints proven to be painful by controlled diagnostic blocks. Thus, correlations might be established with visible morphologic changes and the physiologic perception of pain. In the meantime, however, the diagnosis and treatment of cervical zygapophysial joint pain does not need to await the results of such imaging studies.

REFERENCES

1. Abel MS. Moderately severe whiplash injuries of the cervical spine and their roentgenologic diagnosis. *Clin Orthop* 1958;12:189–208.
2. Abel MS. Occult traumatic lesions of the cervical vertebrae. *CRC Crit Rev Clin Radiol Nucl Med* 1975;6: 469–553.
3. Aprill C, Bogduk N. The prevalence of cervical zygapophyseal joint pain: a first approximation. *Spine* 1992;17: 744–747.
4. Barnsley L, Bogduk N. Medial branch blocks are specific for the diagnosis of cervical zygapophysial joint pain. *Reg Anesth* 1993;18:343–350.

5. Barnsley L, Lord S, Wallis B, Bogduk N. False-positive rates of cervical zygapophysial joint blocks. *Clin J Pain* 1993;9:124–130.
6. Barnsley L, Lord S, Bogduk N. Comparative local anaesthetic blocks in the diagnosis of cervical zygapophysial joints pain. *Pain* 1993;55:99–106.
7. Barnsley L, Lord S, Bogduk N. Clinical review: whiplash injuries. *Pain* 1994;58:283–307.
8. Barnsley L, Lord SM, Wallis BJ, Bogduk N. Lack of effect of intraarticular corticosteroids for chronic pain in the cervical zygapophyseal joints. *N Engl J Med* 1994;330:1047–1050.
9. Barnsley L, Lord SM, Wallis BJ, Bogduk N. The prevalence of chronic cervical zygapophysial joint pain after whiplash. *Spine* 1995;20:20–26.
10. Boas RA. Nerve blocks in the diagnosis of low back pain. *Neurosurg Clin North Am* 1991;2:807–816.
11. Bogduk N. The clinical anatomy of the cervical dorsal rami. *Spine* 1982;7:319–330.
12. Bogduk N, Marsland A. The cervical zygapophysial joints as a source of neck pain. *Spine* 1988;13:610–617.
13. Bogduk N, Aprill C, Derby R. Diagnostic blocks of synovial joints. In: White AH, ed. *Spine care,* vol. 1: Diagnosis and conservative treatment. St Louis: Mosby, 1995;298–321.
14. Bonica JJ. Local anaesthesia and regional blocks. In: Wall PD, Melzack R, eds. *Textbook of pain,* 2nd ed. Edinburgh: Churchill Livingstone, 1989;724–743.
15. Bonica JJ, Buckley FP. Regional analgesia with local anesthetics. In: Bonica JJ, ed. *The management of pain,* vol. 2. Philadelphia: Lea and Febiger, 1990;1883–1966.
16. Clemens HJ, Burow K. Experimental investigation on injury mechanisms of cervical spine at frontal and rearfrontal vehicle impacts. In: *Proceedings of the sixteenth STAPP Car Crash Conference.* Warrendale: Society of Automotive Engineers, 1972;76–104.
17. Dwyer A, Aprill C, Bogduk N. Cervical zygapophyseal joint pain patterns. I: A study in normal volunteers. *Spine* 1990;15:453–457.
18. Fukui S, Ohseto K, Shiotani M, Ohno K, Karasawa H, Naganuma Y, Yuda Y. Referred pain distribution of the cervical zygapophyseal joints and cervical dorsal rami. *Pain* 1996;68:79–83.
19. Jónsson H, Bring G, Rauschning W, Sahlstedt B. Hidden cervical spine injuries in traffic accident victims with skull fractures. *J Spinal Disorder* 1991;4:251–263.
20. Lord S, Barnsley L, Wallis B, Bogduk N. Third occipital nerve headache: a prevalence study. *J Neurol Neurosurg Psychiatry* 1994;57:1187–1190.
21. Lord SM, Barnsley L, Bogduk N. The utility of comparative local anaesthetic blocks versus placebo-controlled blocks for the diagnosis of cervical zygapophysial joint pain. *Clin J Pain* 1995;11:208–213.
22. Lord S, Barnsley L, Wallis BJ, Bogduk N. Chronic cervical zygapophysial joint pain after whiplash: a placebo-controlled prevalence study. *Spine* 1996;21:1737–1745.
23. Lord SM, Barnsley L, Bogduk N. Percutaneous radiofrequency neurotomy in the treatment of cervical zygapophysial joint pain: a caution. *Neurosurgery* 1995;36:732–739.
24. Lord S, Barnsley L, Wallis BJ, McDonald GJ, Bogduk N. Percutaneous radio-frequency neurotomy for chronic cervical zygapophyseal joint pain. *N Engl J Med* 1996;335:1721–1726.
25. Mercer S, Bogduk N. Intra-articular inclusions of the cervical synovial joints. *Br J Rheumatol* 1993;32:705–710.
26. Moore DC, Bridenbaugh LD, Bridenbaugh PO, Tucker GT. Bupivacaine for peripheral nerve block: a comparison with mepivacaine, lidocaine, and tetracaine. *Anesthesiology* 1970;32:460–463.
27. Nowitzke A, Westaway M, Bogduk N. Cervical zygapophyseal joints: geometrical parameters and relationship to cervical kinematics. *Clin Biomech* 1994;9:342–348.
28. Rubin AP, Lawson DIF. A controlled trial of bupivacaine: a comparison with lignocaine. *Anaesthesia* 1968;23:327–331.
29. Spitzer WO, Skovron ML, Salmi LR, et al. Scientific monograph of the Québec Task Force on whiplash-associated disorders: redefining whiplash and its management. *Spine* 1995;20:1S–73S.
30. Taylor JR, Twomey LT. Acute injuries to cervical joints: an autopsy study of neck sprain. *Spine* 1993;9:1115–1122.
31. Taylor JR, Taylor MM. Cervical spine injuries: an autopsy study of 109 blunt injuries. *J Musculoskel Pain* 1996;4:61–79.
32. Watt MJ, Ross DM, Atkinson RS. A double blind trial of bupivacaine and lignocaine. *Anaesthesia* 1968;23:331–337.
33. Wickstrom, J, Martinez JL, Rodriguez R Jr. The cervical sprain syndrome: experimental acceleration injuries to the head and neck. In: Selzer MI , Gikas PW, Huelke DF, eds. *The prevention of highway injury.* Ann Arbor, MI: Highway Safety Research Institute, 1967;182–187.

SECTION 5

Surgical Treatment

Whiplash Injuries: Current Concepts in Prevention, Diagnosis, and Treatment of the Cervical Whiplash Syndrome, edited by Robert Gunzburg and Marek Szpalski. Lippincott–Raven Publishers, Philadelphia © 1998.

23

Surgery after Whiplash Injuries of the Neck: Indications and Approaches[*]

Henry Vernon Crock

H. V. Crock: Spinal Disorder Unit. Cromwell Hospital, London SW5 0TU, United Kingdom.

A patient who sustains a significant neck injury, commonly resulting from a motor vehicle accident, often becomes involved in a sequence of events that may continue over the course of several years as treatment is sought for the resultant, often wide-ranging symptoms. A list of those who will contribute to treatment or will seek to influence it may become very long. The first contact may be with a casualty officer or with the patient's own general practitioner, a day or so after the accident; physiotherapists, chiropractors, and osteopaths may follow before medical or surgical specialists are called in. The order of referral should depend on the advice of the general practitioner, but it is often influenced by that of friends and others. Hence, orthopedic surgeons, neurosurgeons, neurologists, rheumatologists, physiatrists, psychiatrists, pain management specialists, and perhaps insurance assessors of dubious experience become involved. The fate of many of these patients who may require surgery is that they are seen by one after another of the practitioners on this list.

Although the term *whiplash injury* is used widely by the general public in describing the outcome of events, such as collisions between motor vehicles, in which passengers sustain neck injuries, its use within the medical profession is accepted with reluctance. Confusion exists about the mechanism of injury and about the use of this particular terminology. In 1983, the Cervical Spine Research Society published a book, *The Cervical Spine*, in which Hohl's chapter entitled "Soft Tissue Neck Injuries" dealt with clinical aspects of "whiplash, hyperextension, acceleration injury, cervical strain, and cervical sprain," grouping all these terms together as though they were synonymous. Treatment was discussed in just over one page of the text, with no mention of surgery (7). Likewise, in the literature there is a general reluctance to recommend surgery after whiplash injuries of the neck. The Cervical Spine Research Society published another book in 1994, *The Cervical Spine—An Atlas of Surgical Procedures* (9), in which no mention was made of surgical techniques for use in the treatment of whiplash injuries of the neck. In the same year, An and Simpson edited a volume entitled *Surgery of the Cervical Spine* (1), in which there is no reference to the investigation or treatment of whiplash injuries of the neck. In the massive two-volume work, *The Adult Spine—Principles and Practice*, only brief reference is made in one chapter (2) to the use of cervical discography in

---

[*]Figures in this chapter © H. V. Crock.

patients with persisting symptoms after whiplash injuries. In another chapter entitled "Cervical Sprain Syndrome," La Rocca (8) explained that the title was his preferred term "for that cluster of clinical problems attendant upon the sudden application of a propulsive force to the head and neck complex, in which tissue damage occurs directly as the result of the propulsion." He was using the term to mean "the action of driving or pushing forward or onward; the condition of being impelled forward." Its use in that context adds little to the understanding of the whiplash mechanism of injury, and in this chapter, surgical treatment was mentioned in only seven lines of the text.

Whiplash injuries occur in accidents involving the cervical spine when complex extension, flexion, and sometimes rotational forces are applied to the head and neck as a result of rapid acceleration.

Because there is such confusion about the terminology used to describe this mechanism of neck injury, about the explanations proposed for the widespread symptoms afflicting these patients, and about who should treat them, it is not surprising that the role of surgical treatment is controversial.

Despite these difficulties, the indications for surgical treatment after whiplash injuries of the neck can be clearly defined. Specific injuries may follow the extension, flexion, and sometimes the rotational components of the forces that are applied at the time of, and rapidly after the moment of impact. The patterns of these injuries will vary with the state of the patient's cervical spine at the time of the accident. The following classification is useful in identifying indications for surgery.

GROUP 1: YOUNG PATIENTS WITH NORMAL NECK RADIOGRAPHS

These patients are prone to develop nonprolapsing intervertebral disc injuries resulting from damage by the combined forces inflicted on one or more of the cervical discs. Their widespread symptoms of neck pain, occipitofrontal headache, photophobia, hypersensitivity to noise, referred arm pains, lassitude, and irritability fail to respond to conservative treatments.

Investigations

The plain cervical spine x-ray is normal. Magnetic resonance imaging (MRI) of the cervical spine is normal. Computed tomography (CT) of the cervical spine is normal.

Cervical discography is diagnostic for the condition of posttraumatic internal disc disruption (Fig. 1). This test is performed on the lightly sedated but conscious patient. Interpretation of the discogram includes the following:

1. Assessment of the patient's pain response during injection of the radiopaque dye.
2. A record of the volume injected. Only 0.3 to 0.5 mL may be injected painlessly into a normal cervical disc. Injection of a volume in excess of this is abnormal.
3. A measurement of the spread of dye beyond the normal confines of the cervical nucleus pulposus.

Recommended Surgical Treatment

The recommended surgical treatment is anterior disc excision and interbody fusion with autogenous bone grafts.

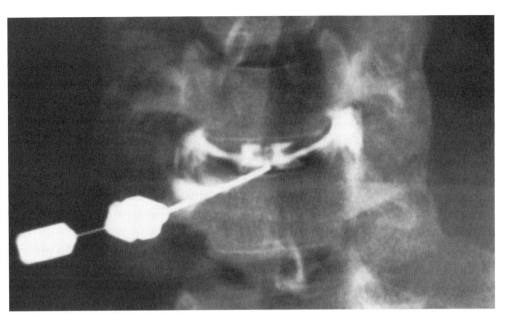

FIG. 1. An anteroposterior radiograph of the cervical spine of a 20-year-old woman after whiplash injury of her neck, showing a discogram between the vertebral bodies of C5 and C6 with marked disruptive changes, the dye leaking transversely across the vertebral interspace towards the uncovertebral joint regions.

GROUP 2: MIDDLE-AGED PATIENTS WITH NORMAL NECK RADIOGRAPHS

These patients may present with two types of cervical disc injury (both of which are rare after whiplash injuries) or with injury to the cervical facet joints.

Cervical Disc Prolapse

These patients present with typical symptoms of brachial neuralgia, with abnormal neurologic findings similar to those found in patients with cervical disc prolapses that have occurred without high-speed trauma to the neck.

Investigations

The plain cervical spine x-ray is usually normal. CT and MRI are diagnostic. In both imaging modalities, the prolapsed disc tissues are easily seen. Cervical discography is not indicated.

Surgical Treatment

Anterior cervical discectomy with interbody fusion using autogenous bone grafts is recommended.

Cervical Vertebral Endplate Cartilage Avulsion

These patients complain of protracted neck pain and head pain with varying degrees of arm pain.

Investigations

Plain x-rays are normal. Flexion and extension x-rays or cine radiography of the neck demonstrate abnormal extensor motion with a widened disc space anteriorly. MRI is not diagnostic. CT is not diagnostic. Cervical discography is unreliable in these cases.

Surgical Treatment

Anterior disc excision and interbody fusion with autogenous bone grafting is recommended.

Cervical Facet Joint Injuries

These patients complain of persistent neck pain, headaches, and brachial neuralgia of varying degrees of severity. These lesions result largely from the flexion phase of neck movement.

Investigations

Plain x-rays are normal. CT may show facet joint injuries, with small fractures or evidence of joint effusions. MRI is not diagnostic. Facet arthrography is diagnostic. Radiopaque dye injected into the affected joints under x-ray control spreads widely beyond the joint capsules.

Surgical Treatment

The treatment of this condition is discussed in Chapter 25 by Dr. Dieter Grob, which outlines the mechanism of production of cervical facet joint injury, and the investigative and clinical methods of identifying these lesions.

GROUP 3: PATIENTS WITH PREEXISTING CERVICAL SPONDYLOSIS

Indications for surgery in this group do not differ from the widely accepted indications for treatment of patients with intractable symptoms of neck pain, occipital headache, and brachial neuralgia caused by degenerative cervical spondylosis (Fig. 2).

Investigations

Plain x-rays are diagnostic. CT and MRI are diagnostic. Cervical discography is not indicated.

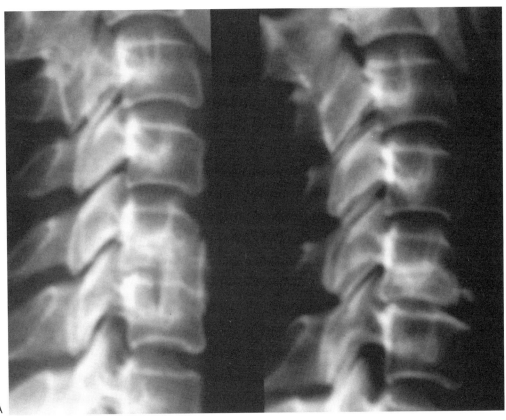

A   B

FIG. 2. A: The postoperative appearance after disc excision, cervical canal decompression, and anterior interbody fusion. **B:** A lateral radiograph of the cervical spine of a 50-year-old woman showing preexisting resorptive-type degenerative change of the disc at C5-6.

Surgical Treatment

Anterior disc excisions and interbody fusion with autogenous bone grafts is the recommended treatment.

GROUP 4: PATIENTS WITH PREEXISTING CERVICAL CANAL STENOSIS

These patients may present after whiplash injuries of the neck with signs of cervical cord irritation that progresses rapidly to clear-cut clinical evidence of cervical myelopathy, which may lead to quadriparesis (Fig. 3).

Investigations

Plain x-rays are not diagnostic. MRI is diagnostic (see Fig. 3). CT is essential for determining the bony dimensions of the cervical canal, which are reduced below the normal values in this condition.

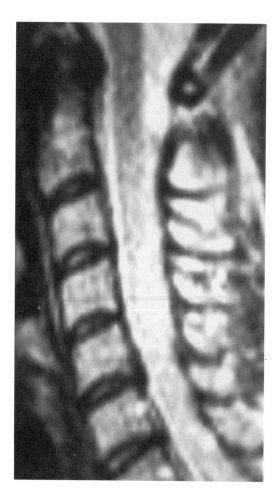

FIG. 3. MRI of the cervical spine of a 36-year-old woman, showing cervical canal stenosis at the C5-6 level. She presented with signs of cervical cord irritation after a whiplash injury to her neck.

Surgical Treatment

In cases of single-level and two-level cervical canal stenosis, anterior interbody fusion, using autogenous bone grafting, combined with decompression of the cervical canal, is appropriate. In cases of three-level cervical canal stenosis, strut grafts with adequate decompression of the cervical canal from the anterior approach may be used. In cases of multilevel stenosis, particularly if more than three levels are involved, a posterior operation of the Hirabayashi (6) open-door laminoplasty type may be indicated.

Anterior Approaches

In most cases, even those involving multilevel cervical canal decompression and interbody fusion, right-handed surgeons are most comfortable using a right-sided hemicollar neck incision. Use of a vertical skin incision running along the line of the anterior border of the sternomastoid muscle is sometimes necessary; however, after its use an ugly keloid scar may develop along its length.

The use of a transverse skin incision followed by a longitudinal split in the platysma muscle leads easily—principally with the use of blunt dissection—to the anterior surface of the cervical vertebral column, without division of any major structures. Occasionally, one of the thyroid arteries or veins may need to be ligated and divided before the midline structures of the esophagus, larynx, and trachea can be retracted to expose the cervical discs.

I have found the tubular cutting system illustrated in Figures 4, 5, and 6 to be very effective in preparing dowel cavities and for harvesting autogenous bone grafts for cervical interbody fusions. Postoperative pain at the iliac donor site is minimal providing the grafts are cut from the inner to the outer table just below the iliac crest, thereby avoiding stripping the tensor fascia lata and gluteal muscles from the outer table of the ilium (4). There is little justification, therefore, for using substitutes such as BOP (biocompatible osteoconductive polymer) or "cages" for cervical interbody fusions on the grounds that they avoid donor site morbidity (5).

Dowel grafting using Cloward's technique (3) also ensures postoperative stability at the graft site, so that the use of bone plates and screws is often not required.

Posterior Approaches

These will be discussed in detail in Chapter 25 by Dr. Grob.

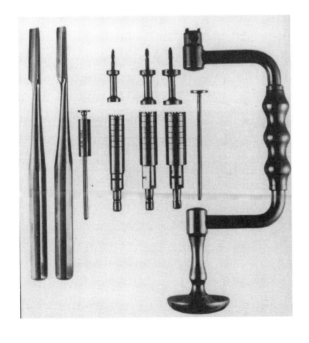

FIG. 4. The Crock instruments used for dowel cutting in the anterior cervical interbody fusion surgery. On the *right* is a Hudson brace with cutters of three sizes, the starter center pieces having been removed from each of these. On the right of the cutters is a pusher, which fits inside the cutters and can be used to eject the starter center pieces or graft bone. On the left of the cutters a pusher is shown with a tubular segment of metal measuring 12.5 mm in depth. When this "dummy" is slotted into the cutter, it acts as a guard, preventing the cutter from penetrating deeper than 12.5 mm into the cervical vertebral bodies. Dummies are provided in three sizes, 10 mm, 12.5 mm, and 15 mm, for use according to the vertebral dimensions in individual cases. On the *left*, two tooled gouges are shown, which fit into the cuts made into the adjacent vertebral bodies and are used to dislodge the bony fragments and intervening disc tissues in the preparation of the dowel cavity. (Reproduced with permission from Crock HV. *A short practice of spinal surgery*. Wein: Springer-Verlag, 1993;238.)

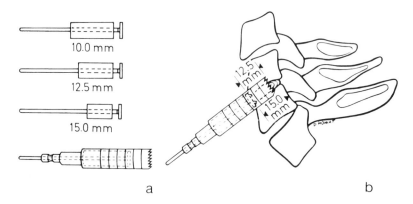

a   b

FIG. 5. A: A drawing to show the range of metal dummies available for insertion into the zero-size cutter, allowing the preparation of dowel cavities of predetermined depth, depending on the depth of the disc space in individual patients. The depth of the space is checked at operation by control x-ray with the use of a needle, the end of which is bent in a Z shape to prevent penetration of the cervical canal. At the *bottom*, note the dummy assembled inside the cutter. **B:** A drawing to depict the cutter in use, demonstrating the safety protection provided by the 12.5-mm dummy which has been inserted after removal of the starter center piece. Note also that the surgeon is able to count the rings on the outer side of the cutter, providing a double safety factor. These rings are separated by 5 mm. This instrumentation has been in use by the author for more than 30 years without any injury to the spinal cord, vertebral arteries, or cervical nerve roots resulting from its use. (Reproduced with permission from Crock HV. *A short practice of spinal surgery.* Wein: Springer-Verlag, 1993;246.)

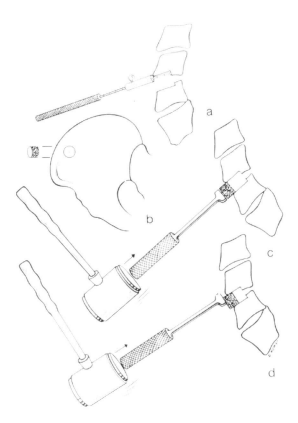

FIG. 6. A: The cervical spine, viewed from the side, showing a prepared dowel cavity between two vertebral bodies with a depth gauge inserted to measure the depth of the cavity before the graft is inserted. **B:** The pelvic crest, showing the site of removal of a plug of bone that is cut from the inner to the outer table. The measurement of this graft between the two cortical surfaces varies depending on the size of the patient's pelvis. Grafts should be trimmed so that the anterior and posterior margins are parallel. The depth of the anterior iliac crest between the inner and outer cortical tables varies between 5 and 15 mm. In patients whose pelvis is thin (3 to 5 mm between outer and inner cortices), it may be necessary to cut grafts vertically downwards from the top of the crest, by the method used in lumbar interbody fusions. **C:** The initial stages of impaction of the graft, the measurement of which has been checked carefully with the measurement of the prepared dowel cavity. At this stage, the anesthetist is asked to elongate the neck by applying traction under the angles of the mandible. **D:** Final seating of the graft is sometimes necessary if the anterior margin is not flush with the vertebral margins after use of the initial impactor, which has a central nipple on it, as illustrated in (**C**). The maneuver shown is performed with a plain-ended impactor, and it is important to note the impactor is placed half way across the graft and half way across the adjacent vertebral body, so that when a blow is struck with the hammer, it is impossible to drive the graft too deeply into the dowel cavity, as the impactor comes to rest on the anterior vertebral margin. Accurate seating of the graft is essential if the complications of graft rotation or postoperative graft prolapse are to be avoided. (Reproduced with permission from Crock HV. *A short practice of spinal surgery.* Wein: Springer-Verlag, 1993;256.)

REFERENCES

1. An HS, Simpson JM. *Surgery of the cervical spine.* London: Martin Dunitz, 1994.
2. Aprill CN. Diagnostic disc injection. In: Frymoyer JW, Ducker TB, Hadler NM, et al., eds. *The adult spine: principles and practice.* New York: Raven Press, 1991;403–419.
3. Cloward RB. Lesions of the intervertebral discs and their treatment by interbody fusion methods. *Clin Orthop* 1963;27:51.
4. Crock HV. *A short practice of spinal surgery.* Wein: Springer-Verlag, 1993.
5. Hafez RF, Crockard HA. Failure of osseous conduction with cervical interbody BOP graft. *Br J Neurosurg* 1997; 11(1):57–59.
6. Hirabayashi K, Toyama Y. Choice of surgical procedure for cervical ossification of the posterior longitudinal ligament. In: Yonenobu S, Sakou T, and Ono K, eds. *OPLL: ossification of the posterior longitudinal ligament.* Tokyo: Springer-Verlag, 1997;135–142.
7. Hohl M. Soft tissue neck injuries. In: Bailey RW, et al., eds. *The cervical spine.* Philadelphia: JB Lippincott, 1983;282–287.
8. La Rocca H. Cervical sprain syndrome—Diagnosis and treatment. In: Frymoyer JW, Ducker TB, Hadler NM, et al., eds. *The adult spine: principles and practice.* New York: Raven Press, 1991;1051–1061.
9. Sherk HH, et al., eds. *The cervical spine.* Philadelphia: JB Lippincott, 1994.

Whiplash Injuries: Current Concepts in
Prevention, Diagnosis, and Treatment
of the Cervical Whiplash Syndrome,
edited by Robert Gunzburg and Marek Szpalski.
Lippincott–Raven Publishers, Philadelphia © 1998.

24

The Diagnosis and Surgical Treatment of Chronic Cervical Whiplash Disc Injuries

E. Jeffrey Donner and Kenneth A. Pettine

E. J. Donner and K. A. Pettine: The Spine Institute, Rocky Mountain Associates in Orthopaedics, Loveland, Colorado 80538.

Serious cervical spine injuries are known to occur after motor vehicle accidents. Less apparent, but still significant, cervical whiplash injuries also occur and account for a majority of patients who visit a physician for treatment of their persistent neck pain and headaches. Cervical whiplash is commonly referred to as acceleration–extension injury of the neck after a rear-end collision. However, in this discussion, it will be defined as any inertial force applied to the head during a motor vehicle accident that results in neck pain (3). Most patients improve over a period of time and resume normal activities with minimal residual symptoms. Those who do not improve can have intense pain and associated symptoms that do not respond to standard non-operative care (22). They may be severely disabled and unable to manage their symptoms despite the use of narcotic medications. It is not uncommon for them to be diagnosed as having a chronic cervical sprain or strain because of the common complaints of muscle pain, spasm, and stiffness. In addition, there is a lack of objective data to confirm that their complaints are related to injuries of more significant structures. Even worse, they become a victim of the system and often carry the burden of proving that they are disabled by their injury and not malingering to reap financial secondary gain.

There is hope for chronic cervical whiplash sufferers, however, because the chronic disabling symptoms can often be diagnosed by cervical discography and treated with anterior cervical fusion. This technique and concept has had some attention in the medical literature but has not become accepted medical care in most treatment algorithms (14–21,28,29). The purpose of this chapter is to attempt to justify both the use of cervical discography to diagnose cervical disc injuries, and the technique of anterior cervical discectomy and fusion to significantly improve the health-related quality of life for chronic cervical whiplash patients.

BACKGROUND INFORMATION

Over 250,000 cervical whiplash injuries occur every year in the United States and in 1992 accounted for 83% of traffic accident medical claims made to insurance companies (3,13). Approximately 25% of these patients go on to have chronic symptoms and 10% to 15% have severe pain (22). Neck pain is often the primary complaint; however, a variety of symptoms are described, including headaches, radiating arm pain, weakness, numbness, paresthesia, dizziness, visual and memory disturbances, and psychological problems (3,12,27).

Routine imaging studies are often normal or demonstrate age-related degenerative changes that are inconsistent with the patient's clinical presentation (6,22). These studies include not only routine x-rays, but also dynamic studies and the more sophisticated myelograms, computed tomography (CT), and magnetic resonance imaging (MRI). Patients who have had an obvious disc herniation and associated neurologic deficit consistent with their symptoms often obtain expedient treatment with a good outcome (8). The majority of the remaining patients have had multiple nondiagnostic studies, and extensive rehabilitation has not significantly improved their symptoms (22).

A recent Québec Task Force study on whiplash-associated disorders published in *Spine* in 1995 extensively reviewed the literature and found that few reports met minimum standards of relevance and scientific rigor (22). Based on the paucity of evidence, they had to retreat to opinion and consensus. They began their own study and their conclusions were as follows:

1. No treatment has been proven effective in the management of whiplash injuries.
2. Whiplash-associated disorders are for the most part mild conditions, self-limiting and of short duration.
3. Of the people with whiplash, 12% lapsed into a chronic state, and these patients accounted for 42% of the cost attributed to that diagnostic class.

Thus, it is clear that we must attempt to further define the pathology that causes the chronic incapacitating symptoms and then direct our treatment and research to this area.

PATHOLOGY

The exact pathology that leads to chronic whiplash syndrome has not been clearly identified. It is reasonable to assume that any structure in the neck that undergoes deformation from a whiplash force is potentially a source of injury and pain. Each anatomic structure has the ability to sustain a variable amount of force before it fails (23). The ability of tissues to heal is also variable, but we know that injured muscles and tendons of the axial skeleton typically heal without long-term sequela. Injured ligaments also have the ability to heal and stabilize; however, there are incidents when the disruption is extensive and chronic ligament instability is possible. This usually leads to some type of instability pattern that can be identified on dynamic flexion and extension views of the cervical spine. The other structures that appear to be more likely associated with chronic pain and are not associated with overt instability are the facet joints and cervical discs (3).

Postmortem pathologic specimens of cervical spines in individuals who sustained fatal injuries in motor vehicle accidents were compared to controls in a study by Taylor and Twomey (24). Clefts in the cartilaginous endplates of the intervertebral discs were identified in 15 of the 16 spines in trauma victims. The findings were quite distinct from the uncovertebral clefts and central disc fissures that were a normal feature of aging in the control group. The authors also observed a significant number of samples of soft-tissue damage at the synovial facet joints, but occult damage to the bone or articular cartilage was unusual. A similar high incidence of potentially deleterious discoligamentous injuries was also identified by Jonsson et al. (9) when they studied 20 traffic accident victims who sustained lethal skull fractures in motor vehicle accidents.

Jonsson et al. (8) also studied 50 consecutive patients who sustained whiplash-type cervical spine distortion injuries over a 13-month period and were followed for 5 years. Twenty-four patients underwent MRI scanning for persistent neck pain or radiating arm pain. On their MRI scans, 13 of these patients were seen to have disc protrusions of varying degrees. Eight patients underwent anterior cervical discectomy and fusion, and all improved immediately after surgery, and at 5-year follow-up they experienced essentially no pain. The authors noted a poor correlation between the radiating pain and the MRI abnormalities. The unoperated symptomatic patients averaged 18 months of cumulative sick leave resulting from their persistent symptoms.

Based on these studies and others, it appears that the cervical disc is commonly injured in whiplash victims and can be a significant source of pain.

DIAGNOSTIC STUDIES AND TREATMENT

The majority of diagnostic studies for cervical whiplash are either normal, or they show age-related degenerative changes and are nondiagnostic (22). There have been multiple studies in the literature that have documented these findings with plain radiographs, CT scans, and MRIs in asymptomatic patients (5,26). Boden et al. (5) demonstrated that there was a 19% incidence of signal changes in the cervical discs associated with slight to moderate disc protrusions in asymptomatic patients.

Discography and anesthetic facet blocks have been demonstrated to be useful in identifying the source of spinal pain. Barnsley found that 54% of patients with chronic cervical whiplash neck pain had painful facet joints based on double anesthetic blocks (4). Lord et al. utilized similar blocks and was able to identify the C2-3 facet joints as the source of pain in patients whose primary symptom after a motor vehicle accident was headache (10). Aprill and Bogduk (1) performed both provocative discography and cervical facet blocks on 56 patients with posttraumatic neck pain and found that 41% had both a symptomatic disc and a zygapophyseal joint at the same segment, 20% had only a symptomatic disc, 23% had an isolated symptomatic facet joint, and 17% had neither symptomatic disc nor facet or zygapophyseal joints. Unfortunately, specific treatment for symptomatic facet joints has been relatively ineffective. Intra-articular steroids are not effective, and facet rhizotomy is only modestly effective (2,11).

There have been many publications that have been favorable and many that have been overtly unfavorable to the use of discography as a means of determining not only the pathology but also its usefulness in making recommendations for surgical treatment (1,3,7,15–21,25). A more recent study by trained specialists in cervical discography has been able to demonstrate its validity (17). In this study, all 10 asymptomatic volunteers had asymptomatic discography. Twenty of the 40 discs tested were normal on MRI and 18 of these 20 proved to have painless annular tears discographically. They also studied 10 chronic neck pain sufferers, and 15 concordantly painful discs were identified. There was no correlation between painful discs and MRI findings or annular tears.

There have been several studies that have confirmed the value of anterior cervical fusion for cervical disc degeneration, but success has been as low as 27% in those without radicular symptoms (28,30). Other studies included discography to determine fusion levels, and surgical success ranged from 70% to 90% (14,29).

STUDY DESIGN AND METHODS

A retrospective study was performed on 39 consecutive patients who sustained neck injuries related to motor vehicle accidents and who underwent anterior cervical fusion over a three-year period (1992–1994). Sixty-two percent were rear-ended and the remaining collisions were passenger's side (16%), rollover (11%), driver's side (7%), and front-end (4%). Eighty-six percent of the patients were drivers, 14% were passengers, and 74% were restrained. All patients had incapacitating symptoms that failed to improve with conservative measures. The average length of symptoms was 35 months, with a range of one month to ten years. Tweny-seven patients had symptoms for over one year.

All but one patient had a preoperative MRI scan and nine were either completely normal or essentially normal. Thirty-six patients underwent cervical discography to identify the source of the symptoms and to determine fusion levels.

Sixteen patients underwent anterior cervical fusion at MRI-normal levels, based on their response to discography. Nineteen patients were fused at MRI-abnormal levels, with the majority of these confirmed with discography. Four patients underwent fusions at MRI-abnormal levels with additional fusions at MRI-normal levels that were symptomatic on discography.

The surgical technique included a left-sided approach to the anterior cervical spine, followed by disc excision and complete removal of the disc material and cartilaginous endplate back to the posterior longitudinal ligament. The disc nucleus and annulus were also removed in the foraminal region on the symptomatic sides. The endplates were prepared by slightly perforating the cortical surfaces. A tricortical iliac crest bone graft was inserted after the disc was extracted. Distraction was then released and anterior plate fixation was added for stability in 35 cases, some of which were second procedures on patients whose fusions were extended or whose pseudoarthroses were repaired. Eight patients had their primary procedure performed without internal fixation.

RESULTS

Thirty-nine patients underwent anterior cervical discectomy and fusion by a single surgeon (EJD) for a motor vehicle accident–related cervical discogenic syndrome. Thirty-seven patients were contacted by a premedical student and queried on their outcome. (Two patients were not reached.) All of the 37 patients contacted improved 50% or more, with an overall average symptom improvement of 77.5%. Ninety-seven percent of the patients felt that their headaches were significantly improved, and 88% felt that their arm pain was significantly improved. Ninety-two percent would repeat the surgery for the same outcome, and 100% stated that they would recommend it to someone else for the same problem. Almost all patients were taking some form of narcotic medications preoperatively, and postoperatively 76% of the patients were taking no medications. There was an average follow-up of 26 months with a minimum follow-up of 1 year.

Table 1 summarizes the outcome data of this study as well as that of all anterior cervical fusions performed by both surgeons in a joint spine practice. Kenneth A. Pettine's outcome data are also presented for comparison. Tables 2 and 3 summarize the fusion levels and work status, respectively. The work status was not positively affected by the surgical procedures. Twenty-six of the 39 patients had significant associated injuries that required additional surgical procedures, which reflects the complexity of managing

TABLE 1. *Data summary for patients undergoing anterior cervical fusion (ACF) for motor vehicle accident–related whiplash injuries*

	Total ACF Patients	Motor vehicle-related patients	
	KAP & EJD	EJD	KAP
ACF patients (contacted/total)	288/313	37/39	61/71
Overall symptom improvement (%)	72	77.5	74
Patients with significant arm pain improvement (%)	68	88	82
Patients with significant headache improvement (%)	60	97	88
Patients who would repeat the procedure (%)	91	92	88
Patients who would recommend the procedure (%)	95	100	96
No medications needed by follow-up (%)	67	76	64
Preoperative MRI abnormality found (%)	77	78	80
Average follow-up (mo)	20	26	25
Average duration of symptoms (mo)	36	35	27

these difficult cases. Table 4 summarizes the additional surgical procedures. Complications included one iliac crest autogenous bone graft site infection. There were three pseudoarthroses in two patients.

After reviewing the data, it was our impression that discography altered the surgical levels in 24 patients, and in 19 patients this occurred in the primary procedure. Five patients who did not undergo discography, and whose surgical level was determined on MRI findings alone, failed to significantly improve. Symptomatic discs were subsequently diagnosed on discography and fusions were performed at these levels with significant (77.5%) overall improvement.

DISCUSSION

Chronic incapacitating neck and radiating arm pain and other associated symptoms are common sequelae of auto accident–related neck injuries. The majority of the patients

TABLE 2. *Spinal level undergoing anterior cervical fusion (ACF)*

One-level	23
C2-3	2
C3-4	3
C4-5	6
C5-6	8
C6-7	4
Two-level	15
C3-5	3
C4-6	2
C5-7	7
C3-6	1
C2-3, C4-5	1
C3-4, C5-6	1
Three-level	1
C4-7	1
Total:	39 ACFs

TABLE 3. *Work status*

Preoperatively	Postoperatively	Patients (N)
Full time	Full time	14
Full time	Part time	3
Not working	Not working	8
Part time	Part time	6
Full time	Unknown	2
Unknown	Unknown	6

eventually recover with the passage of time and non-operative treatment. Ten to 15% of these patients go on to develop chronic incapacitating symptoms, which often go undiagnosed because of the lack of specificity and sensitivity of routine diagnostic studies. These patients become an enormous financial burden to society, accounting for approximately 40% of all costs, most of which are related to reimbursement for lost income. A review of literature indicated that no treatment had been proven to be effective (3,22). The patient often becomes frustrated, depressed, alienated, and labeled as fraudulent or a malingerer.

By utilizing diagnostic blocks and discography, pain generators have been more clearly identified in the cervical spine, which allows for more effective treatment protocols and options for the patients. Although some investigators feel that the cervical facet joint is the main source of whiplash symptoms, the cervical disc has also been identified as a significant source of pain and as amenable to anterior cervical discectomy and fusion (1–4,10). Our present study indicates that the cervical disc can be a significant pain generator that can be documented by discography, and significant improvement in symptoms can be obtained for a majority of patients with anterior cervical fusion. There is obviously a significant learning curve in terms of using discography to identify the source of the pain, which has led many investigators to avoid this technique.

As surgeons, we prefer to perform our own discography to eliminate a potential misinterpretation of the highly subjective discography study. The patient is only slightly sedated, and, because he or she knows the surgeon through previous encounters in the office, he or she is more relaxed. Repeat injections at the level tested are also recommended to ensure that appropriate information is obtained. The feedback the surgeon obtains from performing the discography and surgical procedure allows one to improve one's skills and diagnostic abilities. The good outcome obtained in this study has been shown to be reproducible, in that both surgeons followed the same protocol and the results are essentially equivalent in nearly every category measured.

It needs to be appreciated that this is a very complex condition that requires a multidisciplinary team including psychologists, therapists, and pain management specialists. We feel it is important to clearly identify the pain generators with discography and, if nec-

TABLE 4. *Associated injuries treated surgically*

Procedure	Patients (N)
Lumbar fusion	12
Thoracic outlet syndrome surgery	2
Thoracic fusion	1
Snapping scapula release	1
Lumbar laminectomy	1
Shoulder rotator cuff surgery	9
Extremity nerve decompression	3
Suprascapular nerve release	1

essary, with facet blocks before making a surgical decision. If the patient has one or two levels of pathology, with other normal control levels identified, then a reliably good outcome can be obtained. Multiple-level fusions may also be effective, but less reliable, and we attempt to avoid these if possible. Although not proven by this study, it is our belief that the cervical disc and cartilaginous endplate must be removed as completely as possible back to the posterior longitudinal ligament and nerve roots. A biomechanically sound anterior cervical fusion should be performed, which leads to a solid arthrodesis and relief of the patient's symptoms. We highly recommend use of autogenous bone graft and anterior plate fixation to avoid complications of pseudoarthrosis, graft collapse, and loss of normal lordosis of the cervical spine. Because the average patient has had approximately 3 years of symptoms prior to surgery, the complication of pseudoarthrosis and the need for further surgery needs to be avoided if at all possible.

CONCLUSION

Cervical injuries related to motor vehicle accidents may be associated with cervical disc injuries. Approximately 90% of the chronic whiplash patients in our practice have symptomatic provocative discography. Anterior cervical discectomy and fusion at the symptomatic levels reliably relieved the majority of the symptoms in over 90% of the patients in this study. There is a high patient satisfaction rate and the results are reproducible.

Further research in the area of whiplash injuries is warranted. Prevention is the obvious remedy, but it is unlikely to resolve the problem in the near future and it certainly cannot have any effect on the perhaps millions of patients who continue to suffer from this treatable condition.

REFERENCES

1. Aprill C, Bogduk N. On the nature of neck pain. *Pain* 1993;54:213–217.
2. Barnsley L, Lord SM, Wallis B, Bogduk N. Lack of effect of intra-articular steroids for chronic cervical zygapophyseal joint pain. *N Engl J Med* 1994;330:1047–1050.
3. Barnsley L, Lord S, Bogduk N. Whiplash injury—A clinical review. *Pain* 1994;58:283–307.
4. Barnsley L, Lord SM, Wallis BJ, Bogduk N. The prevalence of chronic cervical zygapophysial joint pain after whiplash. *Spine* 1995;20:20–26.
5. Boden SD, McCowin PR, Davis DO, et al. Abnormal magnetic-resonance scans of the cervical spine in asymptomatic subjects. *J Bone Joint Surg* 1990;72A:1178–1184.
6. Herzog RJ, Guyer RD, Graham-Smith A, Simmons ED Jr. Contemporary concepts in spine care: magnetic resonance imaging. *Spine* 1995;20:1178–1184.
7. Holt E Jr. Fallacy of cervical discography. *JAMA* 1964;188:799–801.
8. Jonsson H, Cesarini K, Sahlstedt B, Rauschning W. Findings and outcome in whiplash-type neck distortions. *Spine* 1994;19:2733–2743.
9. Jonsson H, Bring G, Rauschning W, Sahlstedt B. Hidden cervical spine injuries in traffic accident victims with skull fractures. *J Spinal Disorders* 1991;4:251–263.
10. Lord SM, Barnsley L, Wallis B, Bogduk N. Chronic cervical zygapophyseal joint pain afer whiplash. *Spine* 1996;21:1737–1745.
11. Lord SM, Barnsley L, Bogduk N. Percutaneous radiofrequency neurotomy in the treatment of cervical zygapophyseal joint pain: a caution. *Neurosurgery* 1995;36:732–739.
12. Macnab I, McCulloch J. Whiplash injury of the cervical spine. In: *Backache,* 2nd ed. Baltimore: Williams & Wilkins, 1986:140–159.
13. *The McKee monitor.* Winter, 1996:11.
14. Palit M, Schofferman M, Goldthwaite M, et al. Anterior discectomy and fusion relieves axial neck pain. Presented at a meeting of the North American Spine Society, Vancouver, Canada. Oct. 1996.
15. Parfenchuck T, Janssen M. A correlation of cervical magnetic resonance imaging and discography-computed tomographic discograms. *Spine* 1994;19:2819–2825.
16. Roth O. Cervical analgesic discography: a new test for the definitive diagnosis of the painful-disk syndrome. *JAMA* 1976;235:1713–1714.

17. Schellhas KP, Smith MD, Gundry CR, Pollei SR. Cervical discogenic pain. *Spine* 1996;21:300–311.
18. Shinomiya K, Nakao N, Shindoh K, Mochida K, Furuya K. Evaluation of cervical diskography in pain origin and provocation. *J Spinal Disord* 1993;6:422–426.
19. Simmons E. An evaluation of discography in the localization of symptomatic levels in discogenic diseases of the spine. *Clin Orthop* 1975;108:57–59.
20. Smith G, Nichols P. The technique of cervical discography. *Radiology* 1957;68:718–720.
21. Smith G. The normal discogram. *AJR* 1959;81:1006–1010.
22. Spitzer WO, Skouron ML, Salmi LR, et al. Scientific monolograph of the Québec Task Force on whiplash-associated disorders. *Spine* 1996;20:105–685.
23. Suh J, Kang J, Saito R, Carlin G, et al. Viscoelastic behavior of human cervical FSU in torsion. Presented at a meeting of the North American Spine Society, Vancouver, Canada. Oct. 1996.
24. Taylor J, Twomey L. Acute injuries to the cervical joints—an autopsy study on neck strain. *Spine* 1993;18:1115–1122.
25. The executive committee of the North American Spine Society. Position statement on discography. *Spine* 1988;13:1343.
26. Teres LM, Lufkin RB, Reicher MA, et al. Asymptomatic degenerative disk disease and spondylosis of the cervical spine. MR imaging. *Radiology* 1987;164:834.
27. Wallis B, Lord S, Barnsley L, Bogduk N. Pain and psychological symptoms of Australian patients with whiplash. *Spine* 1996;21:804–810.
28. White A, Southwick W, Deponte R, Gainor S, Hardy R. Relief of pain by anterior cervical fusion for spondylosis. *J Bone Joint Surg* 1973;55A:525–534.
29. Whitecloud T, Seago R. Cervical discogenic syndrome: results of operative intervention in patients with positive discography. *Spine* 1987;12(4):313–316.
30. Williams JL, Allen MB Jr, Harkess JW. Late results of cervical discectomy and interbody fusion. *J Bone Joint Surg* 1968;50A:277–286.

Whiplash Injuries: Current Concepts in Prevention, Diagnosis, and Treatment of the Cervical Whiplash Syndrome, edited by Robert Gunzburg and Marek Szpalski. Lippincott–Raven Publishers, Philadelphia © 1998.

25

Posterior Surgery

Dieter Grob

D. Grob: Spine Unit, Schulthess Clinic, Zürich, Switzerland.

The lesion in whiplash injury of the cervical spine is not fully understood, and it is often difficult or impossible to identify it well enough to proceed with surgical stabilization. Neurologic symptoms and neurophysiologic investigation usually fail to clarify the situation, as no radicular symptoms are present in the classic whiplash injury. The clinical examination and conventional radiologic procedures are perfectly ideal to detect bony or obvious ligamentous lesions, but in most cases of whiplash injury the source of pain remains obscure. Additional investigations by flexion–extension x-rays and magnetic resonance imaging (MRI) are, in the majority of whiplash-injured patients, not sufficient to enlighten the situation (4).

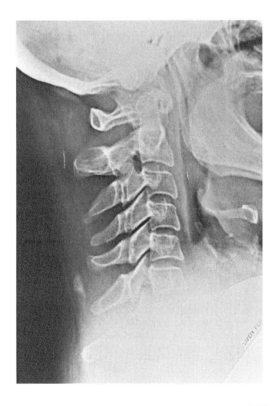

FIG. 1. Posterior calcification of the nuchal ligament in the C5-6 segment of possible traumatic origin. The question remains open if this segment is the source of pain.

Rarely, discrete pathologic changes of traumatic origin can be detected on radiographs of whiplash victims. Calcification in ligamentous structures, mobility at the upper limit of standard deviations (4), or anterior bony ligamentous detachments are then suspect as the source of pain. But the proof remains an unsolved problem, as the specificity of such radiologic findings is low and may not be accepted as an indication for surgery. Therefore, more aggressive diagnostic tools are needed (Fig. 1) that will give more information about the functioning of a potentially painful segment. Once identified, an injured segment may be immobilized, and then the posterior approach is one of the surgical options.

INVASIVE DIAGNOSTICS

Facet Infiltration

Facet infiltration in the cervical spine reveals painful changes of the articular and capsular complex (2). The puncture is done under fluoroscopic control to ensure that the proper segment is approached. The use of dye confirms the correct intra-articular placement of the tip of the needle. A few milliliters of local anesthetics are subsequently injected intra-articularly. It may be assumed that the injected facet represents the cause of pain if pain relief is noted according to the pharmacologic properties of the injected drug. There is, however, controversy about the significance and specificity of this diagnostic procedure, dealing with the polysegmental innervation of the facets. In spite of this, we consider the posterior facet infiltration a useful diagnostic procedure as it should not be used as an isolated indicator but rather in combination with clinical and radiologic investigations.

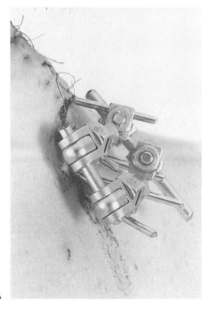

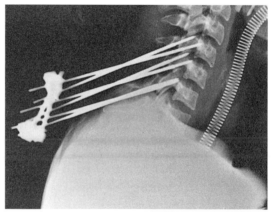

A

B

FIG. 2. Temporary external fixation of the cervical spine in C2. **A:** The threaded K-wires are inserted parallel to the facet plane and diverge 25° to 30°. **B:** The fixation is done by the posterior ends of the K-wires.

Discography

Radiologic changes of the disc are often the only clue to localize the source of pain. MRI reveals and defines most of the alterations in the disc by a noninvasive method. However, the specificity of this investigation is known to be low (1).

Puncture of the disc (discography) can provide further information. A needle is ventrally introduced into the center of the disc under fluoroscopic control. Memory pain may be noted by the patient as the anulus is entered by the tip of the needle. The amount of dye and the resistance during injection, as well as the distribution pattern of the injected dye, provide information about the integrity of the disc and anulus fibrosus.

Temporary Fixation

Temporary external fixation of the lower cervical spine (C2–C7) proved to be a useful tool to identify pain sources of mechanical origin after whiplash injury (6). With a small skin incision, the posterior aspects of the vertebrae involved are exposed. Threaded Kirschner (K-) wires are inserted into the articular masses according to the Magerl technique (e.g., parallel to the facet plane and 25° to 30° divergent). The crossing of the K-wires of each segment is located on the skin level. The posterior part of the K-wires may be alternatively fixed, using the Synthes hand external fixator (Fig. 2). The testing starts

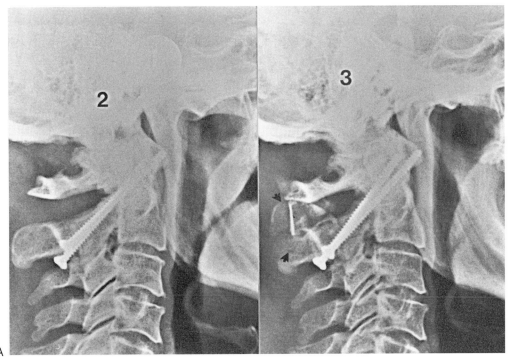

A   B

FIG. 3. A: In a patient with suspected ligamentous lesion of the C1-2 segment, bilateral atlantoaxial screws have been inserted. Ten days after surgery, the patient reports a clear improvement of his previous suboccipital pain. **B:** In a second stage, the posterior bone graft for permanent bony fixation of the atlantoaxial segment has been added.

after the pain of the insertion procedure has calmed down. The segments are alternatively fixed and loosened while the patient is encouraged to communicate pain intensity on a pain scale from 0 to 10. To diminish the placebo effect, the actual configuration of fixation (or no fixation at all) is without the patient's knowledge. Each type of fixation is performed twice to test reproducibility of the pain relief. If a segment can be identified by this temporary immobilization, subsequent stabilization is performed. The anterior approach is preferred, to diminish the risk of infection after removal of the external fixator.

The temporary fixation of the atlantoaxial segment is performed by atlantoaxial posterior screw fixation. The screws are inserted in a first stage without adding the bone graft. To ensure atraumatic surgery, after a midline splitting of the ligamentum nuchae and the trapezoid muscle, no muscle detachment of the deep posterior cervical muscles is performed, as decortication for the bone graft of the midline structures is not necessary. After the screw insertion, the patient is encouraged to walk around in the hospital. If pain relief is reported by the patient, the fixation is completed by adding the bone graft in a second stage, placing it in the midline between the posterior aspect of the atlas and the spinous process of C2. The screws are removed percutaneously if there is no pain relief and therefore no indication for fusion of the segment.

Patient selection for these procedures has to be performed with extreme care, but in desperate cases with no other possibility, these procedures represent a last resort (Fig. 3).

POSTERIOR SURGERY

Upper Cervical Spine

Indications/Diagnostics

Direct visualization of ligamentous injury in the suboccipital area is difficult. Whereas ruptures of the transverse ligament may be detected by flexion–extension radiographs and increased atlantoaxial distance, the injuries of alar ligaments may be diagnosed by functional computed tomography (CT) (4). Temporary internal fixation may be considered in doubtful cases. Surgery is indicated when intractable neck pain exists and conservative management has failed to improve the situation.

Operative Technique

The transarticular atlantoaxial technique according to Magerl provides a reliable three-dimensional stability (7). The patient is placed on the operating table in the prone position. In the case of atlantoaxial dislocation, a reduction is attempted by positioning the patient in a halo-frame or Mayfield-tongue under. The detailed technique of transarticular screw fixation of Magerl has been described (7). The screws are inserted in the posterocaudal portion of the lamina of C2. They cross the atlantoaxial joint on the posterior aspect and penetrate the lateral masses of the atlas. Drilling is preferably performed under fluoroscopic control. For occipitocervical fusions including the occiput, a Y-shaped plate is used. The plate is molded to conform with the occipitocervical anatomy with the head in a neutral position, and it is cut to the appropriate length. The two transarticular screws are placed into the plate. A corticocancellous bone graft is removed from the posterior iliac crest and inserted below the plate. It is first shaped to fit exactly into the space between the occiput, the dorsal arch of the atlas, the spinous process of C2, and the plate. Two 2.5-mm holes are drilled through the proximal holes of the plate into the midline of the skull. By tightening the screws, the graft is firmly fixed between the occiput and the plate. A reliable, immediate stability is achieved.

Plates were used if a fusion had to be extended subaxially. The bent plates are first fixed by atlantoaxial transarticular screws.

Postoperative external fixation was restricted to a soft collar, worn when the patient is out of bed, but only until there is solid fusion, usually radiologically confirmed after 6 to 8 weeks.

Results

In a retrospective study (5), 15 patients with posttraumatic suboccipital pain and pathologic changes of the atlantoaxial segment in the functional CT, but no other bony abnormalities, have been fused by transarticular posterior screw fixation. The average follow-up is 60 months (range, 44 to 84). The average age of the patients (10 women, 5 men) was 35 years (range, 21 to 53). At the follow-up examination, all patients showed a solid bony union of the bone graft and no motion in the flexion–extension radiographs of the cervical spine. The preoperative pain score of 7 (range, 5 to 9) decreased to 4.4 (2.1 to 7.3). No patient was worse. The subjective rating was very good in seven, good in six, and moderate in two patients.

Lower Cervical Spine

Indications/Diagnostics

Mechanical instability of anterior (disc) lesions may be revealed by functional radiographs or MRI. Clinical findings and radiologic changes have to correlate before surgery is indicated. Temporary external fixation is used in doubtful cases.

Persisting pain in spite of adequate conservative management is considered an indication for segmental stabilization.

Operative Technique

The operative technique and internal stabilization has to be performed according to the degree of instability of the injured structures. Simple interspinous wiring may be sufficient for posterior ligamentous instabilities and intact anterior structures (e.g., the anterior longitudinal ligament) (3,9). The stability is ensured by a tension band mechanism. However, posterior screw and plate fixation is recommended in more complex injuries. The screws are placed in the cervical spine in the articular masses according to previously described techniques (8) (not transpedicularly as done in the thoracic and thoracolumbar spine). Through a standard posterior midline approach, the spinous processes and articular masses are exposed. The entry of the drill is into the caudal part at the junction of the lamina and the articular mass. The direction of the drill bit lies in a plane parallel to the facet orientation. Twenty to thirty degrees divergence in relation to the sagittal midline have to be respected to avoid injury of the nerve root or vertebral artery anteriorly.

The Hook-plate is adequate for mono- or bisegmental fixation (8). If longer constructs are desired, 3.5-mm AO reconstruction plates may be used.

To avoid postoperative segmental kyphotic deformity, preoperative MRI is recommended to identify simultaneous disc lesions.

Indications for Posterior Surgery after Trauma to the Cervical Spine

After trauma to the cervical spine, posterior surgery is useful in the following conditions:

1. Insufficiency of posterior tension band mechanism
2. Posterior fracture (–dislocation)
3. Anterior surgery not possible (open injury)
4. Posterior stenosis (ligamentum flavum, foramen)
5. Additional procedure to anterior surgery
6. Salvage procedure (pseudarthrosis after anterior fusion)

CONCLUSIONS

Surgical treatment in whiplash injury is indicated only if the injured level can be clearly identified. For identification of the lesion, invasive diagnostics, such as facet infiltration, discography, or temporary fixation techniques, may be necessary. If the painful segment can be identified, immobilization seems to be justified. Posterior fusion after whiplash injury is indicated in the presence of ligamentous injury of the atlantoaxial segment. In the lower cervical spine, posterior surgery is restricted to isolated posterior soft-tissue injuries.

REFERENCES

1. Boden S, McCowin P, Davis DO, Dina TS, Mark AS, Wiesel S. Abnormal magnetic resonance scans of the cervical spine in asymptomatic subjects. *J Bone Joint Surg* 1990;72A:1178–1183.
2. Bogduk N. The anatomy and pathophysiology of whiplash. *Clin Biomech* 1986;1:92–101.
3. Bohlmann HH. Acute fractures and dislocations of the cervical spine: an analysis of three hundred hospitalized patients and review of the literature. *J Bone Joint Surg* 1979;61A:1119–1142.
4. Dvořak J, Panjabi MM, Novotny JE, Antinnes JA. In vivo flexion/extension of the normal cervical spine. *J Orthop Res* 1991;9:828–834.
5. Ehrat C. Atlanto-axiale Spondylodese bei Patienten mit traumatisch entstandener Bandinstabilität oder Arthrose. University of Zürich. 1997 *(submitted)*.
6. Grob D, Dvořak J, Panjabi MM, Antinnes JA. Fixateur externe an der Halswirbelsäuleein neues diagnostisches Mittel. *Unfallchir* 1993;96:416–421.
7. Grob D, Dvořak J, Panjabi MM, Hayek J. Die dorsale atlanto-axiale Verschraubung. Ein Stabilitätstest in vitro und in vivo. *Orthopäde* 1991;20:154–162.
8. Grob D, Magerl F. Dorsale Spondylodese der Halswirbelsäule mit der Hakenplatte. *Orthopäde* 1987;16:55–61.
9. McAfee PC, Bohlman HH, Wilson WL. The triple wire fixation technique for stabilization of acute fracture dislocations: a biomechanical analysis. *J Bone Joint Surg Orthop Trans* 1985;9:142.

Whiplash Injuries: Current Concepts in
Prevention, Diagnosis, and Treatment
of the Cervical Whiplash Syndrome,
edited by Robert Gunzburg and Marek Szpalski.
Lippincott–Raven Publishers, Philadelphia © 1998.

26

Anterior Cervical Plating: A Historical Perspective and Recent Advances

Peter M. Klara

P. M. Klara: Department of Neurosurgery, Eastern Virginia Medical School, Spinal Research and Education Foundation, Norfolk, Virginia 23502.

Anterior cervical decompression and fusion became a standard surgical approach through the pioneering efforts of Bailey and Badgley (3), Smith and Robinson (21), Cloward (6), and Verbiest (27). This approach was developed in the 1950s, popularized in the 1960s, and began to eclipse the posterior approach in the 1970s for treating traumatic and degenerative lesions (14).

Briefly, the advantages of this surgical approach include the following:

1. Maintenance of the patient in the supine position
2. Anatomic dissection that requires minimal tissue disruption and minimal postoperative pain
3. The ability to obtain anterior decompression
4. Optimal environment for fusion (bone under compression).

The disadvantages of this approach include the risk of damage to mechanisms of speech and swallowing via direct or neural injury.

Furthermore, as the anterior approach became more popular, more aggressive (multi-level) procedures and corpectomy resulted in increased postoperative instability. Pseudoarthrosis (fusion failure) rates were reported to increase proportionally in multi-level procedures (28). As an external orthosis, the Halo provided temporary support and could be used as an adjunct, but this device was inconvenient and had its own set of associated complications (14). Surgeons began exploring internal fixation to reestablish or increase postoperative stability and to improve fusion rates. Internal fixation of long bones was an already recognized and accepted technique.

In 1980, Bohler (4) reported using plates and screws as adjuncts to cervical fusions as early as 1964. Orozco and Llovet-Tapies (16), Herrmann (11), Senegas (20), and Tscherne et al. (23) reported internal fixation of the cervical spine in the decade that followed. These surgeons utilized available bone plates and screws; both unicortical and bicortical bone purchase was accomplished (Fig. 1). Caspar developed an improved set of soft-tissue retractors (Fig. 2C) and a new vertebral body distracter (see Fig. 2B,C) that significantly improved visualization and minimized surgical trauma. Additionally, he developed the first plate and screw system specifically for use in the cervical spine (see Fig. 1B). This plate could be contoured to help reestablish the normal cervical lordosis, and it

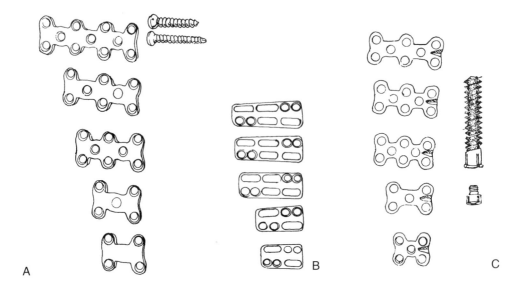

FIG. 1. Anterior cervical plates evolved from long bone plates. In a representation of AO/ASIF cervical plates **(A)**, the screws fix the plate to the spine, but they do not "lock to the plate." The Caspar plates **(B)** were modified to be used specifically in the cervical spine. This plate is non-constrained and uses bicortical screw purchase to minimize toggle and screw loosening. The Morscher plate (CSLP) **(C)** is a constrained system that uses an expansion head to secure the screw to the plate and inhibit screw back-out. The design requires only unicortical screw penetration.

served as an anterior tension band. In this manner, it provided increased stability in the immediate postoperative period.

Early reports were promising. Both standard bone plates (AO/ASIF) and the Caspar plate seemed to offer improved stability, earlier mobilization, and improved fusion (1).

As with any new technology, the indications, contraindications, and utility of a device develop and change with time, as well as the experience of those who use the device. Initially, the most recognized and accepted indication for internal stabilization of the cervical spine was trauma (8). This was not without contention, however. Sutterline et al. (22) cautioned that the Caspar plate did not reestablish adequate stability if significant posterior cervical instability coexisted. A bovine spine model with severed posterior elements was subjected to biomechanical testing. Comparisons were made with posterior constructs, such as the Bohlman triple-wire technique. The conclusion of the authors was that the Caspar construct provided insufficient stability in the presence of concomitant posterior injury and was contraindicated in this situation. Although this study demonstrated that the Caspar construct provided less stability when compared to various posterior constructs, the conclusion made by the authors was presumptuous. The published experience by Caspar et al. (5) demonstrated excellent results in trauma cases, and half of the patients had concomitant posterior instability. This apparent disparity may be resolved by recognizing the limitations of the bovine model used in the biomechanical study. This model fails to adequately reproduce the human condition, as it fails to allow for the role of cervical musculature and the other dynamic processes present in the *in vivo* condition. Other studies conducted with human specimens (7) came to similar conclusions and are subject to similar criticisms. Recently, biomechanical studies by Traynelis et al. (25)

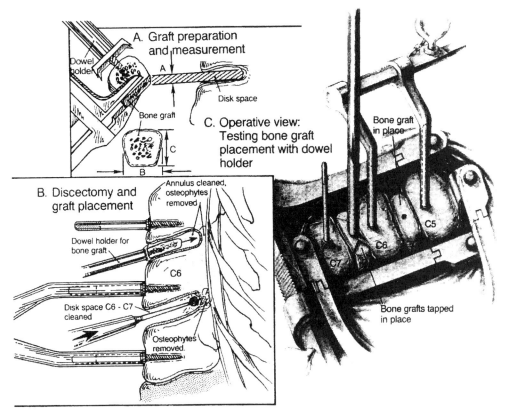

FIG. 2. Caspar modified Cloward's retractors **(A)** and developed a vertebral body distracter **(B,C)**. The distracter provides improved visualization of the disc space and reduced endplate damage. It also allows bilateral tissue removal without repositioning the retractor.

resulted in somewhat different results. They pointed to methodology that may be responsible for these differences. These contentions are supported by other biomechanical studies (18,19,26).

Once the indications for a procedure are developed and relative acceptance of a technique occurs, the safety and efficacy of the technique can be established. Table 1 summarizes the early experience of anterior cervical plating (ACP) in the 1980s and early 1990s.

These results clearly established the utility of ACP. Although the indications for ACP were still being refined, major concerns regarding technique became apparent. They included the following:

1. Insecurity of surgeons with bicortical fixation (drilling through the posterior cortex and possible direct neural injury)
2. Concerns regarding screw loosening and esophageal injury
3. Production of unacceptable magnetic resonance imaging (MRI) artifact by stainless steel plates
4. Uncertainty about indications for ACP.

These concerns led to the development of titanium plates with screws that lock to the plate and require only unicortical penetration (see Fig. 1A). Morscher et al. (15) reported

TABLE 1. *Publications relating the experience and outcome of various systems of anterior cervical plating (ACP)*

Authors (ref.)	Procedures performed *(N)*	Plate used
Tippets and Apfelbaum (24)	28	Caspar
Caspar et al. (5)	60	Caspar
Goffin et al. (10)	41	Caspar
Aebi et al. (1)	86	AO Plate
Illgner et al. (12)	165	AO Plate
Randle et al. (17)	54	Caspar
Garvey et al. (9)	14	Caspar
Lowery et al. (13)	281	Caspar 281
	90	Orozco
	168	CSLP
	157	Orion

their results with such a system, which became available in the United States in the early 1990s. Their system met with widespread acceptance, because it successfully circumvented the concerns mentioned. The system was marketed in the United States as the Cervical Spine Locking Plate (CSLP).

With time and increased utilization of ACP devices such as the CSLP, the strengths and weaknesses of the system became apparent. The CSLP system was originally available with perforated, hollow screws that were plasma coated. This construct had the theoretical advantage of promoting bone ingrowth. Obviously, bone ingrowth occurred over a period of several weeks, and no increase in immediate postoperative stability was to be expected. This ingrowth turned out to be disadvantageous if the implant had to be removed at a later date. Furthermore, the perforations weakened the screws, and increased breakage rates were reported (1).

This product is no longer available in the United States. ACP systems evolved along one of two lines. The Caspar and the CSLP depict the dichotomy of the nonconstrained and the constrained cervical plating systems (Fig. 3). The nonconstrained systems allow for subsidence and theoretically prevent less stress shielding than the constrained systems that are more load bearing and less load sharing (18).

The utility of the overall design of constrained systems is reflected by its wide acceptance. The fixation of the screws to the plate makes unicortical purchase adequate, but it somewhat restricts the surgeon. The screws are convergent with perpendicular screws at the lower end and the superior screws angled 12° toward the head. This is unlike the Caspar system, which has essentially unrestricted screw placement. The result of fixed angulation of screws is that more extensive soft-tissue dissection may be required in longer constructs, and also that the plate may not accommodate optimal placement in the lower cervical spine. The latter situation is somewhat accommodated by inverting the plate. The advantages of titanium were well received, and soon the Caspar plate became available in titanium. One disadvantage of titanium became apparent—notch sensitivity. Unlike stainless steel (but like glass), titanium is subject to breaking along scratch lines. This became apparent with the narrow Morscher plate, which will break through the screw hole portion of the plate, especially if bent or scratched in this region (13).

With the increased utilization of plates and screws, the desirable qualities already available became apparent and were reinforced. These included the following:

Unicortical purchase
Fixation of plate to screw

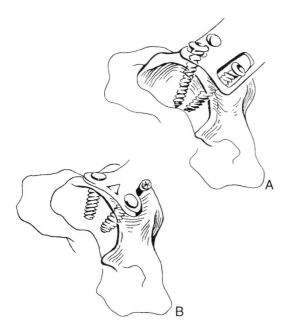

FIG. 3. The Caspar system **(A)** is an unconstrained system, in contradistinction to the CSLP **(B)**, which is a prototypical constrained system.

Titanium construction (MRI compatibility)
Simplicity of use

Also apparent were desirable characteristics that were not available:

Variability of screw placement (superior, inferior, medial, lateral) with maintenance of plate and screw fixation
Option of unicortical or bicortical bone purchase, as necessary
Improved bendability of the plate (decreased notch sensitivity)

Several systems have been marketed since the initial development of the systems of Caspar and Morscher. The Orion plate (Fig. 4A) was the next major improvement to reach the market. It was titanium alloy and allowed for reasonable postoperative evaluation with MRI. The plate was bent to accommodate normal cervical lordosis. Wedge-shaped bone grafts were used to restore lordosis. The Orion plate, which is substantially thicker than the Caspar plate, maintained this posture. Screws were secured to the plate by a locking screw (see Fig. 4B) and these screws could be used unicortically or bicortically. Cephalad and caudad screws were fixed in 15-degree angulation (see Fig. 4C). Although this offered more flexibility than the CSLP, the limited angulation of the Orion system restricted placement in the high and low cervical regions and did not allow the great variability of screw placement as seen with the Caspar system.

Constrained systems such as CSLP and Orion were well received by surgeons, and the most recently developed ACP systems have used this design. Two new systems recently released include the Codman Anterior Cervical Plate System (Fig. 5) and the Smith and Nephews Aline System (Fig. 6). Features of these systems are compared in Table 2. No published experience is available on the Codman system. I have used the Aline system and have had input in its development.

The Aline system was developed in an attempt to afford the following advantages:

Improved variability of screw placement

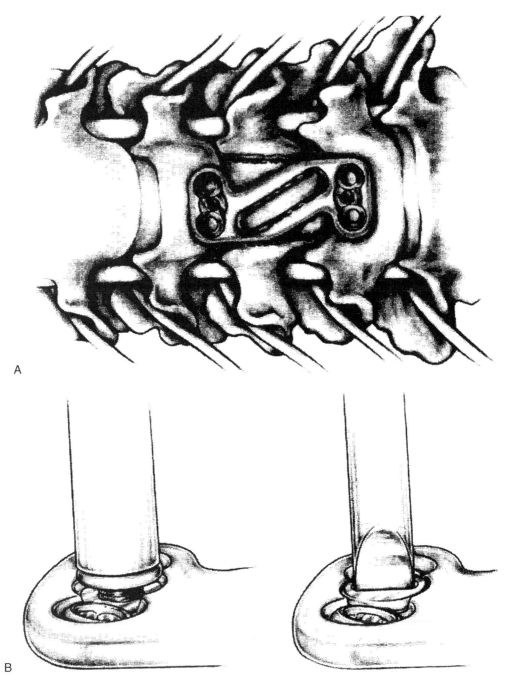

A

B

FIG. 4. The Orion Plate **(A)** is a constrained system that attempted to improve the desirable aspects of the Morscher plate. It was stiffer and has pre-set lordosis. Screws were angled 15° **(C)**, and back-out was inhibited by set-screws **(B)**. *(Continued.)*

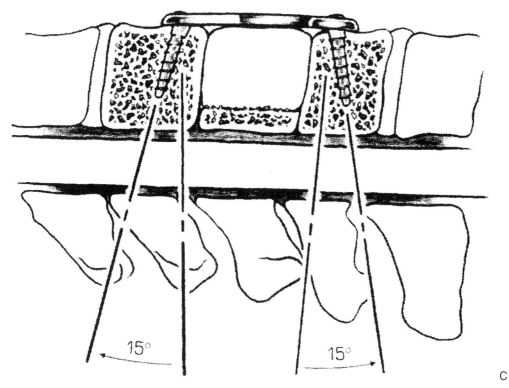

C

FIG. 4. *Continued.*

Both unicortical and bicortical screw fixation
Additional screw placement in cephalad and caudad bodies
The new titanium alloy, to avoid notch sensitivity and debris formation

We have been using the Aline system since September 9, 1995. Between that date and October 10, 1996, we have performed 43 procedures with this system. Patient age ranged from 24 through 74 years, with an average of 45.5 years. There were 19 men and 24 women. Twenty-seven patients presented with radiculopathy and 16 patients presented with myelopathy. The population consisted of patients with degenerative spondylosis (33 patients), trauma (8 patients), neoplasm (1 patient), and infection (1 patient). Surgeries included 8 single-level procedures, 9 corpectomies (considered a two-level procedure, but not included in the two-level count), 20 two-level, 13 three-level, and 2 four-level procedures. This represents a total of 93 operated levels.

Although this study represents preliminary work, it remains promising, as to date there has been no hardware failure, no pseudoarthrosis has been demonstrated, and no patient has returned to the operating room. Two patients experienced temporary vocal cord paralysis, but both problems resolved without sequellae. All patients have undergone flexion and extension x-rays at 8 to 12 weeks and there has been no demonstrable instability. Follow-up will be carried out in excess of 2 years. The Aline system appears user friendly and should be a significant addition to the spine surgeon's armamentarium.

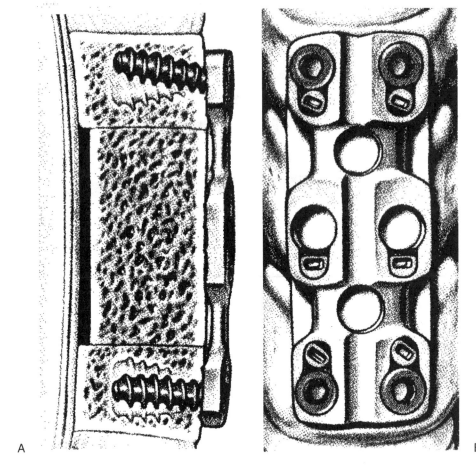

A   B

FIG. 5. The CACPS attempted to improve constrained design by affording variable screw angulation (polyaxial) **(A)**. Screws could be unicortical or bicortical and were secured to the plate with a locking cam **(B)**.

The utility of ACP has been demonstrated. The technical advances in ACP design have made them more user friendly. This has resulted in widespread application of this technique to cervical surgery. Concerns about cost effectiveness and possible overutilization of ACP have resulted in reexamination of indications for ACP. Trauma and instability remain the most accepted applications. Corpectomy and multilevel discectomy for degenerative disease are also acceptable indications (14). Single-level fusion is generally not considered an indication. ACP may have a place when allograft is substituted for autograft in an attempt to obtain higher fusion rates, and it may be indicated in patients who have concomitant problems that adversely affect bone healing. Long-term, prospective studies will be required to address these concerns.

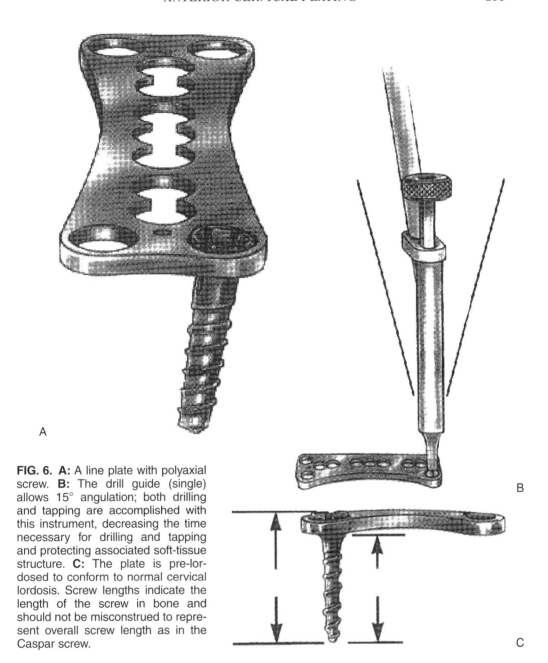

FIG. 6. A: A line plate with polyaxial screw. **B:** The drill guide (single) allows 15° angulation; both drilling and tapping are accomplished with this instrument, decreasing the time necessary for drilling and tapping and protecting associated soft-tissue structure. **C:** The plate is pre-lordosed to conform to normal cervical lordosis. Screw lengths indicate the length of the screw in bone and should not be misconstrued to represent overall screw length as in the Caspar screw.

CONCLUSION

Anterior cervical plating has undergone a rapid evolution since its appearance in the 1960s. Although the tendency of current development seems to favor constrained or semiconstrained systems, nonconstrained systems have unique advantages, and these systems remain in use. The ACP systems available today are improved and more user friendly. Although they have been used infrequently in the treatment of whiplash (2), their indications are relative, and sound clinical judgment should be employed in any

TABLE 2. *Comparison of two new anterior cervical plating (ACP) systems*

Feature	Aline system	Codman system
Titanium	Yes	Yes
Constrained	Yes	Yes
Unicortical	Yes	Yes
Bicortical	Yes	Yes
Variable screw placement	Polyaxial	Polyaxial
Locking mechanism	Expansion head	Cam
Pre-lordosed	Yes	Yes
Bendable	Yes	Yes
Screw diameter	4.0 and 4.35 mm	4.5 mm
Screw length	10–24 mm	10–26 mm
Plate length	28–108 mm	24–110 mm

decision that adds additional risk and cost to a surgical procedure. The surgeon should be trained and familiar with the application of any ACP system chosen. Careful records and patient follow-up are important, to document the effectiveness of ACP. Development will continue and new systems will evolve—such is the nature and the art of medicine and surgery.

REFERENCES

1. Aebi M, Zuber K, Marchesi D. Treatment of cervical spine injuries with anterior plating: indications, techniques, and results. *Spine* 1991;16(3S):S38–S45.
2. Algers G, Petterson K, Hildingsson C, Toolanen G. Surgery for chronic symptoms after whiplash injury. Follow-up of 20 cases. *Acta Orthop Scand* 1993;64(6):654–656.
3. Bailey RW, Badgley CE. Stabilization of the cervical spine by anterior fusion. *J Bone Joint Surg Am* 1960;42A: 565–624.
4. Bohler J, Gaudermak T. Anterior plate stabilization for fracture dislocations of the lower cervical spine. *J Trauma* 1980;20:203–205.
5. Caspar W, Barbier DD, Klara PM. Anterior cervical fusion and Caspar plate stabilization for cervical trauma. *Neurosurgery* 1989;25:491–502.
6. Cloward RB. The anterior approach for the removal of ruptured cervical discs. *J Neurosurgery* 1958;15:602–614.
7. Coe JD, Warden KE, Sutterlin CE III, et al. Biomechanical evaluation of cervical spinal stabilization methods in a human cadaveric model. *Spine* 1989;14:1122–1131.
8. de Oliveira JC. Anterior plate fixation of traumatic lesions of the lower cervical spine. *Spine* 1987;12:324–329.
9. Garvey TA, Eismont FJ, Roberti LJ. Anterior decompression, structural bone grafting, and Caspar plate stabilization for unstable cervical spine fractures and/or dislocations. *Spine* 1992;17(10S):S431–S435.
10. Goffin J, Plets C, Van den Bergh R. Anterior cervical fusion and osteosynthetic stabilization according to Caspar: a prosective study of 41 patients with fractures and/or dislocations of the cervical spine. *Neurosurgery* 1989; 25:865–871.
11. Herrmann HD. Metal plate fixation after anterior fusion of unstable fracture dislocation of the cervical spine. *Acta Neurochir* 1975;32:101–111.
12. Illgner A, Haas N, Tscherne HA. Review of the therapeutic concepts and results of operative treatment in acute and chronic lesions of the cervical spine: the Hannover experience. *J Orthop Trauma* 1991;5:100–113.
13. Lowery G, Appfelbaum R, McDonough R, Allen A. Hardware complications: a review of 700 anterior cervical patients. Proceedings of the 11th annual meeting of North American Spine Society (NASS), Oct. 23–26. Vancouver, BC. 1996;170–171.
14. Meyer PR Jr. Cervical spine fractures: changing management concepts. In: Bridwell K, Dewald R, eds. *Textbook of spinal surgery*. Philadelphia: JB Lippincott, 1991;1001–1080.
15. Morscher E, Sutter F, Jennis M, Olerud S. Die vordere verplattung der halswirbelsaule mit dem hohlschrauben-plattensystem. *Chirurg* 1986;57:702–707.
16. Orozco D, Llovet-Tapies J. Osteosintesis en las lesiones traumaticas y degenerativas de la columna cervical. *Rev Traumatol Cirurg Rehabil* 1971;1:45–52.
17. Randle MJ, Wolf A, Levi L, Rigamonti D, et al. The use of anterior Caspar plate fixation in acute cervical spine injury. *Surg Neurol* 1991;36:181–189.

18. Rapoff A, O'Brien T, Ghanayem A, Heisey D, Zdeblick T. Anterior cervical graft and plate load sharing. Proceedings of the 11th annual meeting of NASS, Oct. 23–26. Vancouver, BC. 1996;284–285.

19. Schulte K, Clark C, Goel V. Kinematics of the cervical spine following discectomy and stabilization. *Spine* 1989; 14(10):1116–1121.

20. Senegas J. Fractures et luxations recent du rachis cervical sans troubles neurologiques. *Rev Chir Orthop* 1972; 58:353–366.

21. Smith GW, Robinson RA. The treatment of cervical spine disorders by anterior removal of the intervertebral disc and interbody fusion. *J Bone Joint Surg Am* 1958;40:607–624.

22. Sutterlin CE III, McAfee PC, Warden KE, Rey RM, Farey ID. A biomechanical evaluation of cervical spinal stabilization methods in a bovine model. *Spine* 1988;13:795–802.

23. Tscherne H, Hiebler W, Muhr G. Zur Operativen Behandlung von Frakturen und Luxationen der Halswirbelsaule. *Hefte Unfallheilk* 1971;108:142–145.

24. Tippets RH, Apfelbaum RI. Anterior cervical fusion with the Caspar instrumentation system. *Neurosurgery* 1988;22:1008–1013.

25. Traynelis VC, Donaher PA, Roach RM, Kojimoto H, Goel VK. Biomechanical comparison of anterior Caspar plate and three-level posterior fixation techniques in a human cadaveric model. *J Neurosurg* 1993;79:96–103.

26. Van Peteghem PK, Schweigel JF. The fractured cervical spine rendered unstable by anterior cervical fusion. *J Trauma* 1979;19:110–114.

27. Verbiest H. Antero-lateral operation for fractures and dislocations in the middle and lower parts of the cervical spine. *J Bone Joint Surg Am* 1969;51A:1489–1530.

28. Zdeblick T, Ducker T. The use of freeze-dried allograft for anterior cervical fusion. *Spine* 1991;16(7):726–729.

Whiplash Injuries: Current Concepts in
Prevention, Diagnosis, and Treatment
of the Cervical Whiplash Syndrome,
edited by Robert Gunzburg and Marek Szpalski.
Lippincott–Raven Publishers, Philadelphia © 1998.

27

Cervical Interbody Fusion with BAK-C Cages

Willem F. Luitjes

W. F. Luitjes: Department of Neurosurgery, Slotervaart Hospital,
Amsterdam, The Netherlands.

The history of operating on the cervical spine is quite long, and a number of historic milestones are worth mentioning. As early as the late 1800s, the techniques of cervical spine surgery were described. Horsley described the posterior approach to the cervical spine in 1892. A few years later in 1895, Chipault described the anterior approach. It was not until the late 1940s and early 1950s that new milestones were reached. Frykholm (24,25), Spurling and Scoville (38) independently described posterior cervical foramino- tomy as a reliable method to decompress cervical nerves and remove free disc fragments or spondylotic spurs.

In the context of this brief history, anterior cervical interbody fusion (ACIF) is a rela- tively recent advance. Bailey and Badgley in 1952 (2), Smith and Robinson in 1955 (37), and Dereymaker and Mulier in 1956 (20) all described methods for fusing the cervical spine by introducing intervertebral iliac crest bone grafts. In 1958, Cloward provided a further advance of this procedure with the introduction of some original instrumentation that allowed for reproducible surgical results (17).

Although the anterior approach to the cervical spine is a well-accepted procedure, the need for interbody implants or fusion at all is still subject to debate (5). Particularly in the case of cervical disc herniation or in cases of spondylosis, the problem is unresolved. Bertalanffy and Egbert reported 85% good outcome with 75% spontaneous fusion of the cervical vertebrae after discectomy without fusion (6,7,19). Bohlman reported good results in 95% despite a 20% radiologic nonfusion rate (9). Epstein (21), Gore and Sepic (26), and Murphy et al. (30) obtained good results without fusion.

The decision to fuse the cervical spine in cases of severe instability, spondylolisthe- sis, or cervical trauma with ligamentous rupture is easier to justify (12,22,23). But when the decision has been made to use an interbody implant for the fusion, there is a wide variety of implant types to consider, including autograft or allograft bone; bone cement; or artificial implants made of carbon fiber, polyethylene, hydroxylapatite, or titanium (10,11,15,16).

The use of bone graft to fuse the spine is associated with secondary problems or com- plications. Harvesting bone graft from the iliac crest can result in graft site pain, infec- tion, hemorrhage, or nerve lesions. Bone harvested from the tibia may cause stress frac- tures at the donor site. When autograft bone is used, the nonfusion rate is approximately

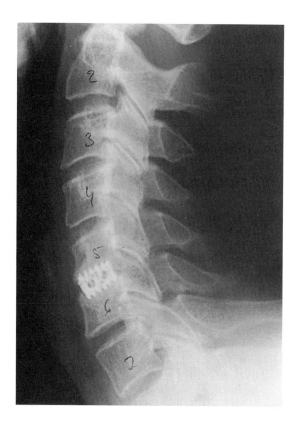

FIG. 1. Implantation of a pair of 8-mm BAK-C cages. Photograph by A. Daemen, Audio Visual Service, Municipal Hospital Slotervaart, Amsterdam, The Netherlands.

20% (8,9,17,26). The use of allograft bone can, in fact, reduce the problems associated with autograft harvest, but the nonfusion rate of allograft implants is approximately 30% (8,32,33,40). Another disadvantage of bone grafts is the risk of collapse of the graft or anterior displacement, although the use of anterior plating systems has minimized these complications. It is also often difficult to obtain the ideal shape for an interbody bone graft.

In spite of these shortcomings, the use of bone graft remains popular, but in the early 1990s, interbody implants made of nonorganic biomaterials began to appear. Bone cement is relatively easy to use, but air inclusion during mixing of the two-component fluid may cause subsequent fracture of the implant. Anterior displacement of this type of implant is another well-known complication. Bone growth into the bone cement is almost nonexistent and the nonfusion rate with a bone cement implant is approximately 30% of all cases (3,4). Implantable devices made from carbon fiber (13), polyethylene (32), hydroxylapatite (35), or titanium represent alternatives for interbody fusion. The majority of manufactured implantable devices are trapezoidal in shape, although some of the more recent titanium implants are cylindrical. When these devices are implanted, they are packed with bone graft, which can either be allograft or autograft.

The BAK-C intervertebral fusion system is the most recent development in the history of anterior cervical fusion. These threaded titanium cylinders have advantages similar to those of the trapezoidal cages with some additional benefits. The BAK-C is manufactured in four different diameter sizes; 6 mm, 8 mm, 10 mm, and 12 mm. The two smaller sizes are designed to be implanted in pairs in a single disc space and the larger two sizes

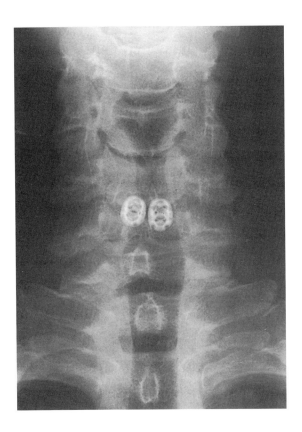

FIG. 2. The patient seen in Figure 1: anteroposterior (AP) view of the implantation. Photograph by A. Daemen, Audio Visual Service, Municipal Hospital Slotervaart, Amsterdam, The Netherlands.

are put in as a single implant. Prior to implantation, the cages are packed with autograft spongiose bone obtained during the drilling of the insertion hole. Additionally, the cages are self-packing: during the insertion process, additional bone is packed inside the cage from the surrounding bone bed. Exploiting the principle of distraction–compression, the BAK-C results in immediate stability of the cervical spine segment, thus creating the environment for bony fusion to proceed (1) (Figs. 1–7).

This report describes the clinical results of a series of 75 consecutive patients who received the BAK-C

STUDY COHORT

Our series of ACIF with the BAK-C cages included 75 patients, of whom 40 were women and 35 were men. Ages ranged from 19 to 72 years, with an overall mean age of 44.3 years. Table 1 shows the number of cases according to each patient's primary diagnosis. The data show that cervical myelopathy occurs more frequently in older patients, whereas instability occurs generally in a younger population.

INDICATIONS

There are a number of different indications for ACIF, including (a) cervical disc herniation with neurologic signs and symptoms, (b) instability or slip of at least 10% of the

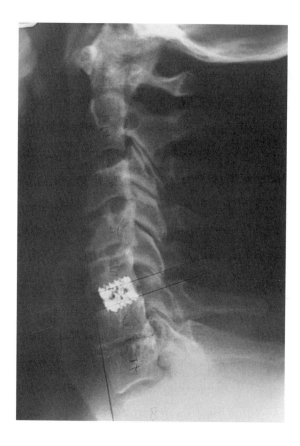

FIG. 3. Correction of the angle of the C5-6 level with a pair of 6-mm cages. Photograph by A. Daemen, Audio Visual Service, Municipal Hospital Slotervaart, Amsterdam, The Netherlands.

vertebral body, (c) cervical myelopathy with no more than two levels involved, and (d) trauma that excludes vertebral fracture (34).

Cervical Disc Herniation

The use of a fusion implant after anterior discectomy performed for cervical disc herniation has been debated by experts for quite some time (41). It is the author's opinion that implantation is becoming increasingly favored, especially those devices that can eliminate bone-graft donor-site complications.

Instability

Anterior cervical interbody fusion is indicated in cases where flexion–extension radiographs demonstrate pathologic movement or a slip of 10% or greater. In these cases, it is important to obtain fusion in an anatomic or near-anatomic shape, thus avoiding additional pressure on the adjacent levels. Overcorrecting disc height may cause additional stress in the posterior longitudinal ligament and the facet joints.

Cervical Myelopathy

Cervical myelopathy is most commonly caused by thickening of the ligamentum flavum and the posterior longitudinal ligament in combination with spondylotic spurs.

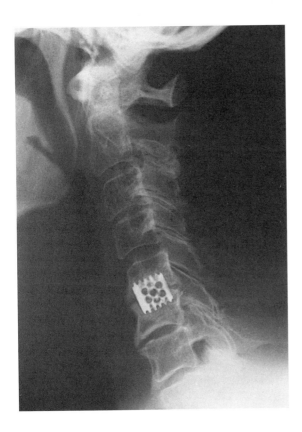

FIG. 4. A case of cervical myelopathy: a single 12-mm cage used as an alternative, instead of the Cloward procedure. Photograph by A. Daemen, Audio Visual Service, Municipal Hospital Slotervaart, Amsterdam, The Netherlands.

Concomitant narrowing of the spinal canal may result in cervical cord compression. To relieve the cord, decompression must be performed. Using a posterior approach, either a laminectomy or a laminoplasty or an open-door technique may be employed. The anterior approach creates the possibility for removal of the spondylotic spurs from the spinal canal and the foramen. In these cases, threaded titanium cylinders, such as the BAK-C, can be used as a modification of the Cloward or Smith-Robinson procedure. The advantages of the cylinder versus a bone dowel are (a) no risk of collapse of the graft, (b) no plating needed, (c) no donor site problems, and (d) no collar needed in the postoperative period.

Trauma

In cases of trauma to the cervical spine, external forces may cause damage to various structures. This damage may be muscular, vascular, or ligamentous, or it may involve bone fractures, disc problems, cord, or nerves. A combination of two or three or more of these problems is possible and, as A. Jung has stated in *The Cervical Spine* (28,29), "The (posttraumatic) cervical syndrome can be isolated, but usually it induces and associates with other complaints of vertebral origin. The localized spinal disturbance is, nevertheless, the indispensable basis of the later radicular, medullar or vertebral artery syndrome." Extension of the cervical spine may cause rupture of the anterior and posterior ligament, disc rupture, and "tear drop" fractures. Flexion trauma may be responsible for anterior and/or posterior ligament rupture, dislocation of the facet

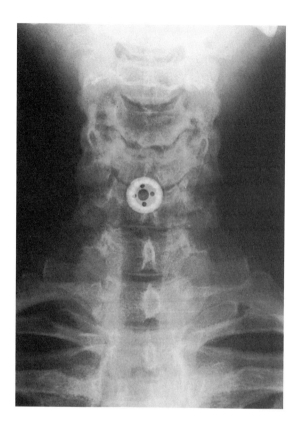

FIG. 5. The patient seen in Figure 4, with an AP view: medial implanted 12-mm cage. Photograph by A. Daemen, Audio Visual Service, Municipal Hospital Slotervaart, Amsterdam, The Netherlands.

joint, disc disruption, and listhesis. Both flexion and extension trauma can result in spinal cord trauma, nerve root involvement, and instability. Vertebral artery insufficiency has been mentioned in some reports as the source of cerebellar and/or cerebral problems caused by extension–flexion trauma.

SURGICAL TECHNIQUES

When there is an indication for an ACIF, the initial part of the procedure is standard. After localizing the operative level by radiographic control, a small incision is made in one of the skin folds. After opening the platysma in a longitudinal fashion, the sternocleido-mastoid muscle is exposed and retracted laterally, along with the carotid artery and veins. Opening of the deep longitudinal ligament and splitting of the prevertebral muscles finally creates exposure of the vertebral bodies and the disc. Before proceeding with the discectomy, it is prudent to verify the level again with a radiograph. After discectomy and decortication of the endplates, free fragments can be removed either from the vertebral canal or the foramen. Foraminal spurs and osteophytes can also be resected. Disc height can be restored to normal dimensions by placement of a distraction plug. After placement and alignment of a drill tube, the distraction plug is removed. After drilling a hole, the BAK-C that has been chosen during preoperative templating is packed with spongiose bone obtained during the drilling. Finally, after tapping the hole, the cage can be inserted. A minimum of pre-packing, and in some cases even no pre-packing, is required because the

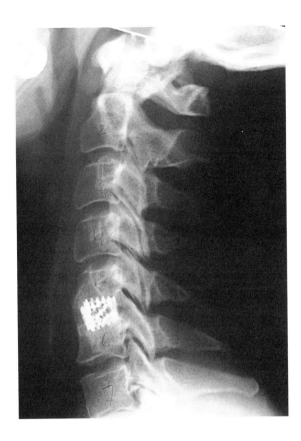

FIG. 6. A double 6-mm implant 3 months after surgery: note the marked bony overgrowth on the anterior side of the cages. Photograph by A. Daemen, Audio Visual Service, Municipal Hospital Slotervaart, Amsterdam, The Netherlands.

cage is self-packing during the insertion into the hole. It should be noted that the entire procedure should be performed under fluoroscopic or radiographic control.

RESULTS

The follow-up period in our BAK-C series varied from 3 months to 1.8 years. Bony consolidation appeared much faster than anticipated, and we now consider 3 months an adequate time period to achieve a stable situation.

Cervical Disc Herniation

Hildingsson et al. suggested that MRI studies show that disc pathology seems to be one contributing factor to the pathophysiology after whiplash injury, and that in some patients this injury is not detectable shortly after the trauma but develops over time (27). The most common indication for anterior cervical discectomy is disc herniation that causes neck and arm pain or compression of the spinal cord. In our series, we followed 23 male and 29 female patients with cervical disc herniation, representing the largest indication for this procedure. Fusion was performed after discectomy with BAK-C cages. The mean age of this group was 44.3 years, with a range from 25 to 63 years. All of the patients had a very good result after discectomy and fusion. Three of the patients developed a new disc herniation one level above the previously operated level. A possi-

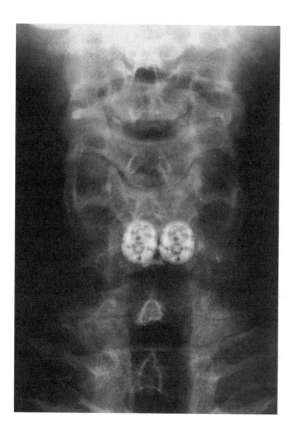

FIG. 7. A pair of 8-mm cages in the AP view: the cages are symmetrically positioned. Photograph by A. Daemen, Audio Visual Service, Municipal Hospital Slotervaart, Amsterdam, The Netherlands.

ble explanation for this result may be that the fusion caused excessive movements in the adjacent levels leading to abnormal pressure and pressure points in that disc with concomitant movement point changes (39).

Instability

Pathologic movement or slip greater than 10% of the vertebral body causing neck pain and/or brachialgia was an indication for fusion in this series. Posterior fixation results in increased forces acting on the screws and results in loss of bone in the pedicles and subsequent loosening of the screws. In contrast, anterior fixation with BAK-C results in an immediately stable situation with bony consolidation within 3 months. Of the three men and five women in this series, six had a perfect result, and there were two failures. These two patients demonstrated a very stable condition with minimal to no motion of flexion–extension on radiographs, yet they complained of neck pain. One of these patients was involved in insurance litigation and one patient was drug addicted.

Cervical Myelopathy

Operative treatment for cervical myelopathy with the BAK-C cage is carried out to prevent progression of the disease. The results with the BAK-C procedure are encouraging. The eight men and four women receiving the BAK-C for cervical myelopathy improved

TABLE 1. *Sex and age distribution according to the patients' primary diagnosis*

	Men *(N)*	Women *(N)*	Mean age (yr)
Cervical disc herniation	23	29	44.3
Instability	3	5	32.1
Cervical myelopathy	8	4	62.2
Trauma	1	2	42.3
Total	35	40	44.3

more than expected. A consistent finding was that the operation resulted in an immediately stable situation, allowing the patient to be mobilized without the need for a cervical collar.

Trauma

The number of patients with a history of previous trauma is limited in our series, there being only one man and two women. These three individuals suffered previous trauma 10 months to 2.5 years before the surgery. All presented with spondylotic spurs. It has been suggested that arthrosis may be posttraumatic if it is localized and the patient is young (28,29). Spondylotic material in our patients was removed from the vertebral canal and the foramen.

DISCUSSION

The use of an interbody graft or device after anterior cervical discectomy has been debated for a number of years. It is clear that when solid fusion and/or maintenance of disc height is required, simple discectomy is insufficient. Epstein (21), Gore and Sepic (26), and Murphy et al. (30) reported 70% fusion rate 2 years after discectomy. (Data about maintenance of disc height in this series was not available.) The use of allograft bone for fusion after discectomy results similarly in a 70% fusion rate (2–4,8). Autograft bone fusion has a slightly better result, with fusion rates of 80% often reported (2,8,9,17,20).

When trapezoidal interbody devices that are pre-packed with allograft or autograft bone are used to assist fusion, late to very late fusion is reported (18,32,33,35,36,42,43). In these cases, allograft bone leads to a higher percentage of nonfusion than autograft bone (4,8,32,33,35,42). The expected late fusions with the use of trapezoid devices requires the patient to wear a stiff collar.

In contrast, the use of the BAK-C threaded titanium cylindrical cage results in an immediately stable situation. Solid bony fusion is obtained within 2 to 4 months and there is no need to wear a collar postoperatively. In our series of 75 patients, the results obtained were extremely good. There were no operative complications and no cases of cage migration, and there was a 100% fusion rate. Nonunion or pseudarthrosis after implantation of autograft or allograft bone in the cervical disc is mainly seen in patients who smoke (8). In our series of 75 patients, 40% smoked cigarettes or shag tobacco, yet our fusion rate was 100%. The negative influence of nicotine appears to be restricted to single autograft or allograft bone implants (8,14).

The advantages of the BAK-C cages are as follows:

1. Ease of handling material
2. Self-packing cages using autograft bone
3. Possibility of correcting the cervical sagittal alignment

4. No donor site problems
5. Elegant approach
6. Short operative time
7. Short hospital stay
8. Relatively minor procedure
9. No postoperative use of a collar without physical therapy
10. Fast return to work and social life

CONCLUSION

Self-packing BAK-C titanium cylinders are, to date, the best option to obtain immediate stability of cervical interbody fusion while avoiding the complications associated with harvesting autograft bone and the use of a postoperative stiff collar. Bony consolidation is obtained within 2 to 4 months and there is a short recovery time for return to work and a normal social life.

REFERENCES

1. Bagby GW. Arthrodesis by the distraction compression using a stainless steel implant. *Orthopaedics* 1988; 931–934.
2. Bailey RW, Badgley CE. Stabilization of the cervical spine by anterior fusion. *J Bone Joint Surg* 1960;42: 565–594.
3. Bent van den MJ. *The use of acrylate in anterior cervical discectomy.* Thesis, Rotterdam 1994.
4. Bent van den MJ, Oosting J, Woude EJ, et al. Anterior cervical discectomy with or without fusion with acrylate. A randomized trial. *Spine* 1996;7:834–840.
5. Berry H. Psychological aspects of chronic neckpain following hyperextension-flexion strains of the neck. In: *Current controversies in neurosurgery.* Philadelphia: WB Saunders, 1976;51–60.
6. Bertalanffy H, Eggert HR. Clinical long-term results of anterior discectomy without fusion for treatment of cervical radiculopathy and myelopathy. *Acta Neurochir (Wien)* 1988;90:127–135.
7. Bertalanffy H, Eggert HR. Complications of anterior cervical discectomy without fusion in 450 consecutive patients. *Acta Neurochir (Wien)* 1989;99:41–50.
8. Bishop RC, Moore KA, Hadley MN. Anterior cervical interbody fusion using autogenic and allogenic bone graft substrate: a prospective comparative analysis. *J Neurosurg* 1996;85:206–210.
9. Bohlman H, Emery S, Goodfellow D, Jones P. Robinson anterior cervical discectomy and arthrodesis for cervical radiculopathy. *J Bone Joint Surg* 1993;75:1298–1307.
10. Boker DK, Schultheiss R, Probst EM. Radiologic long term results after cervical interbody fusion with polymethyl methacrylate (PMMA). *Neurosurg Rev* 1989;12:217–221.
11. Boker DK, Schultheiss R, Roost DV, Osborn JF, Kaden B. Anterior cervical discectomy and intervertebral fusion with hydroxylapatite. Preliminary results. *Acta Neurochir (Wien)* 1993;121:191–195.
12. Braakman R, Penning L. Hyperflexion sprain of the cervical spine. *Radiol Clin Biol* 1968;37(6):309–320.
13. Brantigan JW, Steffee AD, Greiger JM. A carbon fibre implant to aid interbody lumbar fusion. *Spine* 1991;16: 277–282.
14. Broulik PD, Jarab J. The effect of chronic nicotine administration on bone mineral content in mice. *Horm Metab Res* 1993;25:219–221.
15. Bush G. Anterior cervical fusion for cervical spondylosis. *J Neurol* 1978;219:117–126.
16. Clements DH, O'Leary PF. Anterior cervical discectomy and fusion. *Spine* 1990;15:1023–1025.
17. Cloward RB. The anterior approach for removal of ruptured cervical discs. *J Neurosurg* 1958;15:602–617.
18. Cook SD, Reynolds MC, Whitecloud TS, et al. Evaluation of hydroxylapatite graft materials in canine cervical spine fusions. *Spine* 1986;11:305–309.
19. Cuatico W. Anterior cervical discectomy without interbody fusion. *Acta Neurochir (Wien)* 1981;57:269–274.
20. Dereymaker A, Mulier J. La fusion vertébrale par voie ventrale dans la discopathie cervicale. *Rev Neurol* 1958; 99:597–616.
21. Epstein NE. Anterior cervical discectomy and fusion procedures. *Spine* 1991;16:599–604.
22. Frankel VH. Pathomechanic of whiplash injuries to the neck. In: *Current controversies in neurosurgery.* Philadelphia: WB Saunders, 1976;39–50.
23. Frankel VH, Nordim M, Snijders CJ. *Basic biomechanics of the skeletal system.* London: Kimpton, 1980.
24. Frykholm R. Lower cervical vertebral and intervertebral discs. Surgical anatomy and pathology. *Acta Chir Scand* 1951;101:345–359.

25. Frykholm R. Cervical nerve root compression resulting from disc degeneration and root-sleeve fibrosis. *Acta Chir Scand* 1951;160(Suppl):1–47.
26. Gore DR, Sepic SB. Anterior cervical fusion for degenerated or protruded discs. *Spine* 1984;9:667–671.
27. Hildingsson C, Petterson K, Fagerlund M, et al. Disc pathology after whiplash injury. A prospective MRI and clinical investigation. Presented at the 12th annual meeting of the European Cervical Spine Society, 1996.
28. Jung A, Kehr P. Pathologie de l'artere vertebrale et des racines nerveuses dans les arthroses et les traumatismes du rachis cervical. Paris: Masson, 1972.
29. Jung A, Vierling JP, Kehr P. The local cervical syndrome. In: Jung A, Kehr P, Magerl, Weber, eds. *The cervical spine.* Switzerland: Hans Huber, 1974.
30. Murphy GM, Simmons J, Brunson B. Surgical treatment of laterly ruptured disc. *J Neurol* 1973;38:679–683.
31. Penning L. Normal movements in the cervical spine. *Am J Roentgenol* 1978;130:317–326.
32. Robert G, Duplessis E. Preliminary study of a new intersomatic fusion process after cervical discectomy by the anterior approach. *Rachis* 1993;5:261–265.
33. Robert G. Intersomatic fusion with CR cages following cervical discectomy by the anterior approach. Presentation: Gieda rachis, Paris, 1994.
34. Schut CH, Dohan FC. Neck injury to women in auto accidents;a metropolitan plague. *JAMA* 1968;206:2689–2692.
35. Sessa S. Intersomatic cervical cage after anterior discectomy. Presentation to the Groupe d'Etude de Scoliose (GES), Bordeaux, France, 1996.
36. Shono Y, McAfee P, Cunningham B, Brantigan JW. A biomechanical analysis of decompression and reconstruction methods in the cervical spine. *J Bone Joint Surg* 1993;75:1674–1684.
37. Smith GW, Robinson RA. The treatment of certain cervical spine disorders by anterior removal of the intervertebral disc and interbody fusion. *J Bone Joint Surg* 1958;40A:607–624.
38. Spurling RG, Scoville WB. Lateral rupture of the cervical intervertebral discs: a common cause of shoulder and arm pain. *Surg Gynecol Obstet* 1944;78:350.
39. Vortman BJ. Segmental centres of movement of the lower cervical spine. Thesis, Groningen. The Netherlands, 1992.
40. Watters WC, Levinthal R. Anterior cervical discectomy with and without fusion. Results, complications and long-term follow up. *Spine* 1994;19:2243–2247.
41. Yamammoto I, Ikeda A, Shibuya N, et al. Clinical long-term results of anterior discectomy without interbody fusion for cervical disc disease. *Spine* 1991;16:272–279.
42. Zdeblick TA, Ducker TB. The use of freeze-dried allograft bone for anterior cervical fusions. *Spine* 1991;16:726–729.
43. Zdeblick TA, Wilson D, Cook ME, et al. Anterior cervical discectomy and fusion. A comparison of techniques in an animal model. *Spine* 1992;17:S418–425.

SECTION 6

Economic Issues and Prevention

Whiplash Injuries: Current Concepts in
Prevention, Diagnosis, and Treatment
of the Cervical Whiplash Syndrome,
edited by Robert Gunzburg and Marek Szpalski.
Lippincott–Raven Publishers, Philadelphia © 1998.

28

Whiplash Impairment Rating: Guidelines for Measurement

Pierre Lucas

P. Lucas: Department of Legal Medicine, Free University of Brussels, Belgium.

REVIEW OF SOME PRINCIPLES

The sequelae of traumatic lesions caused by a whiplash of the cervical spine may negatively influence the work and economic capacity of the patient. The assessment of those sequelae has to be done *in concreto* by studying the influence of the residual lesions on the ability of the subject to perform his or her profession or to be competitive in the socioeconomic environment where he or she logically belongs according to age, gender, education, and experience. The reference should be either the profession or the general work market (4). In both cases, this personalized assessment needs an understanding of the socioeconomic factors, and most of all it needs to evaluate the compatibilities and incompatibilities between the loads of the workplace and the remaining physical ability of the victim: gestures, movements and their repetitive nature, positions to take or to keep, and weight lifting or carrying. Therefore, one cannot predict on a predefined scale the work or economic incapacity, which varies not only with the sequelae but also with the individual (4).

On the other hand, what *can* be predefined is what is usually called in Belgium invalidity, which describes the real and pure physical disability that I propose to call personal incapacity. Personal incapacity is the functional impairment in daily life, taking into account the decrease in life quality related to the impairment, but without taking into account the professional context. This can be considered identical for all individuals having the same sequelae and, therefore, may be included in a predefined scale. The interest of such a predefined scale is to provide a useful standardization in the quantitative assessment not only when performed by the same physician, but also when performed by different physicians, so that the compensation can also be identical.

Most professions need less and less physical activity and the professional gestures are becoming closer and closer to everyday gestures—just look at the robotized factories—so that a personal incapacity scale can also be a guide in the other disability assessment procedures (7).

Four principles must be systematically applied:

Assess the sequelae, and not the memory of the diagnosis.

Images do not require surgery and, following the same principle, what is compensated is functional sequelae, not the radiograph or the electromyogram (EMG).

Identical sequelae must be assessed identically, whatever their cause.

The original injury and the type of treatment (especially surgical) may influence the medium- and long-term prognosis, and this must be taken explicitly into account.

The major difficulty in compensation of disability is to avoid a double compensation of the same damage and, at the same time, the underestimation of one of the components of the disability when this disability is, as is usually the case, multifactorial.

To avoid these biases, the best technique is to first assess the major sequelae and then to integrate the secondary sequelae. We could, indeed, apply this to the assessment of cervical sequelae of a whiplash injury, but how do we assess those sequelae with the existing scales?

CLASSIC SCALE ASSESSMENT OF SEQUELAE

Are there any predefined scales corresponding to the sequelar reality that enables the physician to assess whiplash trauma sequelae in a standardized, reliable, and reproducible way, determining in this way a fair compensation?

The Barème Officiel Belgedes Invalidités (B.O.B.I.)

The B.O.B.I. (Belgian Official Scale of Impairment), which officially is applied only to civilian and military victims of civic duty, is the most used reference scale in Belgium; furthermore, it is the contractual scale (and thus compulsory) of most of the current individual insurance contracts, nearly system-wide (10). However, the B.O.B.I. describes only three severity levels for cervical spine sequelae, very simply called mild, medium, and severe. No other criterion is described that could help the user to determine an appropriate category. Furthermore, the impairment intervals for the same degree of severity can vary by 10% or even 20% for the cervical spine. Each assessment is therefore influenced by random factors and, thus, debatable.

The European Community Scale

The European Community scale, which is quite precise for other body parts, totally ignores the spine.

The French Scale

The new French scale of functional sequelae in common law (usually called scale of Marin and Muller) (13) assesses the impairment value by referring it to a scale where the sequelae are called light, moderated, medium, more important, very important, and severe. However, those adjectives have no precise definition. This scale is crippled by the same lack of precision as the Belgian B.O.B.I., but it provides for each type of sequela approximate references as to the pain, the functional limitation, and the spinal deformation.

The Melennec Scale (France)

The Melennec scale defines 5 groups:

Group 1. Light troubles, 0% to 5%
Group 2. Moderated troubles, 5% to 15%
Group 3. Medium troubles, 15% to 30%
Group 4. Important troubles, 30% to 60%
Group 5. Very important troubles, more than 60%

It provides for each group quite detailed clinical examples that can be used as a baseline for a reasoned comparison with the actual case being evaluated (9). However, the margin of imprecision remains important.

The New Spanish Scale

The New Spanish scale is of compulsory use in common law (2). It defines different types of clinical settings and provides limits for the impairment quantification. However, those limits are sometimes so wide and the judging criteria so vague that the physician will find only a very wide enclosure, in which there is no problem remaining but in which, also, his problem remains unsolved.

The Society of Automobile Assurance of Québec Scale

The Society of Automobile Assurance of Québec scale is very detailed and purely morphologic (3). It gives very precise quantification corresponding to a vertebral compression: more than 50%, between 25% and 50%, and less than 25%. At each level of the spine, this condition is associated to a fixed quantification. However, this scale refers in no way to the clinical situation: there is no reference to pain or the ability to perform the gestures of daily life. It enables easy quantification of a disability, but without a connection to the reality of the patient's life.

Schedule for Rating Disabilities

The scheme of the Department of Veterans Affairs in the United States classifies ankylosis as favorable and unfavorable, and the limitations of motion as severe, moderate, and slight, without defining the words. The quantification limits may be as wide as 10 or even 20 points. It submits to the same criticism as the Belgian and French scales.

The American Medical Association Scale

The AMA scale (1) for spine impairment is based largely, but very precisely, on range of motion. It gives very precise instructions for the way to measure the range of motion using different types of goniometers. With each range-of-motion value is associated an impairment rate. The method allows standardized assessments. However, it has been shown that relation between range of motion, pain, and disability is very poor, and this method may not accurately reflect impairment in many patients (14).

The Scale of Lucas and Stehman

In agreement with Stehman, I have always advocated that the scale must be the result of a careful listening to and observation of the patient in normal activities, relegating technical investigations to only a confirmational or supplementary status. Thus, in our different studies, we have proposed a functional scale for nearly all parts of the body (6–8).

For the spine, we have proposed a standardized methodology using four variables: pain, daily life activity, static and dynamic study of the spine, and radiologic aspect (8). For each variable, we use four levels of severity, each severity level corresponding to a specific impairment rate value. Each level is illustrated by characteristic examples. The isolated impairment rating values corresponding to the quantification of each variable are eventually added to obtain the global impairment rating value. This is not an inflexible impairment-rating system, but an indication, a guide for the physician. Any sequelar situation that does not fit into the multifactorial description allowed by the examples in our study has to be evaluated using the reasoning and the competence of the examining physician.

Pain

We include local cervical pain and its possible radiation to another site; the true radicular pains are assessed in a specific way.

Level 1

Pain with fatigue
Transient pain occurring with effort and disappearing spontaneously
Rare and short painful crises

   Rating: 0% to 1%

Level 2

Starting pain disappearing after 30 to 60 minutes
Pain after 2 or 3 hours of being in a standing or sitting position
Painful crises lasting a few days

   Rating: 1% to 2%

Level 3

Increase of pain with effort
Pain peaks on a moderate pain baseline
Occasional and short radiations

   Rating: 2% to 4%

Level 4

Important permanent pain
Inability to exert effort
Permanent radiations

   Rating: 4% to 6%

Daily Life Activities

Level 1

Discomfort in daily activities only during significant effort
Discomfort while keeping the same position
Care necessary for lifting and carrying weights

  Rating: 0% to 2%

Level 2

Difficulty in performing heavy tasks
Driving uncomfortable after 300 km
Difficulty keeping the same position for a long time

  Rating: 2% to 3%

Level 3

Inability to perform heavy tasks
Difficulty remaining in a sitting position more than 2 hours

  Rating: 3% to 5%

Level 4

Permanent discomfort and handicap for all activities
Automobile driving difficult
Inability to remain a long time in the same position

  Rating: 5% to 6%

Static and Dynamic of the Spine

Level 1

Unchanged static status
Normal or subnormal mobility

  Rating: 0%

Level 2

Static status slightly modified
Slight stiffness

  Rating: 0% to 1%

Level 3

Moderate static status disorders
Medium stiffness

   Rating: 1% to 4%

Level 4

Significant static status disorders
Significant stiffness

   Rating: 4% to 8%

Radiologic Aspect

Level 1

Absence of traumatic sequelae
Absence of preexisting pathologic status
Preexisting pathologic status not modified

   Rating: 0%

Level 2

Slight traumatic sequelae
Slight worsening of a preexisting pathologic status
Favorable healing of a benign lesion

   Rating: 0% to 2%

Level 3

Moderated anterior or lateral compression
Significant worsening of a preexisting pathologic disorder
Slight to medium posttraumatic arthrosis or curvature abnormality

   Rating: 2% to 4%

Level 4

Important posttraumatic spinal deformation and/or instability
Secondary disorders of global static status
Severe posttraumatic arthrosis

   Rating: 4% to 8%

THE CERVICAL WHIPLASH INJURY

The cervical whiplash injury caused by brutal acceleration and/or deceleration is easily demonstrated by clinical exam, with findings of painful points, muscle contractions, and range of motion limitation (5,11).

The associated ligamentous lesion (if any) is demonstrated by a careful dynamic x-ray investigation (12). The associated symptomatology (e.g., cephalalgia, vertigo, visual disorders, cervicobrachialgia) present if the trauma has involved the vascular and sympathetic structures or has created or worsened a discal lesion, justifies specialized investigations in each of the involved areas to qualify and quantify sequelae (5,7,11).

The Local Cervical Syndrome

The local cervical syndrome is a benign condition if the case is treated correctly and if there is no self-induced pathology (iatrogenic or linked to self-medication). If it is only a contusion or a simple sprain on a radiologically normal spine, with a symptomatology consisting mainly of favorably evolving pain and stiffness, the assessment of disability will be possible after a delay of approximately 1 year. It is conditioned by a dynamic radiograph of the cervical spine, which will be compared to the initial images. If at that time there is no secondary lesion and clinical exam is normal, the subjective symptoms will be rewarded, following the type of accident, the evolution of the case, and unpredictable factors that have to be taken into account by the expert, by an impairment rate of 0% to 3%. If the radiographs show an evolution towards degenerative phenomena, especially in areas that do not correspond to the usual areas of maximal loads, their relation to the accident will be considered confirmed. If all the other factors are normal (e.g., electroencephalogram; ear, nose, and throat; ophthalmology), the local osteoarticular sequelae will be evaluated, following their degree of severity and their handicapping character, at a level approaching that described as "light sequelae" in most of the scales (0% to 10%).

Whiplash injury on a predegenerated spine involves complex medicolegal problems. If the clinical examination shows a limited range of motion and pain, must those phenomena be considered as purely posttraumatic? In which measure must we consider the preexisting condition visible on the initial radiographs?

Only control radiographs taken after 6 to 12 months will show if there was an abnormally fast evolution of degenerative signs, making it possible to identify and compensate the sequelae linked to the whiplash injury (12).

The "Descending" Cervical Syndrome

The descending cervical syndrome is in fact the cervicobrachialgic syndrome, or the cervical sprain accompanied by radiculopathy.

The quantification of radicular sequelae requires the use of medical imaging, specially magnetic resonance imaging (MRI), and a precise clinical and electrophysiologic neurologic study (5,7,11,12). The physician can, however, through the physical examination, develop a valid opinion as to the radicular lesion and its relative importance. After an appropriate delay (1 year minimum, longer after surgery for a slipped disc), the level of impairment is inspired by the impairment scales dealing with cervical sequelae (0% to 20%) and cervical monoradiculopathy (5% to 30%).

We propose, when there is objective cervical radicular symptomatology, and according to pain, sensitivity disorders, mobility disorders, and lack of strength, that a maximum impairment rate of 15% be added to the rate calculated from the pure spinal sequelae tables.

The "Ascending" Cervical Syndrome

The ascending cervical syndrome (or cervicocephalic syndrome, often called posterior cervical syndrome) has become more and more frequent since the compulsory use of the auto safety belt combined with a headrest (the latter being nearly always poorly positioned and totally useless for restraining the violent movement of the cervical spine during the whiplash phenomenon). The wide publicity given to whiplash injuries in automobile collisions has been so important that nearly every subject involved in a frontal or rear collision will speak of "my whiplash" (7).

However, the real cervical ascending syndrome is associated with traumatic causal criteria that justify the need for more complex paraclinical investigations. The impairment rating must take into account a symptomatic whole whose constituents are well defined by a detailed analysis:

Cervical static and dynamic radiographs
Cochlear and vestibular investigations
Ophthalmological investigations
Possible psychiatric disorders

Sequelae in other domains are rare.

An impairment rating in a patient with posterior cervical syndrome will not be attempted before 12 to 18 months after the trauma, especially in the elderly. The cochleovestibular damages may increase with time during neck movements. In this case, the cervicoarthrotic pathology, unco-arthrosis in particular, may have an unfavorable effect as a result of vascular disorders.

The final impairment rating must not be a simple sum of the ratings linked to sequelae in each interested anatomic or functional sphere but must be an intelligent integration (5,7,11). There is no simple recipe of handicap assessment. It is necessary to conduct a rational reflection based on a hierarchy of sequelae and on a realistic synthesis of the corresponding impairment ratings.

Spinal Cord Lesions

A scale of spinal cord lesion sequelae is of little interest (6). Taking the Belgian B.O.B.I. (article 76) as an example, what is there in common between "60% to 80% for a quadriplegic who cannot walk, or who walks only with orthopedic help, accompanied with sensitivity and sphincter disorders" and 65% for the loss of a hand?

Serious sequelae do not coexist well with the logic of rating: all the quantifying scales underevaluate the serious disabilities and overevaluate the more trivial ones.

These sequelae must be characterized by a clear description of the injured person's round-the-clock activity. The British, who do not use these kinds of scales, do it systematically in their disability descriptions by putting forward the description of the problems of daily living.

CONCLUSION

It is always tempting to propose a synthesis in the form of tables with precise scales. This enables us to ensure a standardization of the assessment technique without forgetting any of the important components of disability. The paraclinical investigations bring a necessary moderation.

However, it is always only a basic scheme producing an approximate rating, even when it is as precise as possible.

REFERENCES

1. *American Medical Association: guide to the evaluation of permanent impairment*, 3rd ed. Chicago: American Medical Association, 1988.
2. Borobia Fernandez C. *Valoración de daños personales causados en los accidentes de circulación*, 1st ed. Madrid: La Ley-Actualidad S.A. 1996;223–242.
3. Commission de la santé et de la sécurité du travail. *Règlement annoté sur le barème des dommages corporels.* Québec, 1987:46–53.
4. Fagnart JL. *La réparation du dommage corporel en droit commun.* Bruxelles: Larcier, 1994;149–156.
5. Fournier CL, ed. *Pathologie séquellaire du rachis cervical.* Paris: JB Baillière, 1991;9–48.
6. Lucas P, Stehman M. *Le blessé médullaire.* Bruxelles: Juridoc 1990;219–234.
7. Lucas P, Stehman M. *Syndrome post-commotionnel et syndrome cervical.* Bruxelles: Juridoc 1991;1:121–133.
8. Lucas P, Stehman M. *Hernie discale.* Bruxelles: Juridoc 1993;3:113–130.
9. Melennec L. *Evaluation du handicap et du dommage corporel.* Paris: Masson 1991:211–225.
10. *Ministère de la Santé Publique et de la Famille: Barème Officiel Belge des Invalidités.* Moniteur belge: 1975; 18:09, 1975;04:12, 1976;12:05.
11. Revue Française du Dommage Corporel. *Les séquelles des traumatismes du rachis cervical.* 1982;287–444.
12. Sintzoff S. L'entorse cervicale. *L'imagerie en évaluation du dommage corporel.* France: Springer Verlag, 1993; 157–184.
13. Société de Médecine Légale et de criminologie de France. *Les séquelles traumatiques. Evaluation médico-légale des incapacités permanentes en droit commun.* Paris: Le Concours Médical 1991:21–29,85–94.
14. Wiesel SW, Lowery WD Jr, Horn ThJ, Boden SD. Impairment evaluation based on spinal range of motion in normal subjects. *J Spinal Disord* 1992;5(4):398–402.

Whiplash Injuries: Current Concepts in Prevention, Diagnosis, and Treatment of the Cervical Whiplash Syndrome, edited by Robert Gunzburg and Marek Szpalski. Lippincott–Raven Publishers, Philadelphia © 1998.

29

The Cost of Whiplash-Associated Disorders

Charles S. B. Galasko

C. S. B. Galasko: Department of Orthopaedic Surgery, Hope Hospital, Salford, Manchester, United Kingdom.

Whiplash-associated disorders (WAD) are nonspecific soft-tissue injuries of the cervical spine, excluding fractures, dislocations, and subluxations. Classically, a whiplash is a hyperextension injury following a rear impact. However, soft-tissue injuries to the neck can also occur from frontal or side impacts. These soft-tissue injuries to the cervical spine have also been described by terms such as *neck sprain, neck strain, soft-tissue injury,* and *acceleration–deceleration injuries*.

In 1982, the World Health Authority concluded that previous studies on the costs of road traffic accidents "had been based on the costs of deaths and inpatient treatment, and had neglected to examine the cost of long-term disability to the community" (36).

During the past 12 years, we, together with the Transport Research Laboratories and the Department of Transport in the United Kingdom, have tried to evaluate the cost of road traffic accidents, paying particular attention to WADs. These costs can be broken down into two main categories: (a) the cost to the individual in terms of the residual disability he or she suffers, and (b) the cost to the community in terms of, for example, health care, social services provision, and lost output.

CORRELATION BETWEEN INJURY SEVERITY AND LONG-TERM DISABILITY

Galasko et al. (7) investigated whether there was any correlation between injury severity and subsequent long-term disability, whether long-term disability was a consequence of particular injuries, and whether long-term disability should be included in evaluating the costs of road traffic accidents. They followed (for 6 months) 1,422 consecutive patients who had been seen in an accident and emergency department after a road traffic accident. The study was designed to assess whether there were any changes in lifestyle or occupation, and the effect of the accident/injury on sport, hobbies, or activities of daily living. In this study, long-term disability was defined as a disability persisting for more than 6 months and of sufficient severity to interfere with a job (including housework).

Overall, 25.1% of patients had a residual disability at 6 months. Long-term disability occurred more commonly in pedestrians (30.1%) and least commonly in pedal cyclists (15.9%). It occurred in 24.6% of vehicle occupants and 26.2% of motorcyclists. In each vehicle-user category, patients with a long-term disability were significantly older than those who were left without a residual disability at 6 months.

The patients who were left with a long-term disability required more time off work (71.4 ± 5.0 days versus 15.1 ± 1.3 days; $p < .001$), more time off school/college (32.7 ± 8.5 days versus 11.3 ± 1.2 days; $p < .001$) and were unable to carry out other daily activities for a longer period (53.5 ± 7.7 days versus 10.1 ± 1.5 days; $p < .001$).

The commonest cause of long-term disability in the study was WAD, followed by closed fractures of the long bones (upper limbs and lower limbs).

INCIDENCE OF ROAD TRAFFIC ACCIDENTS AND WHIPLASH-ASSOCIATED DISORDERS

Our studies have shown that there has been an annual increase in the number of patients attending an accident and emergency department, after a road traffic accident, from 1982/1983 (the year prior to the introduction of the compulsory wearing of seat belts in the United Kingdom) until 1991. Thereafter, there was a slight reduction, but throughout this period there has been a progressive increase in the number of patients attending with a WAD (Table 1). There was virtually a threefold increase in the year after the compulsory introduction of seat belt usage, but since then the numbers of injured have increased by an even greater extent. The increase between 1983/1984 and 1994 has been more than fivefold.

One possible explanation for the increased incidence of patients is that patients attend the accident and emergency department for insurance purposes, rather than treatment. However, 99.64% of patients said that they had attended because of their symptoms, and only 0.36% for insurance purposes.

The vast majority of patients claim to have been wearing seat belts at the time of the accident (97.3% of drivers and 99.1% of front seat passengers), but a survey of usage in local roads (excluding motorways and dual carriageways) showed that only 90% of drivers and 86% of front seat passengers were wearing seat belts.

National statistics are taken from police records. In the United Kingdom, the numbers of accident injuries are calculated from Stats. 19, which records fatalities and "serious" and "slight" injuries. The figures are taken from police records, not from hospital records.

Hopkin et al. (12,13) matched the records of 2670 patients seen in three accident and emergency departments with the police records. The study included 1765 patients who had sustained a "slight" injury. For the purpose of this study, WADs were included under

TABLE 1. *Incidence of whiplash-associated disorders[a]*

Year	Number of patients seen after being injured in a traffic accident	Number (%) with WAD
Feb. 1982–Feb. 1983[b]	929	72 (7.7)
Feb. 1983–Feb. 1984	940	193 (20.5)
1988	1,189	372 (31.0)
1990	1,508	564 (37.4)
1991	1,964	709 (36.1)
1994	1,919	1,032 (53.7)

[a] In the Accident and Emergency Department of Hope Hospital, Salford, United Kingdom.
[b] The last year before it became compulsory to wear seat belts in the United Kingdom.

"slight" injuries because they are recorded as such in Stats. 19. There were 799 patients who did not report their injury to the police. There were 966 patients who reported their injury, and of these, 231 were not recorded in Stats. 19, 17 were recorded as "serious," and only 718 were recorded as "slight." In addition, there were 552 patients recorded in Stats. 19 who had not reported to an accident and emergency department. Overall, approximately 45% of patients with WADs were unrecorded.

Using these figures, the current annual incidence in the United Kingdom of WAD is approximately 250,000 new cases per annum (9). Evans (6) estimated that in the United States, the annual incidence of new WADs was approximately 1 million, and Barnsley et al. (2) estimated that the annual incidence was 3.8 per thousand population.

LONG-TERM DISABILITY AFTER A WHIPLASH-ASSOCIATED DISORDER

Although there is no doubt that WADs occur, there is some dispute about their chronicity. Schrader et al. (30) have suggested that disabling or persisting symptoms do not occur as a result of a WAD but that the symptoms are due to expectation of disability, a family history of neck pain, and attribution of preexisting symptoms to the trauma. They based their study on the retrospective analysis of accident victims and sex-matched and aged-matched controls. Awerbuch (1) concluded that WAD was an illness reinforced by legal and social function, rather than a specific injury.

The vast majority of authors who have studied the natural history of WADs have found that a significant minority of these patients are left with a permanent disability, most studies suggesting a figure between 6% and 18%, although some authors quote a higher figure (6,10,11,18,21,25,28). However, most studies have been restricted to small numbers of patients, in many studies a large proportion of the patients were not available for follow-up, and very few studies have continued the follow-up for more than 2 to 3 years. In a 4-year follow-up of 413 patients, we found that the number of patients with a residual disability decreased with time as did the severity of the disability, 8.2% having a residual disability at 48 months (21) (Table 2) (Fig. 1). Palmar and Raymakers (25) studied the natural history in 100 patients and found that at final review (average, 8 years), 14% still had significant pain. Gargan and Bannister (10) reported a 10.8-year average follow-up, but their study was limited to 43 patients. These patients were part of an earlier study, the 2-year follow-up of 61 consecutive patients involved in rear-end collisions reported by Norris and Watt (23), but the study was not confined to patients with soft-tissue injuries and included four patients who had sustained a bony injury. In the 10-year follow-up, Gargan and Bannister (10) reported that only 12% of patients had recovered

TABLE 2. *Long-term disability after a whiplash-associated disorder*

Time after the traffic accident (mo)	Patients with residual disability (%)
6 mo	59.1
12 mo	40.0
18 mo	29.3
24 mo	24.2
30 mo	16.9
36 mo	11.4
42 mo	9.4
48 mo	8.2

$N = 413$.

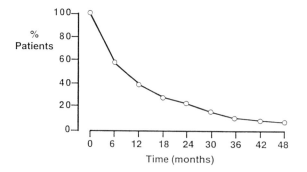

FIG. 1. The percentage of patients with a residual disability after a WAD decreases with time after the causative road traffic accident. At 48 months, 8.2% of patients still have a residual disability.

completely. The residual symptoms were intrusive in 28% and severe in 12%. Of the original 61 patients, five had died and 13 could not be traced at the time of Gargan and Bannister's later follow-up.

Many patients develop neck pain without being involved in an accident. Marshall et al. (19) assessed the relationship between neck symptoms and precedent injury. They found that there was an increase in incidence of neck pain with age, that there was no significant difference between men and women, and that there was no correlation with the physical nature of the work undertaken. Overall, 34% complained of neck discomfort during or after carrying out normal everyday tasks, with an incidence of 23% in the 30- to 39-year age group, 37% in the 40- to 49-year age group, and 44% in the 50- to 59-year age group. In contrast, 80% of patients who had sustained previous neck injury complained of neck discomfort during or after carrying out normal everyday activities ($p < .01$).

Palmar and Raymakers (25) studied the natural history in 100 patients who had sustained a WAD in a rear-impact road traffic accident and who originally had been seen for medicolegal reports. This was less than half of the 204 patients they had initially invited to enter the study. Fifty percent of the patients had significant pain at 8 months, 44% at 1 year, 22% at 2 years, and 18% at 3 years. Their minimum follow-up was 3 years. At final review, which averaged 8 years, 14% still had significant pain.

Whatever the cause of the residual disability, all the studies show that WAD is not necessarily a benign condition: a proportion of the patients will be left with a significant disability that may interfere with their job, their prospects in the open labor market, their everyday activities, and their leisure-time pursuits, although the incidence of long-term disability varies between the different studies. There are several possible reasons for this: most studies have been restricted to small numbers of patients, in many studies a large proportion of the patients were not available for follow-up, many of the studies were retrospective, and many of the studies were based on patients seen for medicolegal reports.

In the majority of patients, the severity of their disability declines with time. Murray et al. (21) developed a method of quantifying the disability, based on an assessment of the residual limitation of movement (such as lifting, bending, walking, sitting, and reaching), the residual limitation in physical activities (such as washing, bathing, dressing, eliminations, and eating), and any residual anxiety affecting daily activities, including recreational activities, occupation, and driving. The maximum disability was 9. There was a progressive reduction in disability during the 4-year follow-up of their patients. At 48 months, the average disability score in the 8.2% of patients with a residual disability was just under 1 (Fig. 2), with a progressive reduction in all three components of the disability score.

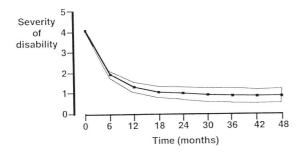

FIG. 2. There is a progressive reduction in the severity of the disability with time after the road traffic accident in which the patient sustained a WAD. The maximum disability score is 9 (21).

There is no good explanation as to why some patients are left with a severe residual disability. It may be the result of an abnormal psychological response to physical and persistent pain. Wallis et al. (35) studied 137 patients with chronic neck pain after a WAD and found a homogeneous pattern of responses characterized by high somatization, obsessive-compulsive behavior, and depression, confirming that the psychological distress exhibited by patients with whiplash was secondary to chronic pain. Other authors have reached similar conclusions (20,27,31,32).

Zygoapophyseal joint pain has been suggested as being the single most common basis for chronic neck pain and may be responsible for many of the headaches (3,16).

Magnetic resonance studies have shown the presence of anterior longitudinal ligament injury, vertebral endplate fracture, disc injuries, and posterior ligamentous injury (5,33), but the changes may be slight, they may be normal variants, and they may be present in asymptomatic individuals (4). MacNab (17) noted that those patients who had injured their wrists or ankles as well as their neck in a rear-impact injury seemed to recover from their limb injuries more readily, leaving them with a neck pain that was difficult to explain in terms of a "compensation neurosis."

It is likely that persistence and severity of symptoms leads to litigation rather than litigation affecting the natural progression of the symptoms, and chronic pain is seen in patients who have not been involved with litigation (6,22,23,25,26,29). Anxiety and depression may result from frustration resulting from the patients' inability to regain their pretraumatic level of physical, social, and professional functioning, rather than causing the chronicity.

FINANCIAL COSTS OF ROAD TRAFFIC ACCIDENTS

Many items contribute to the cost of road traffic accidents. These include the cost of medical treatment, the cost of the social services provided, lost income to the family, a subjective element for pain and suffering, the cost of lost output, the police costs in dealing with the accident and its aftermath, and the cost of damage to property. These have been included in the calculation and have either been taken from our own studies (health care costs, cost of social services provided, and lost income to the family) (21) or from figures provided by the Department of Transport in the United Kingdom (14,24).

There are two methods of measuring the subjective element. Previously, the Department of Transport has calculated a figure based on pain, grief, and suffering. More recently, they have based this figure on the value of avoidance (willingness to pay) (15). The latter is considered to be more accurate and has been used in calculating the costs.

TABLE 3. *Cost[a] of a whiplash-associated disorder*

Health care	300
Social services	355
Lost income	843
Lost output	3,124
Police	200
Damage to property	1,081
Subjective element	4,405
Total	10,308

[a] In pounds sterling—1990/1991 values.

Not all the costs have been included. For example, the calculation has not included the cost of delays to road users as a result of the congestion caused by a road traffic accident, or the cost of caring for someone whose injuries resulted in an extended out-of-work period, in terms of the anxiety, stress, and loss of earnings for the carer. Some of these costs are common to all countries, for example medical costs, lost output, and subjective elements. Holland includes the cost of a house conversion resulting from the disability, and the United States includes funeral costs for fatalities.

We have not included all elements of health care costs. We have included costs of the ambulance service (both the initial journey to the hospital after the accident and any subsequent journeys to the hospital for treatment), the accident and emergency department costs, hospital inpatient costs, hospital outpatient costs, physiotherapy provided by the National Health Service, the cost of any district nurse services, and the cost of any orthoses. The costs of general practice attendances were excluded because general practitioners are paid on a per capita basis and not per treatment. The costs of any private medical care (such as private physiotherapy or private osteopathy) were not included, nor were the costs of pharmaceuticals (including prescription costs and any pharmaceuticals bought over the counter). The costs are, therefore, an underestimate of true costs.

The average health care cost for a patient who sustained a WAD was £300 (in 1991 values). The Social Services cost, which included statutory sick pay and other benefits covering long-term illness and disability, was £355 in 1991 terms. The average number of working days lost after a WAD was 39 days for all patients, with an average loss of income of £843. The average time off work after a WAD for those having work was 81 days. This compares with an absence of 86 days for women and 77 days for men in the Québec study (34). The lost output for WAD was calculated at £3,124. per patient (8).

In reaching the final calculation, the figures quoted by the Department of Transport (in 1990 values) has been used for police costs, damage to property, and the subjective element using the value of avoidance. The average cost per patient is in excess of £10,000. (Table 3). The annual cost, therefore, to the United Kingdom for WADs is £2,553 million. This represents approximately 18% of the total costs of all road traffic accidents and approximately 0.4% of the gross national product.

CONCLUSIONS

Whiplash-associated disorders occur commonly after road traffic accidents. The incidence appears to be increasing, although there may be a slight decrease in the total number of injuries after road traffic accidents. A significant minority of patients are left with permanent disability, and the severity of the disability decreases with time. The causes of the long-term disability are not known.

National statistics underestimate the annual incidence of WAD. WAD not only leaves some patients with severe residual disability that may interfere with their ability to do their job, their prospects in the open labor market, and their everyday and leisure-time pursuits, but it is also a significant cost to the nation. It represents approximately 18% of the total cost of all road traffic accidents and 0.4% of the gross national product.

REFERENCES

1. Awerbuch MS. Whiplash in Australia: illness or injury? *Med J Aust* 1992;157:193–196.
2. Barnsley L, Lord S, Bogduk N. Whiplash injury. *Pain* 1994;58:283–307.
3. Barnsley L, Lord SM, Wallis BJ, Bogduk N. The prevalence of chronic cervical zygapophysial joint pain after whiplash. *Spine* 1995;20:20–26.
4. Boden SD, McCowin PR, Davis DO, Dina TS, Mark AS, Wiesel S. Abnormal magnetic-resonance scans of the cervical spine in asymptomatic subjects. *J Bone Joint Surg* 1990;72A:1178–1184.
5. Davis SJ, Teresi LM, Bradley WG Jr, Ziemba MA, Bloze AE. Cervical spine hyperextension injuries: MR findings. *Radiology* 1991;180:245–251.
6. Evans RW. Some observations on whiplash injuries. *Neurol Clin* 1992;10:975–997.
7. Galasko CSB, Murray PA, Hodson M, Tunbridge RH, Everest JT. Long term disability following road traffic accidents. *Transport Road Research Laboratory research report 59.* Transport Research Laboratory, Crowthorne, TRRL. 1986.
8. Galasko CSB, Murray PA, Pitcher M, et al. Neck sprains after road traffic accidents: a modern epidemic. *Injury* 1993;24:155–157.
9. Galasko CSB, Murray PA, Pitcher M. Whiplash-associated disorders. Proceedings of the 15th International Technical Conference on the Enhanced Safety of Vehicles (ESV), Melbourne, Australia, May 1996.
10. Gargan MF, Bannister GC. Long-term prognosis of soft-tissue injuries of the neck. *J Bone Joint Surg* 1990;72B: 901–903.
11. Hildingsson C, Toolanen G. Outcome after soft-tissue injury of the cervical spine: a prospective study of 93 car-accident victims. *Acta Orthop Scand* 1990;61:357–359.
12. Hopkin JM, Murray PA, Pitcher M, Galasko CSB. Police and hospital recording of nonfatal road accident casualties: a study in Greater Manchester, United Kingdom. *Transport Research Laboratory Project Report, PR/SRC/1/93.* Transport Research Laboratory, Crowthorne, United Kingdom, 1993.
13. Hopkin JM, Murray PA, Pitcher M, Galasko CSB. Police and hospital recording of nonfatal road accident casualties: a study in Greater Manchester, United Kingdom. *Transport Research Laboratory research report 379.* Transport Research Laboratory, Crowthorne, United Kingdom, 1993.
14. Hopkin JM, O'Reilly DM. Revaluation of the cost of road accident casualties: 1992 revision. *Transport Research Laboratory Research Project 378.* Transport Research Laboratory, Crowthorne, United Kingdom, 1993.
15. Jones-Lee MW, Loomes G, O'Reilly DM, Phillips PR. The value of preventing non-fatal road injuries: findings of a willingness-to-pay national sample survey. *Transport Research Laboratory contractor report 330.* Transport Research Laboratory, Crowthorne, United Kingdom, 1993.
16. Lord SM, Barnsley L, Wallis BJ, Bogduk N. Third occipital nerve headache: a prevalence study. *J Neurol Neurosurg Psychiatry* 1994;57:1871–1190.
17. MacNab I. The "whiplash syndrome." *Orthop Clin North Am* 1971;2:389–403.
18. Maimaris C, Barnes MR, Allen MJ. "Whiplash injuries" of the neck: a retrospective study. *Injury* 1988;19: 393–396.
19. Marshall PD, O'Connor M, Hodgkinson JP. The perceived relationship between neck symptoms and precedent injury. *Injury* 1995;26:17–19.
20. Merskey H. Psychological consequences of whiplash. *Spine: State Art Rev* 1993;7:471–480.
21. Murray PA, Pitcher M, Galasko CSB. The cost of long term disability from road traffic accidents. Four year study—final report. *Transport Research Laboratory Project Report 45.* Transport Research Laboratory, Crowthorne, United Kingdom, 1994.
22. Newman PK. Whiplash injury. *Br Med J* 1990;301:395–396.
23. Norris SH, Watt I. The prognosis of neck injuries resulting from rear-end vehicle collisions. *J Bone Joint Surg* 1983;65B:608–611.
24. O'Reilly DM. Costing new traffic accidents: the value of lost output. *Transport Research Laboratory Working Paper WP/SRC.09.* Transport Research Laboratory, Crowthorne, United Kingdom, 1993.
25. Parmar HV, Raymakers R. Neck injuries from rear impact road traffic accidents: prognosis in persons seeking compensation. *Injury* 1993;24:75–78.
26. Pennie B, Agambar L. Patterns of injury and recovery in whiplash. *Injury* 1991;22:57–59.
27. Radanov BP, Di Stefano G, Schnidrig A, Sturzenegger M. Psychosocial stress, cognitive performance and disability after common whiplash. *J Psychosom Res* 1993;37:1–10.

28. Radanov BP, Sturzenegger M, Di Stefano G, Schnidrig A. Relationship between early somatic, radiological, cognitive and psychosocial findings and outcome during a one-year follow-up in 117 patients suffering from common whiplash. *Br J Rheumatol* 1994;33:442–448.
29. Schofferman J, Wasserman S. Successful treatment of low back pain and neck pain after a motor vehicle accident despite litigation. *Spine* 1994;19:1007–1010.
30. Schrader H, Obelieniene D, Bovim G, Surkiene D, Mickeviciene D, Miseviciene I, Sand T. Natural evolution of late whiplash syndrome outside the medicolegal context. *Lancet* 1996;347:1207–1211.
31. Shapiro AP, Roth RS. The effect of litigation on recovery from whiplash. *Spine: State Art Rev* 1993;7:531–536.
32. Shapiro AP, Teasell RW, Steenhuis R. Mild traumatic brain injury following whiplash. *Spine: State Art Rev* 1993; 7:455–470.
33. Silberstein M, Tress BM, Hennessy O. Prevertebral swelling in cervical spine injury: identification of ligament injury with magnetic resonance imaging. *Clin Radiol* 1992;46:318–323.
34. Spitzer WO, Skovron ML, Salmi LR, et al. Scientific monograph of the Québec Task Force on whiplash-associated disorders: Redefining "whiplash" and its management. *Spine* 1995;20(8)(suppl):1S–73S.
35. Wallis BJ, Lord SM, Barnsley L, Bogduk N. Pain and psychologic symptoms of Australian patients with whiplash. *Spine* 1996;21:804–810.
36. World Health Organization. *The epidemiology of accident traumas and resulting disabilities.* Copenhagan: World Health Organisation, WHO Regional Office for Europe. EURO Reports and Studies 57, 1982.

*Whiplash Injuries: Current Concepts in
Prevention, Diagnosis, and Treatment
of the Cervical Whiplash Syndrome,*
edited by Robert Gunzburg and Marek Szpalski.
Lippincott–Raven Publishers, Philadelphia © 1998.

30

Influence of Legislative Changes on Whiplash Injury

Charles G. Greenough

*C. G. Greenough: Department of Orthopaedic Surgery, Middlesbrough General Hospital,
Middlesbrough, Cleveland, United Kingdom.*

The influence of compensation on recovery from whiplash injury has aroused controversy for many years. The proponents of the theory that prolonged disability is purely a result of physical changes have been able to point to an increasing body of research indicating annular tears and more severe disc injuries in victims of whiplash injuries. The suggestion that compensation has any effect on recovery has been usually based on the concept that such an effect results from the patient falsifying either symptoms or their severity, thus leading to an unnecessarily pejorative attitude. Despite many opinions, there is still very little reliable evidence on which to base any conclusions.

There are two questions that need to be addressed when considering the influence of legislative change on whiplash injuries.

1. Do compensation and wage replacement affect the prognosis of whiplash injury?
2. If they do, what are the possible mechanisms?

Some evidence does exist from which tentative conclusions may be drawn. In 1988, an important Australian study was presented by Mitchell on behalf of the Melbourne Motor Accident Board and Transport Accident Commission (11). At the time of the study, patients injured in a road traffic accident could claim compensation and reimbursement of private medical fees from the Board. A population of 600 consecutive claimants were identified and asked to complete an initial assessment of their condition within a maximum of 4 weeks from the accident. There were 496 patients who complied with the initial assessment and were included in the study. Because of the nature of the population, the excluded nonresponders could be compared to the selected study group with respect to demographic details and the number of claims made for treatment after the injury. The excluded patients were not significantly different in profile, but in general they fared much better, with 93% making no late claims for medical treatment.

At follow-up at 9 months, 472 (95%) were interviewed and examined, and, in addition, data from claims were available for analysis. The outcome was assessed by the number of expense claims made between 22 and 39 weeks after the injury. The study defined as "recovered" those who made no claims during this period, as "chronic" those who made between one and five claims, and as "very chronic" those who made six or more claims. Characteristics of patients with a poor outcome were age between 30 and 49; female sex;

TABLE 1. *Association between Zung depression score at 4 weeks and outcome of whiplash injury*

Depression score	Recovered	Chronic/very chronic
Not depressed	75	46
Mild	14	25
Moderate	8	13
Severe	3	12

$p < .000001$

Modified from Mitchell H. *Prospective study of whiplash injury and its outcome in Melbourne.* Melbourne, Australia: Motor Accident Board and Transport Accident Commission, 1988.

being divorced, separated, or widowed; having had primary education only; and being unemployed at the time of the accident.

Factors present at 4 weeks or less from the injury were examined for influence on the prognosis at 9 months. At 4 weeks, 166 (38%) stated that they had no intention of suing for damages, and of these 22% were rated as chronic or very chronic at follow-up. There were 181 (35%) who intended to sue for damages, and 61% of these were chronic or very chronic at follow-up ($p < .001$). Of those unemployed at the time of the accident, 78% were chronic or very chronic as opposed to 39% of employed people ($p < .001$). Depression as measured by the Zung depression scale was associated with a significantly worse outcome (Table 1). Using the Illness Behaviour Questionnaire (14), an increased belief in the existence of physical disease or an increased score on the hypochondriasis scale or the conversion reaction scale was associated with a reduced outcome ($p < .00001$). Of those patients with radiographs taken at the time of injury, 47 showed degenerative changes and 128 did not. No significant difference at review was noted [18 (38%) recovered versus 63 (49%), ns]

In the face of rapidly mounting claims and in the light of the Mitchell study, the Victoria State Government imposed changes in the way claims could be made after whiplash injury. These changes were introduced on January 1, 1987. Prior to the changes, accident victims were entitled to full wage replacement and a full refund of all medical expenses,

TABLE 2. *Injury claims received by the Victoria Motor Accident Board 1983–1995*[a]

Year	Fatalities, N	Whiplash, N (% of all claims)	Other injuries, N
1983	620	5,529 (14)	32,955
1984	633	6,515 (15)	35,638
1985	511	6,726 (16)	35,367
1986	555	6,196 (13)	39,577
1987	619	2,512 (11)	20,025
1988	686	1,824 (9)	18,015
1989	759	1,420 (7)	16,897
1990	544	975 (6)	13,899
1991	543	954 (7)	14,243
1992	459	1,103 (8)	14,475
1993	538	1,198 (7)	16,693
1994	474	1,631 (9)	17,601
1995	520	1,754 (9)	18,578

[a] Legislative changes introduced January 1, 1987.

Modified from McDermott FT. Reduction in cervical "whiplash" after new motor vehicle accident legislation in Victoria. *Med J Aust* 1993;158:720–721; with additional data from the Transport Accident Commission.

TABLE 3. *Time until return to work after whiplash injury,
comparing Victoria with New Zealand*

Time away from work	Victoria (%)	New Zealand (%)
1 wk	173 (11)	67 (29)
1–4 wk	387 (25)	101 (43)
4–8 wk	233 (15)	29 (12)
2–3 mo	145 (9)	9 (4)
3–6 mo	188 (12)	12 (5)
6–12 mo	282 (18)	9 (4)
12–24 mo	149 (10)	6 (3)
Total	1,557	233

$p < .001$

Modified from Mills H, Horne G. Whiplash—man-made disease?. *N Z Med J* 1986;99:373–374.

and they had an unrestricted right to sue for damages. The new regulations required that a police report be obtained before any claim could be made, a $250.00 excess (index linked) was placed on the reimbursement of medical charges, litigation rights were restricted if impairment was rated at less than 30%, and income support ceased at 18 months. The impact on claims is illustrated in Table 2.

Further data were provided by a comparison of the state of Victoria with New Zealand (10). In 1983, compensation and reimbursement of costs for medical treatment were available for whiplash injury in the state of Victoria, Australia, but in New Zealand, compensation was restricted to wage replacement at a level below normal and private medical charges were not refunded. In Victoria, of 15,380 recorded accidents, 2181 were rear-end collisions, whereas in New Zealand, out of 11,173 total accidents only 547 were rear-end collisions ($p < .001$). From these rear-end collisions in Victoria, 4231 cases of whiplash injury resulted, compared to only 422 cases in New Zealand ($p < .001$). Total compensation paid was $5 million in Australia, compared to $440,000 in New Zealand. In Australia, 36% of patients had returned to work within 4 weeks compared to 71% in New Zealand (Table 3).

The incidence of whiplash injury in the United Kingdom has also been rising over the same time period (Table 4) (2). An association with litigation has been noted by Maimaris et al. (7), who noted that 12 out of 32 litigants (38%) recovered compared with 55 out of 70 nonlitigants (79%) ($p < .001$). Such an association, however, was not observed by Pennie and Agambar (13), who found that 98 out of 116 litigants (84%) recovered compared with 26 of 28 nonlitigants (93%) (not a statistically significant difference).

Recently, Schrader et al. reported a retrospective study on occupants of motor vehicles involved in rear-end collisions in Lithuania (15). They identified 202 individuals from police records and compared them to age- and sex-matched controls 1 to 3 years after the accident. The incidence of neck pain and disability were the same in the two groups and there were no reports of pain or disability arising as a result of the accident. Few drivers in Lithuania are covered by insurance and there is little awareness in the general public of the possibility of whiplash injury. Although the study may be criticized for the small number of chronically disabled patients that might be expected to occur from 200 vehicle accidents, this study provides another indication that the compensation structure and social climate may have a very significant effect on the incidence of whiplash injury.

Work performed in controlled groups with nonspecific low back pain have also implicated compensation and wage replacement as a significant prognostic factor for poor out-

TABLE 4. *Incidence of whiplash in the United Kingdom*

Year	Total injuries (N)	Neck sprain (%)
1982	929	7.7
1983	940	20.5
1988	1,189	31.0
1990	1,508	37.4
1991	1,968	36.1

Modified from Galasko C, Murray PM, Pitcher M, et al. Neck sprains after road traffic accidents: a modern epidemic. *Injury* 1993;24:155–157.

come (3,4). Of 72 male claimants, 37 were unemployed at review, compared with 8 of 71 nonlitigants ($p < .00001$). For women, the figures were 29 of 63 and 4 of 55, respectively ($p < .00001$). Highly significant differences were also found in reported pain, disability, and physical impairment.

If, as seems likely, an effect of wage replacement and compensation on the recovery from whiplash injury is present, the mechanism still remains unclear. It is implicit in many analyses that any effect of compensation is a result of malingering, which may be defined as the deliberate falsification of, or exaggeration of, pain and disability for gain. Swartzman et al. (16) studied a group of whiplash litigants, for some of whom claims have been settled and for others claims are on-going. They were able to demonstrate no differences between these groups (Table 5). These findings confirmed those of Norris and Watt (12) who also found no effect of settlement of the claim on recovery from whiplash injuries.

Similar results have been noted in the recovery from nonspecific low-back injury (4). Of 65 claimants whose cases had been settled, 38 (58%) were unemployed, compared with 18 of 30 claimants (60%) in whom litigation was on-going (not a significant difference). Other factors were also unaffected by settlement (Table 6).

If claimants were deliberately falsifying symptoms and disability for gain, then it would be reasonable to expect that once settlement had occurred, they would resume an active lifestyle. This does not appear to occur, and it is unlikely, therefore, that malingering is a significant factor in the association of compensation with poor prognosis.

Possible etiologic factors in the influence of compensation are delay, vindication of innocence, the adversarial system, claim history, and increasing social acceptability. The litigation process has never been noted for brisk efficiency since the days of Jarndyce and Jarndyce (1). The probability of return to work declines with increasing time off work; anything that fosters delay may well have a deleterious effect on the outcome. A number of litigants appear to be more interested in proving the responsibility of a third party and

TABLE 5. *The effect of settlement of litigation on recovery from whiplash injury[a]*

	Settled	Not settled
Number of cases	21	41
Depression score	25.6	26.7
Employment score	2.7	2.4
Activities undertaken	16.9	18.3

[a] The differences were not statistically significant.
From Swartzman LC, Teasell RW, Shapiro AP, McDermid AJ. The effect of litigation status on adjustment to whiplash injury. *Spine* 1996;21:53–58.

TABLE 6. *The effect of settlement of litigation on recovery from low-back injury[a]*

	Settled	Not settled
Number of cases	70	35
Pain scale	5 (1–8)	5 (3–8)
Disability score	36 (8–68)	38 (10–54)
Impairment rating	14 (-2–20)	17 (1–30)

[a] The differences were not statistically significant.
From Greenough CG, Fraser RD. The effects of compensation on recovery from low-back injury. *Spine* 1989;14:947–955.

obtaining a formal acknowledgement of responsibility. These patients can often express outrage at what they see as lack of remorse in the "guilty party" (8). The linking of their recovery to the slow legal process may well be a serious adverse factor.

The adversarial system engenders a team spirit between the patients and their legal advisers. Under such circumstances, there is pressure to maintain the disabled status and to concentrate on remaining areas of disability. The patients may have to recount their symptoms many times to lawyers, doctors, and the courts. In this respect, the system of medical reports may be unsatisfactory, patients expressing great anger at reports that may suggest that they are exaggerating. There is some evidence that medical reports are based on little concrete data: Haddad (6) found in 1818 claims that doctors instructed by the claimants awarded disability in 99.5% of cases, whereas doctors instructed by the insurance companies examining the same patients at the same time awarded disability in only 25% of cases. This gross disparity indicates that there can be little objective evidence of disability that can be reliably obtained by history or clinical examination.

The history of a claim may be detrimental to the chances of obtaining further employment. In addition, the presence of a claim may be a disincentive to employers to provide light-duty jobs that would be of benefit in returning patients to work earlier, as they fear that an exacerbation produced by another incident may lead to a second claim.

It is also possible that the poor prognosis is exacerbated by Health Care Professionals. The care-giver's desire to "do something" may reinforce the belief that significant pathology exists. By continually trying different therapies on an empirical basis, the patient may be led to believe that eventually an effective treatment will be found. Prognostic advice is often negative.

In the study reported by Mitchell (11), those with a poor outcome at follow-up had been subjected to significantly more treatments in the first 4 weeks after the accident (Table 7). Patients initially treated at a hospital had a 60% chance of a chronic result, compared with only 37% in those whose primary consultation was with a general practi-

TABLE 7. *Outcome of whiplash injury related to treatments received in the initial 4 weeks*

Treatment	Recovered	Chronic/very chronic	Probability
Collar	16	36	$p < .00001$
Ultrasound	9	20	$p < .00001$
Short wave	9	24	$p < .00005$
Traction	4	9	$p < .05$
Manipulation	14	21	$p < .05$
Tranquilizers	11	23	$p < .01$

Modified from Mitchell H. *Prospective study of whiplash injury and its outcome in Melbourne.* Melbourne, Australia: Motor Accident Board and Transport Accident Commission, 1988.

tioner ($p < .001$) (but note that patients with other injuries were excluded from the study). Patients who went on to recovery had a mean of 1.38 consultations in the first 4 weeks, compared with 1.85 for chronic and 2.02 for very chronic outcomes ($p < .00001$).

Of course, it remains possible that those with more severe injuries received more treatment and had a worse outcome. Evidence from nonspecific low back injuries suggests this may not be the case. Greenough (3) found that 53% of compensation patients were seen on the day of injury, compared with only 22% of noncompensation patients ($p < .00001$). This was despite the fact that no differences were found in the injury severity scores between the two groups. Of the compensation patients, those initially seen in the first 48 hours had worse results at follow-up than those seen later [36 (range, 6 to 75) versus 46 (range, 20 to 74) ($p < .05$)]. Injury severity scores were again not different between the two groups.

Studies of the lumbar spine have indicated a significant association of spinal muscular decompensation with poor outcome. Active rehabilitation, early return to work, avoidance of rest, and avoidance of passive modes of treatment have all been associated with improved outcomes. Electromyographic studies have confirmed significant changes in spinal muscular function between chronic pain sufferers and normal volunteers (5). It may be that the final common pathway for the action of the etiologic factors important in whiplash injury is the deconditioning of the cervical musculature.

CONCLUSIONS

1. It is likely that compensation and wage replacement have a significant impact on the prognosis after whiplash injury of the cervical spine.

2. This detrimental effect is almost certainly NOT the result of malingering.

3. The effect of settlement is not the same as the effect of compensation, and future studies must clearly distinguish these two factors.

4. Possible etiologic factors in the influence of compensation are delay, vindication of innocence, the adversarial system, claim history, and increasing social acceptability.

5. In part at least, the deleterious effect may be iatrogenic.

6. The final common pathway may be cervical muscular deconditioning.

REFERENCES

1. Dickens C. *Bleak house.* London, 1852.
2. Galasko CSB, Murray PM, Pitcher M, et al. Neck sprains after road traffic accidents: a modern epidemic. *Injury* 1993;24:155–157.
3. Greenough CG. Recovery from low back pain. 1–5 year follow-up of 287 injury-related cases. *Acta Orthop Scand* 1993;64(suppl 254):1–34.
4. Greenough CG, Fraser RD. The effects of compensation on recovery from low-back injury. *Spine* 1989; 14:947–955.
5. Greenough CG, Oliver CW. EMG spectral mapping correlates with chronic low back pain. *J Bone Joint Surg Br* 1994;76B(suppl 2):91.
6. Haddad GH. Analysis of 2932 Workers' Compensation back injury cases. The impact on the cost to the system. *Spine* 1987;12:765–769.
7. Maimaris C, Barnes MR, Allen MJ. "Whiplash injuries" of the neck: a retrospective study. *Injury* 1988;19: 393–396.
8. Mayou R. Medico-legal aspects of road traffic accidents. *J Psychosom Res* 1995;39:789–798.
9. McDermott FT. Reduction in cervical "whiplash" after new motor vehicle accident legislation in Victoria. *Med J Aust* 1993;158:720–721.
10. Mills H, Horne G. Whiplash—man-made disease?. *N Z Med J* 1986;99:373–374.
11. Mitchell H. *Prospective study of whiplash injury and its outcome in Melbourne.* Melbourne, Australia: Motor Accident Board and Transport Accident Commission, 1988.

12. Norris SH, Watt I. The prognosis of neck injuries resulting from rear-end vehicle Collisions. *J Bone Joint Surg Br* 1983;65B:608–611.
13. Pennie B, Agambar L. Patterns of injury and recovery in whiplash. *Injury* 1991;22:57–59.
14. Pilowsky I, Spence ND. *Manual for the Illness Behaviour Questionnaire (IBQ).* Adelaide, Australia: Department of Psychiatry, University of Adelaide, 1983.
15. Schrader H, Obelieniene D, Bovim G, Surkiene D, Mickeviciene D, Mickeviciene I, Sand T. Natural Evolution of late whiplash syndrome outside the medicolegal context. *Lancet* 1996;347(9010):1207–1211.
16. Swartzman LC, Teasell RW, Shapiro AP, McDermid AJ. The effect of litigation status on adjustment to whiplash injury. *Spine* 1996;21:53–58.

Whiplash Injuries: Current Concepts in Prevention, Diagnosis, and Treatment of the Cervical Whiplash Syndrome, edited by Robert Gunzburg and Marek Szpalski. Lippincott–Raven Publishers, Philadelphia © 1998.

31

Automobile Design and Whiplash Prevention

Lotta Jakobsson

L. Jakobsson: Volvo Safety Center, Volvo Car Corporation, Göteborg, Sweden.

Cervical whiplash syndrome (reported as neck injury in accident databases) caused by car collisions has attracted increased attention in recent years. Although usually not life threatening, whiplash injury can have long-term consequences (11), making it one of the most prominent injuries in car accidents.

ACCIDENT STATISTICS

Volvo's traffic accident research team has collected data from Volvo cars involved in accidents, for over 25 years. All new Volvo cars sold in Sweden are covered by a 3-year damage warranty issued by the Volvia Insurance Company. About 10% of these cars are involved in an accident of any kind each year. Accidents in which the repair cost exceeds a specified level (currently over SEK 35.000) are investigated by Volvia's claim assessors. Technical details of the damage, together with accident, occupant, and injury data, are collected in each case and entered to a computer database. The injury data are gathered from medical reports and analyzed by a medical doctor in Volvo's Accident Research Team.

In the database, neck injuries include all neck discomfort and pain, reported by the occupants themselves and in some cases found in the medical records.

Collision Types

The distribution of collision types for neck injuries in the database is shown in Figure 1, where it can be seen that the number of occupants sustaining neck injuries in a frontal impact is twice as high for those riding in a car that is impacted in the rear end. Side-impact and multiple-impact accidents (in the latter, the car has been impacted twice or rolled, together with an impact) also account for many of the occurrences. These data do not cover all incidences. For example, minor accidents, especially rear-end impacts, may occur in which occupants sustain a neck injury, but because of the repair cost selection criterion, they do not show up in the regular accident data.

However, data from several other studies (2,8,10) in which minor accidents *are* considered, confirms that the number of neck injuries in frontal and side impact situations is comparable to those in rear-end impacts. Hence, it is important to consider all crash configurations when investigating whiplash injuries. Still, the risk of sustaining a neck injury

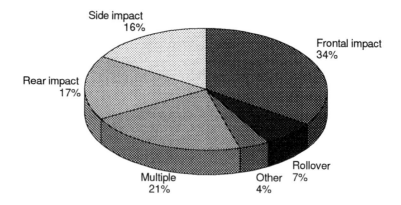

Total 41770 occupants whereof 5566 (13%) with neck injuries

Source: Volvo Accident Data

FIG. 1. Distribution of neck injuries as a function of impact configuration.

is highest if the car is hit from the rear, which is why the main focus is on this crash configuration.

Collision Severity

Neck injuries are reported at all impact speeds. For most other injuries, the risk increases with increased speed. Figure 2 shows the distribution of neck injuries and rib fractures versus impact severity, for frontal impacts.

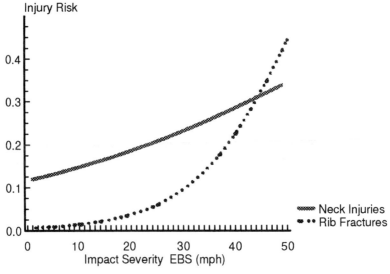

Source: Volvo Accident Data

FIG. 2. Neck injury risk in frontal impacts as a function of impact severity.

Advanced Accident Data Collection

To understand the cause and effect of whiplash syndrome by studying accident data, it is important add a set of parameters to those normally collected in an accident database. Volvo has performed two in-depth studies (6,13) with advanced accident data collection. Some of the additional parameters were primarily related to the risk of injury, such as distance between the head and the head restraint, whether the occupant was turning his or her head to the side at the time of the impact, and detailed information of the car deformation.

POTENTIAL INJURY MECHANISMS

The exact injury mechanism has not yet been established. Several contradictory mechanisms have been suggested by different researchers. Some of them are mentioned below.

The hypothesis formed by researchers at Chalmers University (1,17), which predicts that the volume changes inside the spinal canal may induce injurious mechanical loads to the tissues of the intervertebral foramina, suggests that the injury occurs at the beginning of the rearward motion in a rear-end impact.

On the other hand, the Folksam Insurance Group (19) suggests that the injury mechanism underlying neck injuries both in frontal and rear-end impacts could be considered a frontal mechanism for the occupant, occurring when the occupant is mowing forward and is restrained by the seat belt.

Ono and Kanno (14) performed a series of sled tests using volunteers to demonstrate that the shear force and the axial force on the neck, as well as the neck bending moments and head rotation angle, must be analyzed when evaluating neck responses.

McConnell et al. (9) theorized that forces directed axially through the cervical spine, as a result of the torso ramping up the seat backrest, are injury producing rather than the classic hyperextension–hyperflexion mechanism theory.

Several other studies address the mechanism of the injury. As long as no single mechanism is proven to be the only valid one, it is necessary to take all possible mechanisms into consideration. It is even possible that all mechanisms are valid, for different persons and different crash scenarios.

One way to summarize existing theories is to point out guidelines to follow to be sure that design efforts are purely favorable. Such efforts should (a) attempt to achieve a low *g* level (the occupant should experience as low a change of velocity as possible), (b) minimize movements between adjacent vertebrae (the curvature of the spine should change as little as possible during the crash), and (c) eliminate the rebound into the seat belt in a rear-end impact.

Based on these guidelines, it is possible to suggest design improvements even though the exact mechanism is not established. To be sure that improvements will reduce the occurrences of injured occupants, all the three guidelines should be addressed, because to some extent, they are related to different theories.

CRASH DYNAMICS

In a car collision, the car is subjected to an impact and energy is transferred into the vehicle. All parts play a role in the outcome of the crash. The structure of the car carries the energy and transmits it to the interior. The structure must be plastically deformable (to absorb energy) and also stiff (to avoid a total collapse and maintain the integrity of the vehicle "safety cage"). The interior safety systems, mainly seat belts, which keep the occupants in the vehicle, avoiding ejection, reduce impacts to the interior and offer an extra ride-down. Finally, the interior and the occupant share the final energy, and the interior must, therefore, be designed to absorb as much as possible of the energy to expose the occupant to the least impact.

When the car is being hit from the rear, the occupant will experience a forward force from the seat/car to his or her back. The occupant will start to move rearward relative to the seat. Depending on the seat backrest structure and the distance between the seat backrest and the occupant, the spine's curvature will be changed and most of the time the head will be lagging. When the kinetic energy has reached zero, an opposite motion (rebound) will take part, the amplitude dependent on the seat backrest characteristics.

Existing standard anthropomorphic test dummies, which were primarily designed for high speed frontal impact, are not biofidelic when used in low speed or rear-end impact testing (15,18). To understand the kinematics of the occupant in a rear-end impact, Volvo developed a mathematical model with a segmented spine to simulate a human-like motion (6,7). This model is now used to study the effect of the different parameters in the seat and different impact speeds.

Vehicle Design

Based on statistics, in-depth studies, and biomechanical research, Volvo (3) showed that the occurrence of neck injuries in a rear-end impact is a function of several factors. Vehicle-related parameters, including seat stiffness, and the horizontal and vertical distance between head and head restraint, are important factors, as are individual parameters, such as sex, size, age, awareness of the impending accident, and the ability to endure pain.

The conclusion of a study by Nygren et al. (12) based on accident data is that the vertical position of the head restraint is a major factor in reducing whiplash injuries from rear-end impacts.

An in-depth study by Olsson et al. (13), involving 33 occupants in Volvo cars, indicates that a horizontal distance of more than 10 cm between the head and the head restraint increases the risk of neck injuries in rear-end impacts. The duration of the neck symptoms appear to be a function of the permanent deformation of the impacted car, softer impacts (in which the rear beam structure is not involved) being less likely to result in injury. This study was extended by sending additional questionnaires to 163 occupants in rear-end-impact accidents (6). The latter study supported the findings of Olsson et al. (13). Other factors found to increase the risk of neck injuries were greater seat backrest inclination prior to impact and a stiffer head restraint (without a comfort cushion).

The Québec Task Force (16) has summarized all published whiplash literature and concluded that properly fitted head restraints reduce the severity of whiplash. In rear-end collisions, there is evidence that a head restraint, which is in line with the seat, positioned close to the occupant at the level of occiput, made of the same material as the seat, and strong enough to resist impact but still yielding enough to avoid rebound of the occupant, will reduce the incidence and severity of neck injuries.

In a recently published study (4), it was shown with volunteers that parameters such as vertical and horizontal distance between head and head restraint, as well as design and adjustment of seat and head restraint, greatly influence the injury risk in a rear-end impact.

Based on the facts that whiplash can occur in any crash situation at any speed, and that several injury mechanisms are probable, it is emphasized that the design of the whole car must be considered in the ambition to reduce the number of whiplash incidences (Fig. 3).

Car Body Structure

The structure of the car should absorb energy in a plastic way even at low velocity impacts.

Seat and Head Restraint Design

Over the years, a head restraint with certain characteristics was believed to be the solution to the whole problem. Studies have shown that a high and fixed-in-position head restraint, positioned close to the head, is favorable. Volvo models have been equipped with such head restraints as standard equipment in the front seat, for over two decades. In 1995, Volvo head restraints were recognized with the highest scores in a whiplash study by Insurance Institute for Highway Safety (5).

The head restraint should be considered an integrated part of the seat backrest. The characteristics of the seat backrest and head restraint should be similar, offering the whole spine and head comparable support in case of a rear-end impact. For frontal impacts, the same guidelines would be beneficial.

The seat backrest should offer energy absorption to reduce the rebound in a rear-end impact. The question of height-adjustable head restraints is of secondary importance. A misuse factor needs to be accounted for. It would be preferable to have the seat and head restraint designed to fit all occupant sizes, offering close and high enough support for as many occupant sizes and seating postures as possible.

Seat Belts and Inflatable Restraints

The role of seat belts for neck injuries has not been clarified. There are suggestions from the literature that seat belts may increase the incidence of neck injuries in rear-end impacts (16). This increase is minor and not scientifically proven, and it is largely offset

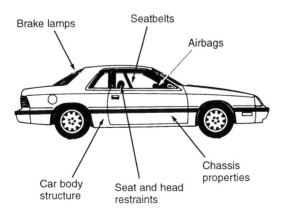

FIG. 3. Car design areas that are important to consider when investigating whiplash.

by the demonstrated effectiveness of seat belts in decreasing overall fatality and the incidence of severe head, face, and other injuries.

When the seats are designed to be less elastic, the rebound in rear-end impacts will be reduced or diminished, and then the role of the seat belt in rear-end impacts will be less important. In a frontal impact, the effect of the seat belt is probably more important, but this area is in need of more research.

There are no known studies of how air bags or other automatic protection devices influence the frequency and severity of whiplash (16). Complementary restraint systems are important to look at to more effectively give the occupant a smooth ride-down.

Collision Avoidance Systems

The ultimate prevention is a system that helps the driver avoid the accident, such as improved chassis properties for better handling and high-mounted brake lamps.

DISCUSSION

This chapter does not offer the ultimate whiplash solution. There are still many areas of uncertainty and important issues that need more research, such as the main injury mechanisms. The attempt here is to suggest guidelines for various design areas that, based on today's knowledge, are helpful in mitigating whiplash. It is important to work with a broad perspective to significantly reduce the incidence of whiplash. As whiplash is a very complex injury, so too is whiplash prevention by car design.

It is possible that the ongoing development of new cars has, in some ways, a negative effect on this problem. Cars are becoming smaller to reduce weight and lower fuel consumption. The ambition to enable a soft car crash pulse in low-velocity impacts, in order to reduce whiplash, is in conflict with the size of the car and the goal of maintaining a safety cage in a high-velocity impact. Also, seat backrests are becoming stiffer to carry more cargo load in a frontal impact and to eliminate the risk of seat backrest collapse in a high velocity rear-end impact. It is not certain that a stiffer seat backrest is necessarily worse for whiplash, but a seat backrest designed to withstand high forces tends to give a greater rebound which, based on some theories (19), could be injury producing.

The human factors are very important issues. Apart from the individual differences in sustaining, evolving, and recovering from the injury, the fact that occupants not sitting properly are subjected to a higher risk (at least for rear-end impacts) makes it very hard to really be able to predict the benefit for different designs. To cope with this problem, it is necessary to offer easily adjustable seats and also to inform about the importance of using them correctly. In some situations, it will be difficult to easily reduce the incidences, such as when the occupant is leaning forward or turning his or her head to the side to see the surrounding traffic.

CONCLUSIONS

Whiplash can occur in all crash situations and at all speeds. The exact injury mechanism has not yet been established, and it is possible that whiplash can be caused by several different mechanisms. This chapter suggests that the design of the whole car must be taken into consideration to significantly reduce whiplash. It is not necessary that improvements be made in all design areas, but it is important to understand the effect of the different designs on mitigating whiplash.

The following improvements would help to reduce whiplash:

1. The *car structure* should be energy absorbent even at low velocity crashes.

2. The *seat design* should preferably support the occupant's whole spine and head. The *head restraint* should be regarded as the upper part of the seat backrest, both when geometry and characteristics are concerned. In a rear-end impact, the seat backrest should be plastically energy absorbing and not give a forward rebound. The occupant's seating posture and the position and angle of the head at impact are very important to benefit from an improved seat design.

3. The effect and best design of *seat belts and inflatable restraints* are not known for certain. There is probably a big potential for improvements in this area, primarily to reduce the whiplash incidences in frontal impacts.

4. The ultimate safety systems are *systems that help the driver to avoid the accidents*: improved chassis properties for better handling and high-mounted brake lamps.

REFERENCES

1. Aldman B. An analytical approach to the impact biomechanics of the head and neck. Proceedings of the 30th annual American Association for Automotive Medicine (AAAM) conference, 1986;439–454.
2. Björnstig U, Hildingsson C, Toolanen G. Soft-tissue injury of the neck in a hospital based material. *Scand J Soc Med* 1990;18(4):263–267. Also in: Hildingsson C. Umeå University Medical Dissertations, new series no. 296, 1990.
3. Carlsson G, Nilsson S, Nilsson-Ehle A, Norin H, Ysander L, Örtengren R. Whiplash injuries in rear end car collisions: biomechanical considerations to improve head restraints. Proceedings of the International Council on Biokinetics of Impacts (IRCOBI) conference, Göteborg, Sweden, 1985, 277–289.
4. Deutscher C. Movement of car occupants in rear-end accidents. Paper no. 96A5016, International Conference on Active and Passive Automobile Safety, Capri, Italy, Oct. 1996.
5. Insurance Institute of Highway Safety. Special issue: whiplash injuries, status report. 1995;30(8).
6. Jakobsson L, Norin H, Jernström C, Svensson S-E, Johnsén P, Isaksson-Hellman I, Svensson MY. Analysis of different head and neck responses in rear-end car collisions using a new humanlike mathematical model. Proceedings of IRCOBI conference on biomechanics of impacts, Lyon, France, 1994;109–125.
7. Jernström C, Nilson G, Svensson MY. A first approach to an implementation of a human body model for rear-impact modelling. Proceedings of the 4th international Madymo Users meeting. Eindhoven, Netherlands, September 6 and 7, 1993.
8. Maimaris C, Barnes MR, Allen MJ. Whiplash injuries of the neck: a retrospective study, *Injury* 1988;19: 393–396.
9. McConnell WE, Howard RP, Guzman HM, Bomar JB, Raddin JH, Benedict JV, Smith HL, Hatsell CP. Analysis of human test subject kinematic responses to low velocity rear end impacts. In: *Vehicle and occupant kinematics; simulation and modeling (SP-975)*. Society of Automotive Engineering technical paper series 930889, SAE International Congress and Exposition: March 1–5 1993, Detroit, MI, Warrendale, PA: pp. 21–30.
10. Morris AP, Thomas P. A study of soft tissue neck injuries in the UK. Paper no. 96-S9-O-08, 15th enhanced safety vehicles conference, Melbourne, Australia, May 1996.
11. Nygren Å. Injuries to car occupants—some aspects of the interior safety of cars. *Acta Otolaryngol* 1984;(suppl 395).
12. Nygren Å, Gustafsson H, Tingvall C. Effects of different types of head restraints in rear-end collisions. 10th international conference on experimental safety vehicles, NHTSA, 1985;85–90.
13. Olsson I, Bunketorp O, Carlsson G, Gustafsson C, Planath I, Norin H, Ysander L. An in-depth study of whiplash injuries in rear end collisions. Proceedings of IRCOBI conference on the biomechanics of impact, Bron, France, 1990;269–280.
14. Ono K, Kanno M. Influence of the physical parameters on the risk to whiplash injuries in low speed rear-end collisions. Proceedings of IRCOBI conference on the biomechanics of impact, Eindhoven, Netherlands, 1993; 201–212.
15. Scott MW, McConnell WE, Guzman HM, Howard RP, Bomar JB, Smith Hl, Benedict JV, Raddin JH, Hatsell CP. Comparison of human and ATD head kinematics during low-speed rearend impacts. Society of Automotive Engineering paper no. 930094, 1993.
16. Spitzer WO, Skovron ML, Salmi LR, et al. Scientific monograph of the Québec Task Force on whiplash-associated disorders: redefining whiplash and its management. *Spine* 1995;20(8S).

17. Svensson MY, Aldman B, Hansson HA, Lövsund P, Seeman T, Sunesson A, Örtengren T. Pressure effects in the spinal canal during whiplash extension motion—a possible cause of injury to the cervical spinal ganglia. Proceedings of IRCOBI conference on the biomechanics of impact, Eindhoven, Netherlands, 1993;189–200.
18. Szabo TJ, Welcher JB, Anderson RD, Rice HM, Ward JA, Paulo LR, Carpenter NJ. Human occupant kinematics response to low speed rear end impacts. In: *Occupant containment and methods of assessing occupant protection in the crash environment, SP 1045*, Society of Automotive Engineering technical paper series 940532, SAE International Congress and Exposition, Detroit, MI, 1994;23–35.
19. von Koch M, Kullgren A, Nygren Å, Tingvall C. Soft tissue injury of the cervical spine in rear-end and frontal car collisions. Proceedings of IRCOBI conference on biomechanics of impacts, Brunnen, Switzerland, 1995; 273–283.

*Whiplash Injuries: Current Concepts in
Prevention, Diagnosis, and Treatment
of the Cervical Whiplash Syndrome,*
edited by Robert Gunzburg and Marek Szpalski.
Lippincott–Raven Publishers, Philadelphia © 1998.

32

Saab Active Head Restraint System

Seat Design to Reduce the Risk of Neck Injuries

Kristina Wiklund

K. Wiklund: Saab Automobile AB, Trollhättan, Sweden.

Injury statistics indicate that almost every fourth injury to car occupants is related to rear-end crashes, and that three quarters of these injuries involve the neck (1,2). Neck injuries in rear-end collisions occur primarily in impacts with velocity changes (Δv) of 20 km/hr or less (7,17,19,21), and they are mostly classified as AIS 1 (1–3,6,18). However, they cause significant harm to society because almost 10% of the AIS 1 neck injuries occurring in rear-end collisions have been found to lead to permanent disability (disability degree, 10%) (15,16).

Rear impacts also involve serious or fatal injury, in addition to the many minor injuries (1,2). Such injury is generally associated with large changes in velocity of the struck vehicle, seat-back deflection, and head impact. In a series of sled tests, Viano found that the occupant surrogate was retained on the seat if the seat-back angle with respect to vertical stayed below 60° (29). When the seat-back deflection exceeded 70°, the occupant was translated rearward, with potential impact against interior components of the car.

Although the relationship between kinematic and kinetic parameters of the head–neck motion and the risk of sustaining neck-injury in a rear-end impact is not fully known, previous research indicates that the initial, linear motion is critical for the occurrence of injury symptoms. Thus McConnell et al. produced mild, transient, and clinically classic neck discomfort symptoms in volunteers who experienced substantial linear displacement between head and shoulders, but only small cervical spine extension (8,9). In the tests, the volunteers were seated in car seats with head restraints and exposed to staged rear-end collisions at low-impact velocities. These results are in agreement with results obtained by Svensson (25), who found clinical evidence of nerve root injuries in pigs that had been exposed to swift linear displacement of the head relative to the upper torso. Nightingale et al. demonstrated in a series of drop tests with cadaver head-and-necks onto oblique planes that injuries to the bones and ligaments also occur at the initial, linear displacement of the head relative to the torso, and also that there is only weak correlation bewteen the type of injury and the direction of motion of the head (14).

The importance of controlling head motion during rear impact had already been demonstrated by Mertz and Patrick (12,13), who found no evidence of injury in a volunteer whose head was in contact with the seat back during rear-end impact sled tests at velocity changes (Δv) of up to 30 km/hr. These results are corroborated by field data, which show a low incidence of cervical spine injuries in children (i.e., occupants whose heads are normally supported by the seat back) (Tingvall, personal communication, 1996).

Melvin, McElhaney, and Roberts identified four factors as being important in reducing potential injury in rear impacts: (a) head displacement, rotation, and acceleration; (b) differential motion of the head and torso into the deflected seat back; (c) occupant ramping up the deflected seat-back; and (d) occupant rebound (11).

States et al. suggested elastic rebound of the seat back could be an aggravating factor for the whiplash-extension motion (23). According to this hypothesis, the rebound of the seat back can push the torso forward relative to the vehicle at an early stage of the whiplash extension motion. This in turn would increase the relative linear and angular velocity of the head relative to the upper torso and could at the same time delay contact between the head and the head restraint, thus increasing the maximal displacement and extension angle. Other studies support this theory (3,10,20,21,27,28). If, on the other hand, the seat back collapses or yields plastically during a rear-end collision, the elastic seat-back rebound is eliminated or reduced. In fact, seat-back collapse may decrease the risk of neck injury in rear-end collisions (3,23).

The aim of the present study was to analyze the relative rearward and forward motions between head and torso that occur in a rear impact, and to evaluate means of eliminating swift relative motion between head and torso in low- and medium-speed rear impacts.

MATERIALS AND METHODS

A series of rear impact sled tests (HyGe) were carried out. In the tests, a 50th percentile Hybrid-III dummy (4) was used. In all tests except high severity tests with the dummy out-of-position, the Rear-Impact Dummy (RID) neck replaced the standard

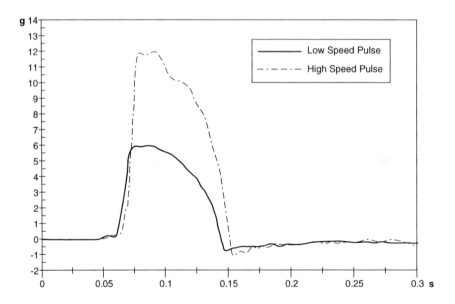

FIG. 1. The sled acceleration pulses for the 12.5 km/hr *(solid line)* and 25.8 km/hr *(dotted line)* impact.

TABLE 1. *Text matrix*

	12.5 km/hr		25.8 km/hr	
	ip	op	ip	op[a]
Concept	x	x	x	x
Baseline	x	x	x	x

[a]Hybrid-III neck.
ip, in-position; op, out-of-position.

Hybrid-III neck. The RID neck was developed and validated in 1992 (26), because the neck of the Hybrid-III dummy had been found to generate too high a torque during extension for a human-like response in the sagittal plane (3,22). Another advantage of the RID neck compared to the Hybrid-III neck is that it has more articulations (the same number as the human cervical spine), and therefore it has a lower resistance to translational displacement between head and torso without head rotation. This has recently been shown to improve neck biofidelity in low-severity rear impacts (5).

The dummy was seated with lower arms resting in the lap. The rubber was removed from the thighs of the dummy, to uncouple upper body rotation from leg rotation. The dummy was equipped with accelerometers in the head, chest, and pelvis, and with force-moment transducers at the upper neck (R. A. Denton, type 1716).

A production bucket-seat was used as reference (baseline) seat. Various elaborations on the prototype seat were carried out, with the aim of developing a concept seat that would eliminate relative motion between head and torso for normally seated occupants in rear impacts. Another design criterion for the concept seat was that it should in no case worsen the situation for the occupant compared to the reference seat.

The final concept seat accommodated a large extent of torso penetration into the seat back, with maintained seat back strength and exterior. The torso penetration exerted force on a movable plate, which in turn moved the head restraint upward and forward. Thus, the head was supported earlier than what was possible with a fixed head restraint.

Tests were run at 12.5 and 25.8 km/hr Δv, with acceleration pulses of about $6g$ and $12g$, respectively (Fig. 1). Each of the impact velocities was run with the dummy seated in two different initial positions, referred to as in-position (ip) and out-of-position (op). When in-position, the back of the dummy was aligned with the seat-back, which in turn was angled 21° rearward with respect to vertical. In the out-of-position case, the dummy was instead leaning slightly forward, and the H-point was 50 mm more forward with respect to the seat back than in the in-position case. This placed the back of the head 300 mm away from the headrest, compared with 30 mm in the in-position seating. The neck was slightly more flexed in the op posture. At the higher test speed, the

TABLE 2. *Head rearward displacement with respect to torso*

	12.5 km/hr		25.8 km/hr	
	ip	op	ip	op[a]
Concept	19	270	55	n.a
Baseline	34	310	99	n.a

[a]Hybrid-III neck.
ip, in-position; op, out-of-position.

TABLE 3. *Neck extension angle (degrees)*

| | 12.5 km/hr | | 25.8 km/hr | |
	ip	op	ip	op[a]
Concept	0	8	0	31
Baseline	6	47	22	50

[a]Hybrid-III neck.
ip, in-position; op, out-of-position.

regular Hybrid-III neck was used for the op tests. The test matrix is shown in Table 1. Criteria measured in the tests were head linear (x direction) and angular displacement with respect to the chest, and shear and tension/compression force, as well as bending moment in the upper neck (C1 to head joint).

DISCUSSION

Although a generally accepted injury mechanism for the so-called whiplash syndrome is yet to be found, recent research points out swift linear displacement between head and torso as being a critical process for the cervical spine. Such motion is generated in rear-end car collisions when the upper torso, but not the head, is pushed forward by the seat back. For comfort reasons and in order not to obstruct the field of view of car occupants, the top of current seat backs typically reaches the shoulder region of seated adults. For comfort reasons, there must also be a gap between the head and the head restraint, or the head restraint would repeatedly hit the head during the ride. The distance required to avoid the head restraint bumping into the head varies from seat to seat, but it is rarely less than 30 mm. Thus, the torso is generally engaged early when the car is impacted from behind, whereas the head is unsupported until the head restraint has bridged at least this "comfort gap." This difference in support time causes rearward motion of the head with respect to the torso (neck retraction), which in turn may be the cause of the whiplash syndrome (28). The neck retraction can also increase after the head has contacted the head restraint, if the torso is rebounded (i.e., moving away from the seat-back) before the head has been fully accelerated forward. Differential motion in the opposite direction (head forward with respect to torso, with neck protraction) can occur if the rebound motion of the torso is stopped, for instance by the seat belt, while the head continues its unsupported travel. Rebound requires that there be some elastic energy stored in the seat back. However, the vast majority of current

TABLE 4. *Neck moment rearward bending (C1)*

| | 12.5 km/hr | | 25.8 km/hr | |
	ip	op	ip	op[a]
Concept	3.1	2.6	2.2	27
Baseline	2.9	6.8	7.9	35

[a]Hybrid-III neck.
ip, in-position; op, out-of-position.

TABLE 5. *Neck shear force (head rearward with respect to torso) (C1)*

	12.5 km/hr		25.8 km/hr	
	ip	op	ip	op[a]
Concept	21	271	46	349
Baseline	24	264	85	224

[a]Hybrid-III neck.
ip, in-position; op, out-of-position.

seats do store more or less of the incoming energy of a low or medium severe impact in the seat back-frame or suspension.

In this study, the comfort gap between the head and the head restraint was bridged on impact by means of a plate system in the seat back. Load generated between the upper torso of the dummy and the seat back was exerted on a movable plate that pushed the head restraint upward and forward. The load required to activate the plate was barely higher than loads occurring during normal ride, and motion of the system started within a few millseconds (0 to 5 ms) after the first signs of load between the upper torso of the dummy and the seat-back.

A concept seat equipped with the active head restraint substantially reduced neck retraction and extension compared to the baseline seat in the impact situations tested, and also neck loads (Tables 2 to 6). This effect of bridging the comfort gap is additionally demonstrated in Figure 2, which shows that the concept seat accelerates the neck in one homogeneous motion, whereas the baseline seat produces a substantial delay between lower and upper neck accelerations, and also a difference in magnitude. Furthermore, the concept seat generally reduced other neck loads such as bending moment, shear, and tension. The numbers for relative displacement between head and torso are with respect to the sled. Thus, in the tests where the head of the dummy was far away from the head restraint at t = 0 (op), and the neck was consequently in flexion prior to impact, the relative displacement was far larger than the actual neck retraction. However, the observed reduction in relative displacement should be attributable to reduced retraction more or less in full, because the "free flight" kinematics of the dummy were not much affected by differences in upper seat-back design.

CONCLUSIONS

A seat design that offers distributed and simultaneous support for the upper body, including the head, significantly reduces neck retraction and extension compared to a

TABLE 6. *Neck tension force (C1)*

	12.5 km/hr		25.8 km/hr	
	ip	op	ip	op[a]
Concept	270	800	449	2088
Baseline	417	1127	598	2553

[a]Hybrid-III neck.
ip, in-position; op, out-of-position.

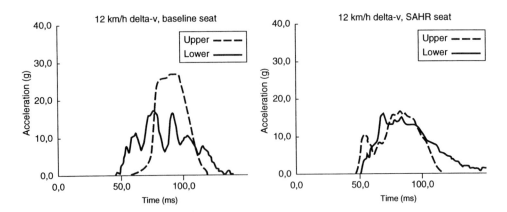

FIG. 2. The *x* axis acceleration of the lower *(dotted line)* and upper *(solid line)* part of the neck in a low-speed, in-position test, with the baseline and the concept seat, respectively.

baseline seat, and thus it can potentially reduce the risk of whiplash injury in rear impacts of moderate and medium severity. Such a design can be achieved with maintained comfort and appearance, and without adversely affecting other aspects of occupant safety.

REFERENCES

1. DataLink Inc. Car crash outcomes in rear impacts, *appendix A to current issues of occupant protection in car rear impacts*. Washington, DC: DataLink, 1989.
2. DataLink Inc. Current issues of occupant protection in car rear impacts, *prepared for the Office of Crashworthiness, Rulemaking, National Highway Traffic Safety Administration, docket 89-20-NO1-021*, Washington DC: DataLink, 1990.
3. Foret-Bruno JY, Dauvilliers F, Tarriere C, Mack P. Influence of the seat and head rest stiffness on the risk of cervical injuries in rear impact. Proceedings of the 13th ESV Conference, Paris, France, paper 91-S8-W-19, NHTSA, USA, DOT HS 807 991, 1991.
4. Foster JK, Kortege JO, Volanin MJ. Hybrid III—A biomechanically based crash test dummy. Proceedings of the 21th STAPP Car Crash Conference, SAE Inc., New York, LC 67-22372, 1977;973–1014.
5. Geigl B, Steffan H, Dippel C, Muser MH, Walz F, Svensson MY. Comparison of head-neck kinematics during rear end impacts between standard Hybrid-III, RID neck, volunteers, and PMTOs, Proceedings of 1995 International IRCOBI Conference on the biomechanics of impacts, Brunnen, Switzerland, 1995.
6. James MB, Strother CE, Warner CY, Decker RL, Perl TR. Occupant protection in rear-end collisions: 1. Safety priorities and seat belt effectiveness. Proceedings of the 35th STAPP car crash conference, SAE/P-91/251, Society of Automotive Engineers paper no. 912913, 1991.
7. Kahane CJ. An evaluation of head restraints—Federal Motor Vehicle Safety Standard 202. *NHTSA Technical Report, DOT HS-806 108*, National Technical Information Service, Springfield, VA, 22161, 1982.
8. McConnell WE, Howard RP, Guzman, et al. Analysis of human test subject responses to low velocity rear end impacts. SP-975, Society of Automotive Engineers paper no. 930889, pp. 21–30, SAE Inc., 1993.
9. McConnell WE, Howard RP, Poppel JV, et al. Human head and neck kinematics after low velocity rear end impacts—understanding "whiplash." SP-975, Society of Automotive Engineers paper no. 952724, pp. 215–238, SAE Inc., 1993.
10. McKenzie JA, Williams JF. The dynamic behaviour of the head and cervical spine during whiplash. *J Biomech* 1971;4:477–490.
11. Melvin JW, McEnhaney JH, Roberts VL. Improved neck simulation for anthropometric dummies. Proceedings of the 16th STAPP car crash conference, SAE Inc., New York, LC 67-22372, 1972;45–60.
12. Mertz HJ, Patrick LM. Investigation of the kinematics and kinetics of whiplash. Proceedings of the 11th STAPP car crash Conference, Anaheim, CA, SAE Inc., New York, LC 67-22372, 1967;267–317.
13. Mertz HJ, Patrick LM. Strength and response of the human neck. Proceedings of the of 15th STAPP car crash conference, SAE Inc., New York, LC 67-22372, 1971;207–255.

14. Nightingale RW, McElhaney JH, Richardsson WJ, Myers BS. Dynamic responses of the head and cervical spine to axial impact loading. *J Biomechanics* 1996;29(3):307–318.
15. Nygren Å. Injuries to car occupants—Some aspects of the interior safety of cars. *Akta Otolaryngol* 1984;suppl 395.
16. Nygren Å, Gustafsson H, Tingvall C. Effects of different types of headrests in rear-end collisions. 10th international conference on experimental safety vehicles, NHTSA, 1985;85–90.
17. Olsson I, Bunketorp O, Carlsson G, Gustafsson C, Planath I, Norin H, Ysander L. An in-depth study of neck injuries in rear end collisions. International IRCOBI conference on the biomechanics of impacts, Bron, Lyon, France, 1990;269–282.
18. Ono K, Kanno M. Influences of the physical parameters on the risk to neck injuries in low impact speed rear-end collisions. International IRCOBI conference on the biomechanics of impacts, Eindhoven, The Netherlands, Sept. 8-10, 1993;201–212.
19. Parkin S, Mackay GM, Hassan AM, Graham P. Rear end collisions and seat performance—To yield or not to yield. Proceedings of the 39th AAAM conference, Chicago, Oct. 16-18, 1995;231–244.
20. Prasad P, Mital N, King AI, Patrick LM. Dynamic response of the spine during -Gx acceleration. Proceedings of the 19th STAPP car crash conference, SAE Inc., 1975;869–897.
21. Romilly DP, Thomson RW, Navin FPD, Macnabb MJ. Low speed rear impacts and the elastic properties of automobiles. Proceedings of the 12th international technical conference ESV, U.S. Department of Transportation, NHTSA, 1989;1199–1205.
22. Seemann MR, Muzzy WH, Lustick LS. Comparison of human and Hybrid III head and neck response. Proceedings of the 30th STAPP car crash conference, paper 861892, Society of Automotive Engineers/P-86/189, 1986;291–312.
23. States JD, Korn MW, Masengill JB. The enigma of whiplash injuries. *N Y State J Med* 1970;70(24):2971–2978.
24. Strother CE, James MB. Evaluation of seat-back strength and seat belt effectiveness in rear end impacts. Proceedings of the 31st STAPP car crash conference. Society of Automotive Engineers technical paper no. 872214, 1987.
25. Svensson MY. Neck injuries in rear-end car collisions—sites and biomechanical causes of the injuries, test methods and preventive measures. Doctoral thesis, Department of Injury Prevention, Chalmers University of Technology, Göteborg, Sweden, 1993.
26. Svensson MY, Lövsund P. A dummy for rear-end collisions—Development and validation of a new dummy-neck. Proceedings of the 1992 International IRCOBI Conference on the biomechanics of impacts, Verona, Italy, 1992;299–310.
27. Svensson MY, Lövsund P, Håland Y, Larsson S. Rear-end collisions—A study of the influence of backrest properties on head-neck motion using a new dummy neck. Society of Automotive Engineers paper no. 930343. In: *Seat system comfort and safety*, SAE/SP-93/963, LC 92-63161, 1993;129–142.
28. Svensson MY, Lövsund P, Håland Y, Larsson S. The Influence of seat-back and head-restraint properties on the head-neck motion during rear-impact. Proceedings of the 1993 International IRCOBI Conference on the Biomechanics of Impacts. Eindhoven, The Netherlands 1993;395–406 (Submitted to *Accid Anal Prev*)
29. Viano DC. Restraint of a belted or unbelted occupant by the seat in rear-end impacts. Society of Automotive Engineers paper no. 922522, Proceedings of the 36th STAPP car crash conference, 1992;165-178, Society of Automotive Engineers/P-92/261.

Whiplash Injuries: Current Concepts in Prevention, Diagnosis, and Treatment of the Cervical Whiplash Syndrome, edited by Robert Gunzburg and Marek Szpalski. Lippincott–Raven Publishers, Philadelphia © 1998.

33

Insurance Perspectives on Managing Soft-Tissue Disorders

Marie Dayton

M. Dayton: Insurance Corporation of British Columbia, Bodily Injury and Rehabilitation Services, North Vancouver, British Columbia, Canada.

Whiplash-associated disorders cost the motorists of British Columbia (B.C.) about half a billion dollars annually. The Insurance Corporation of British Columbia (ICBC), charged with collecting premiums and disbursing claims, is actively involved in recovery management programs and other strategies that will lower the fiscal and social costs associated with this type of injury. This chapter discusses the economic and social climate within which the Corporation functions, and it explores the specifics of the corporation's recovery management initiatives.

ICBC is a provincial Crown Corporation. Established 22 years ago to provide universal vehicle-related insurance, it collects premiums from more than 2 million motorists. The premiums are invested so that funds are available to provide benefits for its clients and victims of crashes.

All motorists in the province are required to buy a basic package of Autoplan insurance that includes accident benefits to help with the immediate needs of crash victims, third-party legal liability protection for motorists who injure someone else or damage another's property, and underinsured motorist protection. Extended third-party legal liability and other optional insurance plans are also offered in an environment that offers retail competition for this particular range of coverage.

ICBC operates on a nonprofit, break-even basis. Premiums are not set nor do they discriminate on the basis of age, sex, or marital status. A claim-rated scale gives discounts to motorists who do not cause crashes and applies surcharges to the premiums of those who have at-fault claims.

The Corporation has 50 drive-in claim centers throughout the province and it employs a staff of about 4,000. Claim adjusters investigate, evaluate, negotiate, and settle claims both for at-fault parties and for those who are entitled to sue for such damages as pain and suffering, and wage loss.

THE PROBLEM

More Accidents Costing More Money. The provincial vehicle crash rate is 25% higher than the national average and 65% higher than our neighboring province. Whatever the reasons for this (climate, topography, lifestyle, etc.), the end result is a staggering escalation of costs. Automobile insurance costs have risen from 1.2% of gross provincial product in 1980 to 2.4% in 1995. ICBC's overall claims costs are now over 2 billion dollars annually!

Since 1990, the costs of settling bodily injury claims have nearly doubled while the number of such claims has risen about 7%. The number of injuries only partially accounts for the significant increases in claim payments. General damage payouts (primarily for pain and suffering) increased by 81% between 1990 and 1995. In the same time frame, past and future wage loss disbursals increased by 102% and 129%, respectively.

Increase in Soft-Tissue Injuries. A major contributor to these rising costs is the number of soft-tissue injuries. They account for approximately 70% of the injury-related claims and 50% of the payouts. Since 1985, B.C. has outpaced the rest Canada in the number of litigated claims involving syndromes such as fibromyalgia, fibrositis, and chronic pain, to name but a few. Most relevant in this explosion is that a half billion Canadian dollars is paid out each year for soft-tissue neck and back injuries.

The Legal and Social Environment. We are becoming a litigious society. The motto seems to be, "When in doubt sue," or at the very least make a claim against the insurance company. The Corporation must initially accept claims on face value, just as doctors have to believe their patients when they say they hurt. But both diagnoses and claims settlements are based on subjective symptoms that can provide an avenue for insurance fraud or exaggeration.

Equally concerning are the high costs of legitimate claims, in terms of patient suffering, recovery, and delays in return to work. Customers whose soft-tissue injuries prevent them from resuming their lives keep presenting themselves. If they fall into a chronic category, the Corporation finds it extremely difficult to break the cycle and help them return to their pre-crash condition. Many of these people are willing to try various treatments that promise some kind of temporary relief and hope for recovery. Each year, ICBC pays for 20 million dollars' worth of physiotherapy, chiropractor, and massage treatments.

The chain of events attached to the injury–compensation–return to work cycle was just not working. Working in an adversarial system that gauged a person's pain and suffering to the length of time they were off work or not able to resume their normal activities appeared to promote a get-rich scheme.

From both the social and economic perspective, the dynamics of getting clients with whiplash-associated disorders (WADs) on their feet and fully functioning are complex and require a team approach. Resolution of those dynamics are clearly in the best interest of the client, the Corporation, and the premium payers.

THE SOLUTIONS

ICBC has recently merged with the province's Motor Vehicle Branch, consolidating authority for the prevention of accidents and injury. Strategic prevention initiatives continue to be a priority.

Prevention

Mass advertising has a twofold purpose. It is used to convince people to slow down and concentrate on better driving behavior, and more importantly to ensure there is public support for better enforcement of speed limits. To make the point graphically, real people are used in the advertising spots, including an emergency room physician, a coroner, and a paraplegic crash survivor, among others.

Education about whiplash is another feature of our prevention initiatives. Much effort has been directed to getting motorists to properly position their head restraints. Particularly appreciated have been the Corporation's efforts to provide this information to motorists while they are on the road. Border crossings and ferry line-ups have provided useful points of intervention.

The Corporation has a Material Damage Division whose Research Centre has examined the effectiveness of various head restraint systems. This work, used in conjunction with Dr. Svensson's examination of the biomechanics of head restraints (1), have enabled us to publish a booklet called *How to Buy a Better Auto.* Educating consumers in this way pushes manufacturers to develop better safety devices.

As a result of their head-restraint studies, the Research Centre developed a piece of equipment that allows standardized measurement of head restraint positioning, something the Corporation is now selling to those auto makers who need to build improved restraints.

Incentives

To stem the tide of claims where there are no objective signs of injury, we have instituted a "no crash, no cash" policy. Usually, such claims involved rear-end collisions with little or no damage to the vehicle. Given the minimal nature of impact forces in such a collision and what we regard as the unlikelihood of injury, we require some evidence of preexisting problems or some other factor that would explain injury in those circumstances. In the absence of such a factor, the Corporation will not pay the claim. Although controversial, and challenged in the courts, for the most part the "no crash, no cash" policy has been successful.

Motorists also respond to lower premiums, and those with long track records of safe driving are so rewarded. It is important to send the right signals that safe driving behavior will be recognized. But, of course, where prevention has not succeeded and accident and injury do occur, then early intervention in the recovery process is key.

The Recovery Management Program

At the heart of Corporation's initiatives is its Recovery Management Program, launched in January of 1995. It is based on the widely respected original Québec Task Force Study conducted by Dr. W. O. Spitzer and his associates at McGill University in Montreal.

Following the Québec model, the program adheres to these principles:

- Early intervention.
- Injured patients should be active, and return to work (paid employment or unpaid homemaking) as soon as possible.
- Pain must be acknowledged, but patients need to be encouraged to work through discomfort to improve function.
- The treating physician (in B.C., this includes chiropractors) is the medical manager, and a case coordinator is used to keep every aspect of recovery on track.
- A flexible recovery program is set in place, using community resources, with patients as active participants in their recovery.

Distribution of the Québec Task Force report on whiplash-associated disorders in April of 1995 reinforced the ICBC's own Recovery Management Program.

Bodily injury adjusters have been trained to identify, as soon as possible after injury, clients with the potential of developing chronic problems. Signs include bed rest longer than 2 to 3 days; no reduction in pain or increase in functional ability at the end of 30 days; continuing reliance on medication, supports, braces, and collars; and a prior disability or claims history.

If such signs persist, the adjuster will refer the case to a case coordinator, who is an occupational therapist or specially trained physiotherapist. The therapist will then meet with the treating physician to obtain a referral for an active recovery program. If the client is represented by a lawyer, the lawyer will be informed of the plan. The program typically includes assistance in returning to work and a specific self-guided activation program.

After 30 days participation in the recovery program without a return to work, there may be a referral to a medical specialist. Further medical interventions may be brought into play at the 3-month and 6-month marks in cases proving difficult to resolve. However, most files should not stay open this long. With its emphasis on early active intervention, we anticipate most people will return sooner to an active, fulfilling life.

That is the theory on which the Corporation based its actions when it took on Recovery Management in earnest. The road to implementation took on some formidable obstacles.

IMPLEMENTATION CHALLENGES

The Corporation was faced with several challenges when it accepted the challenge of implementing a formal Recovery Management Program. It was clear that nothing could be accomplished without the support and participation of all the health care providers. Up to that point, communication with the medical community at local levels had been inconsistent.

For our claims staff, an intervention model meant a fundamentally new approach to handling claims. Instead of adjusters waiting to settle a claim, they now had to be encouraged to promote and pay for special intervention early in the life of the claim. The focus changed from compensation to rehabilitation.

To tackle both these challenges, individual staff members in each claims office were appointed as focal points for this program. They became very active in organizing community meetings with physicians, chiropractors, and physiotherapists. As we started to talk with the physicians, we learned that they were frustrated with soft-tissue injures and we confirmed there was no consistency in the treatment of these injuries. It was equally clear that the primary care physician should play the central role in the management of the patient's recovery from injury.

A presentation script was developed to ensure the key steps were well communicated. There was room to change the script to suit the community needs and the presenter's style. Within the first 6 months, over 2000 doctors met with us to talk about their frustration in dealing with whiplash-associated disorders and to hear how we wanted to implement the new program.

During this communications phase, the Recovery Management Program was piloted in 1994 in four communities in the province. It quickly won the support of physicians, therapists, lawyers, and injured clients. People were starting to get better and to return to work sooner.

With the assistance of some respected community physicians, the program was not being seen as corporate, but community based. The program was providing doctors with support for their own patients, and from there the program's credibility in the medical community grew. This endorsement provided the support our claims handlers needed in taking a proactive approach, helping them establish rapport with injured customers.

Case Coordinators. There had been a lack of communication between care givers. As a resource who could be a liaison between the primary treating physician and the care givers, occupational therapists (OTs) turned out to be a good choice, because they had training in functional assessment and return-to-work strategies. They provided us a method to talk to physicians, allowed for work site visits, and motivated the injured person.

In some cases, there were not enough OTs to support the program. Because we believed that all injured clients had the right to the program's benefits, approved physio-therapists, trained in ergonomics and work capacity, were assigned to work in these areas.

Some 200 independent OTs and physiotherapists now work in this network. These case coordinators are assigned to claim offices within their communities to reduce traveling time, use their knowledge of local facilities, and help in the building of relationships between adjusters and therapists.

The role of the case coordinator is to focus on what intervention the client needs to recover, to provide objective information on the client's progress, and to identify potential difficulties. It is necessary to look beyond the physical factors to recognize the cultural, environmental, and psychosocial challenges individuals may face in their attempts to resume their pre-accident lives.

Performance Standards. Performance standards were developed jointly with the case coordinators and ICBC, with emphasis on good communication, client-centered goals, and effective plans of intervention.

Reports. The case coordinator is responsible for providing a report outlining the plan of intervention, who will be performing the treatment, for what period of time, and at what cost. This report is directed to the medical manager and all team members are provided with copies.

Consultation Fees. Everyone's time and participation is critical for the success of this program, and that costs money. Among other things, we asked the treating doctor to speak with the case coordinator to approve the treatment plan, and ICBC has agreed to pay a consultation fee of $46.00 for this service.

Grading of WADs. Our claims staff had used the terms mild, moderate, and severe to help determine the dollar value of whiplash claims. To introduce the new grading system of WAD 1, 2, 3, and 4, we worked with the Medical Association of B.C. to design a new medical report to assist physicians in the diagnosis and treatment management plan, parallel to the Québec Task Force recommendations. We are working on changing our claims evaluation policies to reflect this.

Training. For the Recovery Management Program to reap benefits, we had to invest in the person's recovery up front and not wait to pay the bills at the time of settlement. This required a major shift on how we handled claims.

To ensure a focus on early intervention, ICBC claim handlers had to change attitudes and look for ways to assist the person with their injury. We needed to train almost 1000 claims staff who deal with injuries, spread across a million square kilometers. The travel, time, and expense implications were daunting. Another solution was sought.

Working in a partnership, ICBC and the Open Learning Agency (a provincially funded education institution) designed a program that met ICBC's training needs. Utilizing their broadcast facilities, training was delivered in 2 days at 17 sites around the province via video teleconferencing. Two 1-day training sessions allowed ICBC to keep half its adjusters working each day, while ensuring our people were getting top-notch instruction. The fast-paced interactive program was delivered by the best subject experts available and backed by video presentations. Each site had a facilitator and a focal point to lead the training. The intensive province-wide delivery of training fostered a corporate spirit and a sense of common goals that translated into a high compliance rate among employees, improving ICBC's service to the public.

Does Recovery Management Work?

Because the Recovery Management Program has been in place for only a relatively short time, comments on success or failure are tenuous at best. Trends show that doctors are making referrals to the program, that people are getting better faster, and that wage loss costs are moving downwards.

Having said that, some growing pains have become evident.

Data collection has been a problem. The lack of firmly established benchmarks make firm conclusions difficult. The Corporation is now examining the preliminary data and determining what further statistics need to be collected to ascertain the benefits of the program. A conceptual data model that includes information from external partners is being built. It will provide various departments within ICBC with accurate data. However, the building of an ideal system will take time. We are determining the best methods to collect data from our external partners as well.

Adjusters must recognize the potential of assisting a claimant within 30 days of the crash. Without early referrals, the success of returning the person to regular employment is compromised, with related costs associated with delay much greater. Currently, workloads and procedural constraints can affect an adjuster's ability to make those early referrals. As well, further ongoing education is required to ensure all adjusters recognize the benefits of and the need for early interventions.

Other Problems. There are no treatment protocols yet in place. And some proven interventions are not yet compensable under our fee-for-service system. Finally, we do not yet have the performance standards in place to assist practitioners in recognizing when their interventions are no longer helpful.

Other Initiatives/Other Partners

B.C. Whiplash Initiative. The Physical Medicine Research Foundation and other partners in the medical profession are spearheading the British Columbia Whiplash Initiative. It is a multi-agency project dedicated to developing a multifaceted continuing medical education program on the diagnosis and management of patients presenting with whiplash-associated disorders.

In concert with doctors' organizations and the medical school at our largest university, this initiative aims to provide education to all emergency room, family, and sports physicians as well as updating the medical school curriculum. It will utilize the best evidence-based synthesis on WAD, as well as recent systematic reviews of effective continuing medical education interventions, to create and deliver a comprehensive and effective education program. The research component of this project is to monitor changes in physician behavior as reflected in changes in diagnostic investigations, and pharmaceutical and therapeutic interventions.

The Initiative has several different delivery mechanisms in the works, and starting in the fall of 1997, doctors will be able to attend 1-hour sessions or 1-day symposia on this issue. There will also be a World Wide Web site where they can get this instruction. The address for this site will be http://www.health-sciences.ubc.ca/whiplash.bc/home.html and it should be accessible early in 1997. The site is interactive, and various branches can be followed to review the BC Whiplash Initiative Syllabus and the Québec Task Force (QTF) guidelines. The site also provides the opportunity to discuss WAD with colleagues.

National Institute for Disability Management and Research. The Corporation strongly supports the work of the National Institute for Disability Management and Research. It is a joint union–management body aimed at ensuring that there is knowledgeable support within companies that will help disabled workers return to employment. When we help soft-tissue-injured people return to function, it is very helpful to have that person's co-workers and bosses ready, willing, and able to assist them back on the job.

CONCLUSION

We have learned that any recovery management program is a work in progress—and probably always will be. To be successful, it must contain a number of elements including fast and accurate data collection, end-to-end treatments with measured best outcomes, and education of the family and the workplace.

Most important of all are changes in attitude focusing on wellness and not disability.

REFERENCES

1. Svensson MY. Neck injuries in rear-end car collisions—sites and biomechanical causes of the injuries, test methods and preventive measures. Doctoral thesis, Department of Injury Prevention, Chalmers University of Technology, Göteborg, Sweden, 1993.

*Whiplash Injuries: Current Concepts in
Prevention, Diagnosis, and Treatment
of the Cervical Whiplash Syndrome,*
edited by Robert Gunzburg and Marek Szpalski.
Lippincott–Raven Publishers, Philadelphia © 1998.

34

Implementing the Recommendations of the Québec Task Force on Whiplash-Associated Disorders[*]

Marc Giroux, Christiane Beauchemin, and Claire Desbiens

*M. Giroux, C. Beauchemin, and C. Desbiens: Direction of Policy and Programs for
Accident Victims, Société de l'assurance automobile du Québec, Québec, Canada.*

A BRIEF LOOK BACKWARD

During the 1980s, Québec's automobile insurance corporation, the Société de l'assurance automobile du Québec, saw that whiplash was becoming a widespread problem. Some 20% of all claims submitted to the Société included such a diagnosis, which in most cases should be a relatively benign injury but quite often ended up being a chronic condition. The average length of disability for whiplash and related disorders rose from 72 days in 1987 to 95 days in 1988, and to 110 days by 1989. The cost in terms of reimbursement of expenses and income compensation amounted, for 1987, to over 18 million dollars.

The Société also noted that whiplash was a type of injury poorly understood by health care professionals:

- The diagnosis was used for very many cases, and far too imprecisely.
- Because the natural history of the disorder was not well-known, long disability periods ensued.
- Treatment prescribed varied greatly from one therapist to another.

IN 1991

In light of these observations, in 1991 the Société mandated a task force composed of internationally renowned experts (Table 1) to conduct a study on whiplash-associated disorders.

One of the goals of this Québec Task Force was to improve knowledge of preventive and therapeutic strategies for cervical sprains, so that accident victims who sustain this type of injury could receive the most appropriate care.

---

[*] © Société de l'assurance automobile du Québec, 1996.

TABLE 1. *Composition of the Task Force, under*
Dr. Walter O. Spitzer, MD, MPH, FRCPC, Chairman

Member	Specialty	Location
Duranceau, Jacques, MD, FRCPC	Physiatrist	Québec
Suissa, Samy, PhD	Biostatistician	Québec
Salmi, L. Rachid, MD, PhD	Epidemiologist	France
Skovron, Mary-Louise, DrPH	Epidemiologist	New York
Abenhaim, Lucien, MD	Epidemiologist	Québec
Bouvier, Guy, MD	Neurosurgeon	Québec
Cassidy, J. David, DC, PhD, FCCSC	Chiropractor	Saskatchewan
Dionne, Jacques, MD, FRCSC	Otorhinolaryngologist	Québec
Dupuis, Pierre, MD, FRCSC	Orthopedic surgeon	Québec
Grantham, Harry, MD, FRCP, FAPA	Psychiatrist	Québec
Leclaire, Richard, MD	Physiatrist	Québec
Liang, Matthew H., MD, MPH	Rheumatologist, general internist	Massachusetts
Nordin, Margareta, Med DrSci	Ergonomist, physiotherapist	New York
Nygren, Åke, MD	Physiatrist	Sweden
Thompson, Lloyd, Ing, BA, PhD	Engineer	Québec
Veilleux, Martin, MD	Neurologist	Québec
Wood-Dauphinée, Sharon, PhD, PT	Physiotherapist, epidemiologist	Québec
Villeneuve, Claire	Observer, the office des professions	Québec

IN 1992

While the study was under way, the Société examined the data from road accidents occurring in 1992. The data showed that 6669 persons sustained at least whiplash in an accident in 1992, or 26.8% of accident victims, compared to 20% in 1987. This increase of 6.8% translates into 1903 persons more than in 1987. To date, claims from 1992 account for over 25 million dollars in income compensation and payment of accident-related expenses.

TASK FORCE REPORTS IN 1995

At a press conference for the media and health care professionals held on May 1, 1995, the Québec Task Force delivered its report on whiplash-associated disorders.

TABLE 2. *Proposed clinical classification of*
whiplash-associated disorders

Grade	Clinical presentation
0	No complaint about neck No physical sign(s)
I	Neck complaint of pain, stiffness, or tenderness only No physical sign(s)
II	Neck complaint AND musculoskeletal sign(s)
III	Neck complaint AND neurologic sign(s)
IV	Neck complaint AND fracture or dislocation

From Spitzer WO, et al. *Scientific Monograph of the Québec Task Force on Whiplash-Associated Disorders.* © Société de l'assurance automobile du Québec, 1995.

The official report, entitled *Whiplash-Associated Disorders (WAD)*, presents a best-evidence synthesis on the risks, diagnoses, treatments, and prognoses of whiplash-related problems. The experts also examined whiplash injury mechanisms and prevention measures. Overall medical literature on the subject was reviewed, including basic science in anatomy, physiology, and semiology.

To get a better understanding of the epidemiology of whiplash-related disorders, the Task Force also studied a cohort of patients who had experienced cervical problems after car accidents in 1987. This patient sample was drawn from the base of claims filed with the Société by the victims themselves.

The recommendations arising out of the work of the Task Force touch on six main aspects:

- Social impact of whiplash-associated disorders
- Prevention
- Diagnosis
- Treatment
- Current practice
- Training for health care professionals

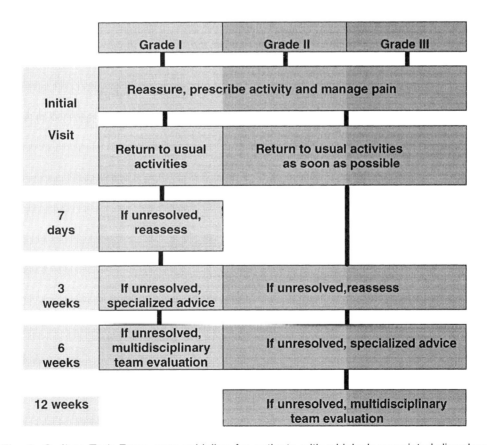

Fig. 1. Québec Task Force care guideline for patients with whiplash-associated disorders. From Spitzer WO, et al. *Scientific Monograph of the Québec Task Force on Whiplash-Associated Disorders.* © Société de l'assurance automobile du Québec, 1995.

THE QUÉBEC CLASSIFICATION OF WHIPLASH-ASSOCIATED DISORDERS AND PATIENT CARE GUIDELINES

The Québec classification of whiplash-associated disorders proposed five grades, from 0 to IV, with 0 corresponding to "no complaints about the neck" or "no signs", and with IV corresponding to bone-tissue injury such as fracture or dislocation (Table 2).

A patient care guideline was proposed by the Task Force, taking into account the length of time that has elapsed since the moment of injury (Fig. 1).

THE SOCIÉTÉ'S ACTION PLAN (1996)

Before developing its plan for action, the Société spelled out the objectives it sought to reach, and it determined which groups would be affected, so as to then be in a better position to implement measures.

The Objectives

- To enhance clinicians' knowledge of care for patients with whiplash-related disorders.
- To ensure a prompter response for persons afflicted with these disorders and the application of a treatment plan better adapted to this type of injury.
- To avoid the serious consequences to accident victims and society as a whole of chronicity by accelerating the resumption of work or usual activities.
- To reduce the average length of disability resulting from this type of injury, which will lead to lower compensation costs.

The Approach Chosen for Smooth Implementation

Many people are affected by the recommendations of the Task Force: close to 15,000 health care professionals and 5000 accident victims yearly (Table 3). The Société decided to work in a concerted fashion with the people directly concerned by whiplash.

TABLE 3. *The target clientele*

Category	(N)
Accident victims	5,000/yr
General practitioners	
Front-line physicians	8,223
Physicians in family practice	
Emergency physicians	
Other health care professionals	
Physiotherapists	3,000
Chiropractors	859
Occupational therapists	1,500
Specialists	
Orthopedic surgeons	371
Physiatrists	90
Rheumatologists	95
Neurosurgeons	84
Neurologists	225
Société staff processing accident victims' claims	200
Total	19,647 persons

A committee was formed, with a representative from each of the following groups: accident victims, general practitioners, specialist physicians, and other health care professionals. The committee defined the needs of the clientele, and the interventions and/or activities to be done, taking into account the reality and work context facing each professional.

Representatives spoke about the particular interests of their group, and together they settled on a strategy based on raising the awareness of, and informing and training, health care professionals. The ultimate goal is to have health care professionals subscribe to what is currently recognized as the scientifically based treatment, so that an accident victim can be given a plan tailored to his or her condition.

The First Phase: Awareness in Organizations

Professionals in Québec are governed by separate organizations—professional corporations that have a right to oversee anything concerning the profession. Those organizations play an important role in the eyes of the public, because, in the area of health care, they have a duty to protect people and promote the better health of all Quebecers. They include the following:

- Collège des médecins,
- Ordre professionnel des chiropraticiens,
- Ordre professionnel des physiothérapeutes, and
- Ordre professionnel des ergothérapeutes.

The Société has developed a partnership with those professional corporations, meeting with most of them to make them aware of the report. They have approved the action plan to implement the recommendations, and they have assured the Société support for any initiatives it might take with their membership and the general population.

The cooperation of the two federations representing general practitioners and specialists has been secured.

The Second Phase: Information for Professionals, the Public, and Accident Victims

Each health care professional was sent a letter signed by his or her professional corporation and federation, and by the Société, describing the main elements in the report and the work of the Task Force on whiplash-associated disorders. Articles will be published regularly in the professional bulletins to maintain interest and convey timely information. Conference speakers will be promoting the report at annual meetings and conventions of professional associations.

Daily newspapers will publish articles on the steps being taken to care for a patient with a cervical spine problem, and articles that will remind the public of the importance of staying active and doing exercise.

Automobile accident victims who sustain whiplash will receive a folder from a compensation officer as soon as they file a claim with the Société. The folder will bear the logos of the Collège des médecins, both medical federations, and the Société.

The Third Phase: Training for Professionals

The Task Force's report noted instances of serious lack of knowledge on the part of physicians and other health care professionals about problems linked to whiplash. Representatives of professional groups who collaborated with the Société in developing the action plan also recognized that the education of physicians and students in the health sciences is deficient about care to be administered to patients with whiplash, resulting in a decreased effectiveness in treating the condition.

Therefore, the Société asked Laval University to work in conjunction with the sister institutions of McGill, Montréal, and Sherbrooke to design a course on whiplash for medical students and health care professionals across Québec. The result is a 3-hour course that will be basic training for all health care professionals. The professional corporations will be urging their members to take the course for the benefit of their patients.

Subsequently, an in-depth, 2-day training course will be offered to all professionals who want to give specialized advice and take part in multidisciplinary assessments under the patient care guideline.

Taking its inspiration from the data forms devised by the Task Force, the Société developed a form for clinicians' use in collecting information at the time of examination of a patient with a problem in the area of the cervical spine. After each of the patient's visits, the clinician will be required to send the completed form to the Société for compensation file management.

The Fourth Phase: Specialized Advice and Multidisciplinary Assessment

A list of professionals capable of proffering specialized advice and taking part in multidisciplinary assessments will be compiled and given to all clinicians. An accompanying guide will specify the way to obtain the opinion of the professionals consulted within the time allowed under the patient care guideline. The patient's attending physician will initiate the referral for specialized advice to the professional selected from the list.

When an assessment from a multidisciplinary team is required, the attending physician will also make the referral, on the basis of the biological, psychological, and social condition of the patient, to the appropriate specialties. The opinion of at least two health care professionals is necessary. More complex cases will require the input of a larger number of professionals working in different areas.

Whatever the stage of the patient's whiplash, the assessment report from the multidisciplinary team must be complete and detailed, relating the case history, physical examination, any test results, and specific diagnosis for each speciality involved. The synthesis of data gathered and the discussion must rest on verifiable premises supported by objective reasoning. Recommendations will have to be clearly set forth and will emerge from a consensus of all members of the multidisciplinary team.

Patients with a Chronic Condition

The report of the Task Force explains that patients who still show symptoms of whiplash or disability 6 months after the injury should be considered "chronic." With the help of the attending physician, the Société will have to identify those accident victims who have not responded adequately to treatment, before the 6-month term is up, and direct them into a rehabilitation program that encompasses dynamic intervention based on a multidisciplinary approach.

Postimplementation Phase: Guideline Evaluation

The Société plans to evaluate the patient care guideline after a few years of use. An analysis will be done of the information contained in the reports filled out by clinicians, making it possible to see whether diagnoses have become more precise or not, and if treatments prescribed do indeed follow the recommendations of the Task Force. A comparison can then also be made between the data on the length of disability and the patient cohort figures studied by the Spitzer team (see reference in Table 1) to see if patient recovery and economic efficiency have improved.

*Whiplash Injuries: Current Concepts in
Prevention, Diagnosis, and Treatment
of the Cervical Whiplash Syndrome,*
edited by Robert Gunzburg and Marek Szpalski.
Lippincott–Raven Publishers, Philadelphia © 1998.

35

Whiplash: Can the Cost to Society Be Diminished?

Michael Sullivan

*M. Sullivan: Department of Orthopaedics, London University,
Royal National Orthopaedic Hospital, London, United Kingdom.*

The costs of whiplash and its associated disorders are those to society in general and the cost to the individual patient. This is probably best looked at under seven headings:

At the level of the public
1. Increased road safety
2. Increased car safety

At the level of the individual
3. Diminished cost of litigation
4. Removal of the adversarial system of litigation
5. Incentives to return to work
6. Pre-set payout for particular injuries
7. Early treatment of the injury

At the national level, car safety and road safety are quite definitely improving. In 1995, the cost of road traffic accidents in the United Kingdom was £13.25 billion, of which £9.5 billion was attributable to personal injury accidents, with damage-only accidents accounting for the remainder. The average cost of a single accident where there is a fatality is £950,000, but taken as a single casualty it is £810,000, the difference being that in fatal accidents there are usually a number of other vehicles involved in which there may be no casualties. The average cost of a serious accident is £110,000, and of a slight accident, £11,000. There are no accurate figures on the cost of whiplash injury, but it is probably around £50,000 (2).

The actual accident rate has steadily declined from 1985 to the present time (Table 1).

TABLE 1. *Rate of accidents per 100 million vehicle · kilometers*

Year	All roads	Motorways	Built-up roads
1985	84	13	133
1988	67	11	111
1990	62	11	102
1992	56	11	93
1994	55	11	89
1995	53	10	87

From these figures, it would seem that it is possible to reduce the number of accidents by having motorways rather than routine built-up roads. This, of course, is the steady expectation around the world.

There is no doubt about the increased safety of motor cars with air bags and proper head restraints. Air bags come into effect only with front-end impact and these do not normally cause whiplash injuries: rear-impact accidents cause whiplash injuries. In this case, it is most important to have good, well-formed head restraints that do in fact support the head rather than use the neck as a fulcrum for hyperextension.

At the single-patient level, the cost of litigation is usually twice as much as the award to the patient. There are two reasons: in our adversarial system of litigation, it behooves each side to employ experts to write medical reports, and, as a corollary, this system takes a great deal of time, it being not unusual for a simple whiplash injury case to be settled 5 years after the accident. This not only increases the legal costs but, inevitably, both sides insist on updated medical reports on a yearly basis.

Lord Woolf, who is the present Master of the Rolls and the second most senior judge in Britain, has produced a document, "Access to Justice" (1). His idea is that there should be a panel of experts who could be asked very early in the litigation to give an opinion. These two experts would be expected to meet and to sort out the medicolegal work between them. If there is continued disagreement, the court could call a third expert. Lord Woolf's preferred option would simply be to have one expert who gave an opinion for both sides. This is seen as unacceptable by both the medical and the legal fraternities. It has been estimated that about 25% of the income of orthopedic surgeons in the United Kingdom is from medicolegal reports, predominantly arising from rear-end motor vehicle collisions. Neither of these two professions is prepared to give up such a large proportion of their practice.

If all litigation could be sorted out within 1 year, there would be a higher expectation of these litigants returning to work. If patients do not return to work within a year, they have very poor expectation of ever returning to full employment.

This is also tied up with the long-term results of whiplash injury. Squires et al. (5), studing whiplash injuries at Bristol, found that at the 15-year follow-up, 70% of the patients continued to have symptoms, frequently long after payment from litigation. However, 52% of the symptomatic patients had evidence of psychological disturbance, which is presumed not to have been present prior to their accidents. An interesting point is that between the 10-year follow-up and the 15-year follow-up, 18% of the patients improved, whereas 28% deteriorated. The commonest symptom was neck pain, but low back pain was present in 50% of the sample and this is often the cause of failure to return to work.

That the problem of litigation is more complex is shown by the paper by Schrader et al. (4) on "Disability in Lithuania." In that country, there is no litigation for road traffic accidents in the Western sense of the word. Schrader et al. found that the incidence of chronic symptoms was no more than one would expect from the past history and expectations of the patient.

Only two countries have managed to cut down the figures of sickness rate for back pain. The first of these is Sweden, where, on January 1, 1993, as it was about to enter the European Community, the ccountry cut the disability compensation because it could no longer afford the high cost to the gross national product (GNP) (6). Prior to 1993, sickness benefit was paid at 90% of salary from day 1, indefinitely. After that January 1, the claimant would get nothing for the first day of illness, 70% of salary for the next 3 days, and then 80% of salary from the 5th day onward. As most episodes of back pain are very short lived, the maximum loss was in those early days. The figures before and after 1993 showed a 25% reduction in the general illness rate but a 50% reduction in days lost due to spine-related illness.

The other country that seems to have solved this problem to some extent is Singapore. In that country, 40% of the GNP is saved for every worker up to the age of 55. The employee and the employer each pays 20% of the worker's salary into a central provident fund, so that 40% of the salary is saved. The money is paid into the named person's provident fund rather than going to the general exchequer to be treated at will by the government of the day (3). Not only is this beneficial to the worker, but it has an enormous advantage to the country, in that 40% of salary is saved as compared with 20% in the United Kingdom.

This sum of money is available to the whole family to be used for health care, unemployment benefit, and pension. However, if this fund reaches a minimum level (which is slightly variable depending on the job of the wage earner), it may be used for certain other luxuries, such as buying a flat or private education for children, but not for buying motor cars. The result is that there is enormous family pressure not to be out of work for long, because they then must draw not from the exchequer but from the family next egg.

In conclusion, it is possible to have fewer accidents. It is much more sensible to have motorways than fast two- and three-lane roads, especially in and around cities. If accidents continue to occur, as they will, at least the cars can be made safer with properly designed seats. If litigation is inevitable, it can be sorted out more quickly with a minimum of medicolegal reports (preferably only one). If patients can be back to work as early as possible, there is less likely to be long-term ill health. There will be long-term neck problems, but no more than in the general population, as has been shown by the Lithuanian experience. There should be no financial incentive not to return to work or to have long-term ill health.

REFERENCES

1. Lord Woolf. *British Orthopaedic News* 1996;13:3.
2. Department of Transport statistics 1996, *Highways Economic Note number 1.*
3. *Daily Mail.* Leading article, January 9, 1996.
4. Schrader et al. Natural evolution of late whiplash syndrome outside the medico-legal context. *Lancet* 1996;347: 1207.
5. Squires, Gargen, Bannisters. Soft-tissue injuries of the cervical spine. *J Bone Joint Surg* 1996;78B:955.
6. Stromquist B. Personal communication, 1996.

Subject Index